Contemporary Pediatric and Adolescent Sports Medicine

Series Editor
Lyle J. Micheli

More information about this series at http://www.springer.com/series/11729

Michael O'Brien • William P. Meehan III
Editors

Head and Neck Injuries in Young Athletes

Springer

Editors
Michael O'Brien, MD
Division of Sports Medicine
Childrens Hospital Boston
Boston, MA, USA

William P. Meehan III, MD
The Micheli Center for Sports Injury Prevention
Waltham, MA, USA

ISSN 2198-266X ISSN 2198-2678 (electronic)
Contemporary Pediatric and Adolescent Sports Medicine
ISBN 978-3-319-79497-6 ISBN 978-3-319-23549-3 (eBook)
DOI 10.1007/978-3-319-23549-3

Springer Cham Heidelberg New York Dordrecht London

Softcover re-print of the Hardcover 1st edition 2016

Printed on acid-free paper

Springer International Publishing AG Switzerland is part of Springer Science+Business Media (www.springer.com)

The Micheli Center for Sports Injury Prevention

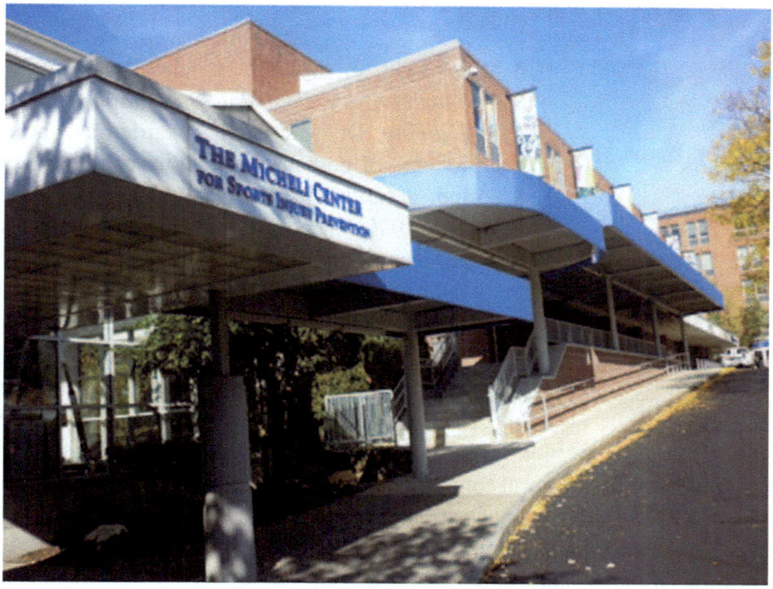

The mission of the Micheli Center for Sports Injury Prevention is at the heart of the *Contemporary Pediatric and Adolescent Sports Medicine* series.

The Micheli Center uses the most up-to-date medical and scientific information to develop practical strategies that help young athletes reduce their risk of injury as they prepare for a healthier future. The clinicians, scientists, activists, and technologists at the Micheli Center advance the field of sports medicine by revealing current injury patterns and risk factors while developing new methods, techniques, and technologies for preventing injuries.

The Micheli Center had its official opening in April 2013 and is named after Lyle J. Micheli, one of the world's pioneers in pediatric and adolescent sports medicine. Dr. Micheli is the series editor of *Contemporary Pediatric and Adolescent Sports Medicine*.

Consistent with Dr. Micheli's professional focus over the past 40 years, The Micheli Center conducts world-class medical and scientific research focused on the prevention of sports injuries and the effects of exercise on health and wellness. In addition, the Micheli Center develops innovative methods of promoting exercise in children.

The Micheli Center opens its doors to anyone seeking a healthier lifestyle, including those with medical conditions or illnesses that may have previously limited their abilities. Fellow clinicians, researchers, and educators are invited to collaborate and discover new ways to prevent, assess, and treat sports injuries.

Series Editor Biography

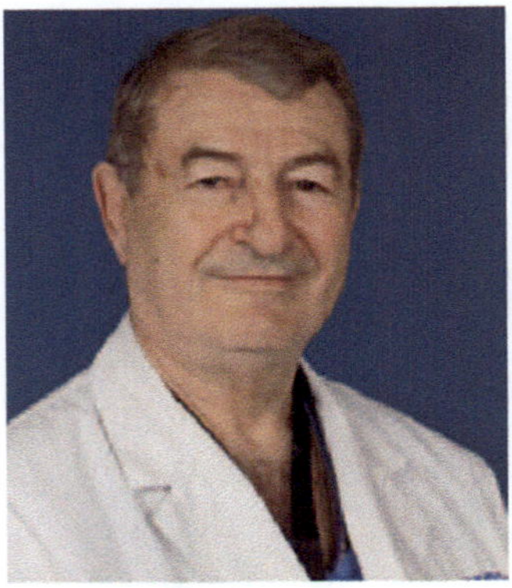

Dr. Lyle J. Micheli is the series editor of *Contemporary Pediatric and Adolescent Sports Medicine*. Dr. Micheli is regarded as one of the pioneers of pediatric and adolescent sports medicine, a field he has been working in since the early 1970s when he co-founded the USA's first sports medicine clinic for young athletes at Boston Children's Hospital.

Dr. Micheli is now director of the Division of Sports Medicine at Boston Children's Hospital, and Clinical Professor of Orthopaedic Surgery at Harvard Medical School. He is a past president of the American College of Sports Medicine and is currently the Secretary General for the International Federation of Sports Medicine. Dr. Micheli co-chaired the International Olympic Committee consensus on the health and fitness of young people through physical activity and sport.

In addition to many other honors, Dr. Micheli has served as Chairperson of the Massachusetts Governor's Committee on Physical Fitness and Sports, on the Board of Directors of the United States Rugby Football Foundation, as Chairman of the USA Rugby Medical and Risk Management Committee, and on the advisory board of the Bay State Games. He has been the Attending Physician for the Boston Ballet since 1977 and is Medical Consultant to the Boston Ballet School.

Dr. Micheli received his undergraduate degree from Harvard College in 1962 and his medical degree from Harvard Medical School in 1966. As an undergraduate student, Dr. Micheli was an avid athlete, competing in rugby, gridiron football, and boxing. Since graduating, Dr. Micheli has played prop for various Rugby clubs including, the Boston Rugby Football Club, the Cleveland Blues Rugby Football Club, Washington Rugby Club, and Mystic Valley Rugby Club where he also served as team coach.

Dr. Micheli has authored over 300 scientific articles and reviews related to sports injuries, particularly in children. His present research activities focus on the prevention of sports injuries in children. Dr. Micheli has edited and authored several major books and textbooks.

Foreword

It gives me great pleasure to be writing the foreword for this excellent book on head and neck injuries in young athletes.

The problem of head and neck injuries has been cast into sharp relief the last few years. The focus has shifted from professional adult athletes to young athletes. Fortunately, our profession has responded with research into not just the most effective diagnosis and treatment but also into identifying the most common risk factors for these injuries. Identifying and addressing these risk factors is the most successful way to prevent them.

It is notable that the editors of this latest volume in the series Contemporary Pediatric Sports Medicine chose to include a chapter on injury prevention and make it the very first chapter in the book. This is in keeping with philosophy of the sponsoring institution for the book series, The Micheli Center for Sports Injury Prevention.

The Micheli Center hosts one of the first Concussion Clinics for young athletes in the country, and the co-editors of this book have been instrumental in making it one of the best possible resources for athletes who sustain these kinds of head injuries.

As an examination of the Table of Contents reveals, this is a comprehensive volume with authors drawn from the top ranks of their respective fields. The information you will find in these pages is first-rate. As such, it deserves a place on the bookshelf of anyone with an interest in sports medicine in young athletes.

Congratulations to the editors for their efforts at creating a very important new contribution to the literature.

Lyle J. Micheli, MD
Division of Sports Medicine
Children's Hospital Boston
Boston, MA, USA

Preface

Head and neck injuries are among the most serious injuries in sports. They are responsible for greater incidences of disability and fatality in athletes than sports injuries of any other body parts. Increasingly, these injuries are a source of concern among parents who see the media scrutiny over head and neck injuries and ask the question, "Is my child at risk?" and "Should I let me child play sports?"

In particular, there is a lot of attention focused on the long-term implications of concussions sustained by athletes engaged in collision sports such as football, ice hockey, and rugby.

The good news is that serious head and neck injuries are rare in all sports, youth sports included, even in those sports with the potential for falls and collision. When a serious head or neck injury occurs, however, the consequences are profound and far-reaching. The implications may extend beyond the health of the child to the well-being of the child's family, school, fellow athletes, and the community at large.

With all this in mind, we set about to create a book that contained the most up-to-date information about the head and neck injuries sustained by young athletes. We are fortunate to have attracted some of the preeminent names in the field.

Our authors were able to provide a thorough review of several complex and emerging issues for adolescent athletes. Some chapters expand on previous treatment guidelines, like encouraging some early cognitive activity in concussion management, while others attempt to summarize the current evidence of topics that are still incompletely understood, like chronic traumatic encephalopathy. We have striven to make this book complete with practical information that ranges from the sideline assessment of injuries, to the safe transport of athletes, to the theory of a stepwise approach to rehab and return to sports.

In addition to addressing the kinds of head and neck injuries one might ordinarily expect to see in a sports medicine book with an orthopedic orientation, we were also able to enlist the expertise of authors to write about important related issues such as visual dysfunction and protective equipment. We felt it was important to include practical information for the sports medicine physician on topics that are often treated by specialists in other fields such as dental and ear injuries. The inclusion of these chapters makes this book all the more comprehensive and useful.

It goes without saying that our stellar authors are busy people, and we thank them for taking time out of their busy schedules to share their expertise in the chapters they contributed.

With head and neck injuries increasingly in the spotlight, the time is right for a new book that covers the important subject matter. We are pleased to share with you this new addition to the literature. We are proud of the amount of time and effort that went into this book by so many people and trust that you will find such effort reflected in the finished product.

Boston, MA
Waltham, MA

Michael O'Brien, MD
William P. Meehan III, MD

Contents

Contributors

Muhammad M. Abd-El-Barr, MD, PhD Brigham and Women's Hospital/Boston Children's Hospital, Harvard Medical School, Boston, MA, USA

Purnima Bansal, MD Jennie Stuart Medical Center, Hopkinsville, KY

Laura S. Blackwell, PhD Center for Neuropsychology, Boston Children's Hospital, Boston, MA, USA

Robert V. Cantu, MD, MS Dartmouth Hitchcock Medical Center, Lebanon, NH, USA

Robert C. Cantu, MD, FACS, FACSM Emerson Hospital, Concord, MA, USA

Children's Hospital, Boston, MA, USA

Pierre A. d'Hemecourt, MD Division of Sports Medicine, Boston Children's Hospital, Boston, MA, USA

Emilie Dolan, BS Rhode Island Hospital, Providence, RI, USA

Kate Dorney, MD Division of Emergency Medicine, Boston Children's Hospital, Boston, MA, USA

Ian F. Dunn, MD Department of Neurosurgery, Brigham and Women's Hospital, Boston, MA, USA

Courtney Gleason, MD Division of Sports Medicine, Rhode Island Hospital, Warren Alpert School of Medicine, Brown University, Providence, RI, USA

David Howell, PhD Division of Sports Medicine, Department of Orthopaedics, Boston Children's Hospital, Waltham, MA, USA

The Micheli Center for Sports Injury Prevention, Waltham, MA, USA

Kevin T. Huang, MD Department of Neurosurgery, Brigham and Women's Hospital/Harvard Medical School, Boston, MA, USA

David Alexander Keith, DMD, BDS Department of Oral and Maxillofacial Surgery, Massachusetts General Hospital, Boston, MA, USA

Hamish A. Kerr, MD Department of Internal Medicine and Pediatrics, Albany Medical College, Albany Medical Center, Latham, NY, USA

Peter Kriz, MD Rhode Island Hospital, Providence, RI, USA

Preetha A. Kurian Department of Internal Medicine and Pediatrics, Albany Medical College, Albany Medical Center, Latham, NY, USA

Deborah I. Light, MD Department of Internal Medicine and Pediatrics, Albany Medical College, Albany Medical Center, Latham, NY, USA

Anthony Luke, MD, MPH Department of Orthopaedic Surgery, University of California, San Francisco, San Francisco, CA, USA

James P. MacDonald, MD, MPH Division of Sports Medicine, Department of Pediatrics, Nationwide Children's Hospital, Dublin, OH, USA

Rebekah Mannix, MD, MPH Department of Emergency Medicine, Boston Children's Hospital, Boston, MA, USA

William P. Meehan III, MD Division of Sports Medicine, Department of Orthopaedics, Boston Children's Hospital, Waltham, MA, USA

The Micheli Center for Sports Injury Prevention, Waltham, MA, USA

Andrew F. Miller, MD Division of Emergency Medicine, Department of Medicine, Boston Children's Hospital, Harvard Medical School, Boston, MA, USA

Michael O'Brien, MD Division of Sports Medicine, Childrens Hospital Boston, Boston, MA, USA

Mark R. Proctor, MD Vice-Chair of Neurosurgery, Boston Children's Hospital/ Harvard Medical School, Boston, MA, USA

Aparna Raghuram, OD, PhD Boston Children's Hospital and Harvard Medical School, Boston, MA, USA

Marcus Robinson, BASc, MASc, MD, CCFP, Dip Sport & Exercise Medicine, Calgary, Alberta, Canada

Jane P. Sando, MD Department of Pediatric Emergency Medicine, Johns Hopkins Hospital, Baltimore, MD, USA

Ankoor S. Shah, MD, PhD Department of Ophthalmology, Boston Children's Hospital and Harvard Medical School, Boston, MA, USA

Andrea Stracciolini, MD Division of Sports Medicine, Department of Orthopaedics, Boston Children's Hospital, Boston, MA, USA

Division of Emergency Medicine, Department of Medicine, Boston Children's Hospital, Boston, MA, USA

Harvard Medical School, Boston, MA, USA

Alex M. Taylor, PsyD Department of Neurology, Boston Children's Hospital, Boston, MA, USA

Brain Injury Center, Boston Children's Hospital, Boston, MA, USA

Lisa M.G. Vopat, MD Orthopedics/Division of Sports Medicine, Boston Children's Hospital, Boston, MA, USA

Mariusz Kajetan Wrzosek, DMD, MD Department of Oral and Maxillofacial Surgery, Massachusetts General Hospital, Boston, MA, USA

1 Head and Neck Injury Prevention

David Howell and William P. Meehan III

Introduction

In high school athletics, concussion comprises more than 10 % of sport-related injuries [1]. Approximately 7 % of paraplegia or quadriplegia cases occur during sport participation [2]. More than a third of life-threatening injuries to the head and neck sustained by children are sport-related, and 12 % of those sustained by adults are sport-related [3]. This includes nearly a quarter of cervical spine fractures sustained by children [3]. Therefore, seeking out proactive methods for preventing head and neck injuries sustained during sports is crucial to preserving the safety of young athletes. Although the prevention of head and neck injuries has proven a difficult task, substantial gains have been made over the last 50 years. Although there are no empirically proven methods to eliminate head and neck injury risk, researchers have employed various intervention programs and treatment protocols in order to investigate the best ways to keep athletes safe. Thus, the purpose of this chapter is to briefly review the mechanism and epidemiology of common head and neck injuries sustained during sports participation and discuss various proposed methods for preventing those injuries.

D. Howell, PhD (✉) • W.P. Meehan III, MD
Division of Sports Medicine, Department of Orthopaedics, Boston Children's Hospital, 9 Hope Ave, Waltham, MA 02453, USA

The Micheli Center for Sports Injury Prevention, Waltham, MA, USA
e-mail: David.Howell2@childrens.harvard.edu

M. O'Brien, W.P. Meehan III (eds.), *Head and Neck Injuries in Young Athletes*, Contemporary Pediatric and Adolescent Sports Medicine,
DOI 10.1007/978-3-319-23549-3_1

Concussion

Biomechanics and Pathophysiology

Concussion is defined as a traumatically induced alteration of mental status that may or may not involve loss of consciousness [4]. When an external force is applied to the head, neck, or elsewhere on the body, it may result in an impulsive force which acts on the head [5]. This force creates a sudden acceleration or deceleration of the brain within the cranium causing a temporary disruption of the axons [6]. Correcting axonal function requires adenosine triphosphate. There is, however, a simultaneous alteration of blood flow to the brain after concussion that leads to a mismatch of energy supply and demand. This mismatch is thought to underlie the common signs and symptoms associated with a concussion [6, 7].

Recovery times after concussion vary widely, and the duration of time that is needed for the brain to fully heal after injury is unknown. Oftentimes parents, coaches, athletic trainers, or other clinicians rely on symptom reporting when determining when to return an athlete to play. But this can be problematic because objective impairments resulting from a concussion have been reported to require a longer duration of recovery than self-reporting symptoms in some athletes [8–12], and returning to play too early may put an athlete at an increased risk for a subsequent injury [13, 14].

Epidemiology

Over the past decade, an increased rate of diagnosed concussions [15] and concussion-related emergency room visits [16] indicate that either more individuals are sustaining concussions or that the awareness of concussions has recently increased. The diagnosis and management of the injury still remains controversial and variable among healthcare professionals [17]. Although several prevention strategies have been theorized, no overwhelming evidence has demonstrated clear efficacy for a specific type of intervention to reduce the risk of concussions.

In addition to high incidence rates, anatomical, physiological, and biomechanical factors may put younger athletes at an increased risk of sustaining a concussion. Factors such as the relative size of the head and neck compared with the body, the degree of myelination of nerves, and the shape of the skull have all been identified as reasons which may contribute to worse outcomes following head injuries for children [18]. As a vulnerability to concussive injuries may exist for youth athletes [18, 19], there is a need to identify and test potential strategies which help to reduce the risk of suffering a concussion.

Proposed Methods of Concussion Prevention

Previously, epidemiological studies have identified a higher concussion injury risk for those who previously suffered a concussion compared with those who did not [13, 20]. The factors which contribute to this risk, however, are not fully understood.

Due to the metabolic vulnerability in brain tissue following a concussion, a second insult of modest intensity before full recovery may cause further neuronal impairment, delay recovery [6, 21, 22], or result in cerebral edema and permanent neurological injury, a rare but devastating entity known as second impact syndrome [23]. Thus, proper management of a concussion and appropriate timing of returning to sports may be the primary key to reducing the risk of a secondary injury. Currently, many athletes fail to report concussion symptoms to medical personnel or other responsible adults, leaving many concussions unreported [24, 25]. Educating athletes about the signs and symptoms of concussion as well as the risk of returning to play prior to full recovery may decrease the incidence of recurrent injuries and second impact syndrome [26].

Motor deficits have been reported to persist in some adolescent athletes beyond symptom resolution [12]. If these motor abilities are compromised, the athlete may possess a decreased ability to properly orient their body in space in response to an oncoming impact, thus increasing the likelihood of sustaining a concussion [27]. In a study conducted by Mihalik and colleagues, youth hockey players who anticipated an oncoming collision were able to adequately position their body and brace for the impact [27], thereby decreasing their risk of sustaining a concussion, while unanticipated collisions were more likely to result in a concussion. Such abilities require proper motor function and awareness, both of which may provide a crucial role in preventing a concussion. Thus, identification of complete motor and cognitive recovery following concussion or training interventions aimed to increase awareness and improve technique may be beneficial in reducing the risk of recurrent and secondary concussion injuries. Similarly, the adequate tracking of neurocognitive function may decrease the risk of early return to play and associated secondary injuries, as some studies have shown incomplete cognitive recovery in some athletes, even when they report being symptom-free [9, 28]. Thus, the assessment of cognitive function as one of several determinants of recovery may also decrease the risk of additional, secondary injuries, prior to full recovery.

Specific strengthening protocols may be also beneficial. Different research groups have investigated interventions which may strengthen neck muscles in order to better stabilize the head and neck together during an impact. No reports up to this point, however, have identified an effective, easily implementable, and cost-effective prevention protocol [29]. Two studies employed an 8-week resistance training program targeted at increasing neck strength and reported modest improvements in the overall strength of neck muscles, but no muscle activation or movement pattern changes [30, 31]. Neck strength may be a key factor in the odds of sustaining a concussion, as recent epidemiological evidence suggests that greater neck strength may be associated with reduced odds of sustaining a concussion in contact sport athletes [29]. This indicates that targeted neck strengthening protocols may provide a feasible mechanism to reduce the risk of concussion for adolescent athletes and warrants further exploration. Neuromuscular training regimens may also help to enhance the dynamic response of the head during an impact, as this type of training has been reported to reduce odds of sustaining a high magnitude impact to the head [32]. Thus, a combination of strength and proper neuromuscular response training may reduce the risk of sport-related concussion.

Researchers have investigated new and innovative head and neck protective equipment hoping to reduce concussion risk [33–35]. Within the context of sport-related concussion, however, little reliable evidence exists to support the idea that a helmet can effectively decrease injury risk. Instead, helmets have been designed to prevent serious head trauma such as skull fractures, rather than concussion, and they have been highly successful in reducing injuries such as fractures and severe traumatic brain injury [36]. However, for most sports, there is sparse evidence reporting any changes in the incidence of concussion due to different helmet types. Mouth guards have also been proposed as a type of equipment to prevent head injuries, but little reliable evidence exists to support their efficacy for any protection against concussion [35].

Rule changes, however, have been documented to positively influence behavior and may reduce concussion rates [37]. In ice hockey, rule changes encouraging "fair play" have been observed to reduce aggressive, dangerous behavior [38] as well as the number of face lacerations and time-loss injuries [39]. Therefore, although hope remains for development of protective equipment that will effectively reduce the risk of concussion, protective equipment may not provide the best way to prevent a concussion. Instead, focusing efforts on proper conditioning and training along with appropriate rule changes and enforcement may best prepare athletes to safely compete in sports.

Catastrophic Head Injury

Biomechanics and Pathophysiology

Catastrophic head injury is a serious and potentially life-threatening form of brain injury which may occur during athletic participation. By definition, a catastrophic injury results in death or permanent neurologic sequelae. Although catastrophic injuries occur much less frequently than concussion, the consequences are devastating [1, 40].

Intracranial hemorrhages result from a high velocity impact which damages arteries (epidural) or veins (subdural) causing an accumulation of blood within the cranial vault. Although initial symptoms may be subtle, intracranial hemorrhages can result in rapid deterioration and eventual coma or death [23]. To rule out this type of injury, removal from the field of play and evaluation by medical personnel are recommended for all athletes that sustain a head injury during sports, especially when symptoms persist and worsen over time or neurological findings are detected [23].

As noted above, "second impact syndrome" [41] has been documented throughout a series of case studies since the 1980s. Second impact syndrome occurs when an athlete sustains a head injury, followed by a second head injury prior to symptom resolution, and results in rapid deterioration and eventually permanent disability or death [23]. The majority of cases of second impact syndrome involve athletes who are adolescents [42]. Although the mechanism underlying this pathological condition remains unknown, it is hypothesized that the loss of cerebral blood flow autoregulation leads to unrestricted swelling of the brain within the cranium [23]. This condition has been reported to result in a mortality rate of 50 % and a morbidity rate of 100 % [2]. Thus, while it may occur rarely, due to its catastrophic nature, prevention is of utmost importance.

Epidemiology

Due to their rarity [23], it is difficult to properly study and reliably estimate the incidence of catastrophic head injuries. The available evidence suggests the incidence is low, even in high risk sports such as American football, where the incidence may be higher in the adolescent population than in the young adult population [40]. Although the exact mechanism for this increased incidence is not clear, multiple possibilities have been identified. The brain is not fully developed during adolescence, and due to ongoing development, the threshold for injury may be decreased [40]. The ongoing development of the brain may also affect brain blood vessels, which may be more likely to tear during adolescence than during adulthood [40]. Further, high school events often have less medical coverage than professional or collegiate sporting events. Therefore, there may be limited recognition and immediate treatment of neurological injuries resulting in worse outcomes, including an increased risk of second impact syndrome [42], as athletes with unrecognized concussions return to play.

A study conducted by Boden and colleagues reported that among those who sustained a catastrophic head injury, 71 % reported that they suffered a concussion earlier in the season, indicating a potential risk factor [40], a finding that has been reported subsequently as well [43]. Thus, due to this increased risk of reinjury, all states in the USA have enacted legislation to reduce the likelihood of an adolescent athlete continuing to play while still experiencing head injury symptoms [44, 45]. However, this type of legislation still relies on accurate recognition and reporting. As such, proper education and medical personnel presence remain critical components in reducing the risk of subsequent injury.

Proposed Methods of Injury Prevention

Since the addition of helmets with a hard plastic shell to American football in the 1950s, severe head injuries and associated fatalities have decreased, due, in part, to the regulatory body which oversees equipment regulation and inspection: the National Operating Committee on Standards for Athletic Equipment (NOCSAE), as well as improved medical care [46]. Initially, the implementation of helmets was associated with a dramatic increase in catastrophic spinal cord injuries, outlined in the next section of the chapter. Consequently, helmets may be effective at reducing the risk of a catastrophic head injury but may also lead to a more aggressive, dangerous playing style, potentially predisposing athletes to vulnerable postures leading to neck injuries.

Other than equipment, measures exist which may assist to prevent serious head injuries. The pre-participation examination allows a physician to understand the athlete's injury history, including instances where the athlete may still be suffering from any previous head-related trauma, and may help to identify if an athlete is not ready to begin participation in a sport [2, 47]. Once competition begins, proper on-site medical personnel, ideally including a certified athletic trainer and a physician, may improve outcomes by identifying those who should be removed from play, initiating early medical care, and referring players with potentially severe injuries promptly to a hospital [2, 47]. Proper coach training and the hiring of coaches who can teach proper fundamental skill acquisition are another imperative aspect to the safety of the adolescent athlete, as improper teaching may increase risk for a direct catastrophic injury [47, 48].

Cervical Spine Fracture and Quadriplegia

Biomechanics and Pathophysiology

The cervical spine is an area of the body that performs a variety of complex movements while protecting the fragile spinal cord. As a result, trauma to the spinal cord at the neck may result in devastating and irreversible consequences [49]. Although advances in rules, training, and equipment may have helped to reduce the overall incidence rates of cervical spine fractures and quadriplegia, it is still a complex condition that must be recognized properly and managed appropriately to avoid further damage [49].

Cervical spine injuries most often occur when a compressive force is applied to the top of the head in a downward direction [50]. Events such as being driven into the mat in wrestling, tackling headfirst in American football, or getting knocked into the boards headfirst during ice hockey place the cervical spine in a vulnerable position [47, 50]: directly between the rapidly decelerating mass of the body and a fixed mass such as the dasher boards or wrestling mat or an oncoming mass such as an opposing player [51, 52]. The type and severity of the injury that results depends on the position of the individual's neck at the time of impact. In its usual resting position, the cervical spine of most athletes has a lordotic curve. This positioning allows the cervical spine to extend slightly as a force is applied to the top of the head and allows force to be absorbed, in part, by the cervical musculature. The most vulnerable position when an impact occurs to the top of the head is when the neck is flexed forward and aligns the spinal column into a straight line. When this happens, the force from the impact is directed straight down the spinal column, which is poorly equipped to withstand these forces [50]. Further, this position decreases the efficacy of the neck musculature, which typically serves to dissipate forces imparted to the head–neck segment [52].

If forces imparted to the spine are high enough, a fracture or dislocation may occur, leading to a risk of bony impingement into the cervical canal. When the cervical spine is fractured, bone fragments may intrude into the spinal canal, injuring the cord and may lead to permanent disability (quadriplegia) or death [49].

Epidemiology

In the context of American football, technology and equipment regulations have appeared to dramatically influence the rate of catastrophic cervical spine injuries. In the 1950s, when face masks were not a part of the standard equipment in football, athletes primarily initiated contact with the shoulder during a tackle [53]. But the introduction of the face mask resulted in athletes more readily initiating contact with their heads first, leading to a high rate of death or disability [53]. Following this rise, helmets were regulated, beginning in 1978 at the collegiate level and in 1980 at the high school level [53]. While these changes led to a dramatic decrease in fatalities caused by catastrophic head injury, they may have led to an increase in neck injuries. In addition, the scalp, which typically is highly sensitive to trauma, is protected by the hard plastic shell of the helmet. Thus, techniques such as butt blocking and spear tackling, in which the athlete initiates contact with the top of the head as opposed to the shoulder, became more common after the introduction of the hard plastic shell helmets with face masks. This led to an increase in cervical spine injuries and quadriplegia.

In the early 1970s, there were 259 documented cases of cervical fractures or dislocations in the National Football League, which primarily occurred due to an axial loading of the neck [50]. In response to such a high incidence rate, headfirst contact was banned from American football in January 1976 [49]. Following this rule change, a substantial decrease in the number of cases of cervical fractures, dislocations, and subluxations occurring in American football was observed (see Fig. 1.1). Although improvements in conditioning, education, equipment, and technique may have also contributed to this decrease, the rule change to disallow headfirst tackling appears to have had the biggest impact on the reduction of catastrophic cervical spine injuries [50]. Proper coaching of tackling technique may continue to keep the rate of this type of injury low in the high school athlete population.

Proposed Methods of Injury Prevention

Anatomical factors may play a role in the risk of cervical spine fracture or quadriplegia. Individuals with cervical spine stenosis, narrowing of the cervical spinal canal, have an increased risk for suffering permanent neurological injury [50, 54]. Further, the combination of anatomy and playing style may increase the risk for cervical spine fracture or dislocation. The combination of spinal stenosis, persistent straightening of the typically curved cervical spine, radiographic abnormalities, and a history of headfirst tackling has been termed "spear tackler's spine," and, in the athletic setting, may present for an increased risk for cervical spine fracture [52].

Once headfirst tackling was banned from American football in 1976, the rate of catastrophic cervical spine injuries steadily decreased (see Fig. 1.1) [55]. Further, the removal of the word "intentional" in 2005 made any type of headfirst tackling illegal and allowed referees to call a penalty without having to interpret intention of the player, creating a safer playing environment [56]. While these rule changes have

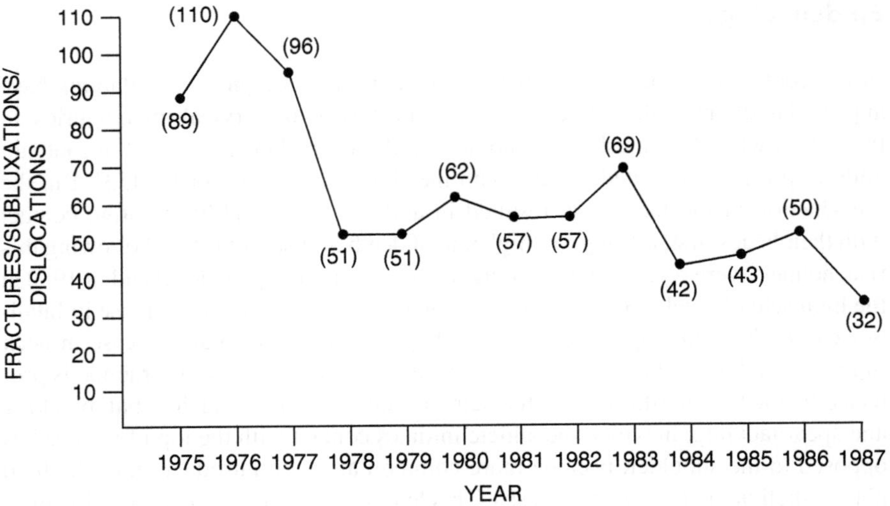

Fig. 1.1 Cervical spine fractures, dislocations, and subluxations for high school, collegiate, and professional football players decreased substantially beginning in 1977 as a result of rule changes implemented in 1976, which banned head-first blocking, tackling, and spearing. From Torg et al. [51] © 1990, reprinted by Permission of SAGE publications

been effective in reducing the incidence of cervical spine fractures and quadriplegia, proper instruction remains a key component in preventing catastrophic injuries. A poorly executed block or tackle may be one cause of cervical spine fractures [47], so coaches play a pivotal role in athlete protection. Avoidance of any repeated posture which creates a vulnerable position for an athlete, including leading with the top of the head or an impact that combines a headfirst and slightly flexed neck posture, should be stressed by all coaches in all sports.

Burners and Stingers

Biomechanics and Pathophysiology

Burners and stingers are typically transient events involving sensory and/or motor function loss in the arms resulting from a rapid stretch of the brachial plexus or compression of the exiting nerves to the upper extremity [54]. During a collision, particularly those involving younger athletes, the shoulder nerves may stretch when the head is abruptly flexed laterally while simultaneously the shoulder is displaced in a downward direction, stressing the nerves that travel from the cervical spine into the upper extremity, resulting in a burning sensation down the arm [50]. This injury is always unilateral and rarely persists beyond 30 min but has been documented to go on for days to months in rare circumstances [50]. For a further discussion of burners and stingers, please see the chapter by Kerr et al.

Epidemiology

Various risk factors have been explored related to the occurrence of a burner or stinger. It appears that they take place most often during participation in American football or wrestling [50]. As with cervical spine injuries, burners or stingers have been implicated to occur more frequently in athletes with a spinal stenosis [50]. Continued presence of this injury may be indicative of a lesion in the brachial plexus or underlying dislocation of the shoulder joint [57], and a physician referral should be made if stingers or burners are experienced frequently.

Proposed Methods of Injury Prevention

Of particular importance following a burner or stinger is proper management, including ruling out any cervical spine or spinal cord injury, which may be the cause of the reported pain [54]. But as no randomized control trials exist examining this type of injury, strong evidence to support prevention measures is sparse [54]. Expert opinion has identified risk factors following the first burner or stinger, which may help to prevent further burners or stingers. Following any type of cervical spine injury, an athlete should not return to play until they have demonstrated full strength and full range of motion in the injured areas [54]. By identifying residual symptoms, neck pain, or incomplete strength or range of motion, the healthcare provider may help to allow time for proper recovery and reduce the risk of sustaining a future burner or stinger.

The use of proper fitting protective equipment such as shoulder pads, cowboy collars, and neck rolls may reduce the risk of these injuries [58], but there is little currently available evidence supporting their use [57, 59, 60]. However, adherence to proper equipment regulations, instruction of proper tackling technique, and appropriate conditioning are all currently employed in order to reduce the likelihood of sustaining a burner or stinger.

Conclusion

While it may be impossible to completely eliminate the risk of injury, reducing risks of all types of injury, from severe to mild, may be achievable with proper education, training, equipment, and medical management to reduce the likelihood of a repeat injury. Future research should prospectively examine each of these components individually and when performed in conjunction with each other in order to identify how well these strategies help reduce head or neck injury rates. In addition, research will help advance the development of innovative and clinically implementable ways to proactively help athletes compete in sport activities in a safer manner.

References

1. Gessel LM, Fields SK, Collins CL, Dick RW, Comstock RD. Concussions among United States high school and collegiate athletes. J Athl Train. 2007;42:495–503.
2. Mueller FO. Catastrophic head injuries in high school and collegiate sports. J Athl Train. 2001;36:312–5.
3. Meehan WP, Mannix R. A substantial proportion of life-threatening injuries are sport-related. Pediatr Emerg Care. 2013;29:624–7.
4. Broglio SP, Cantu RC, Gioia GA, Guskiewicz KM, Kutcher J, Palm M, et al. National Athletic Trainers' Association position statement: management of sport concussion. J Athl Train. 2014;49:245–65.
5. Broglio SP, Surma T, Ashton-Miller JA. High school and collegiate football athlete concussions: a biomechanical review. Ann Biomed Eng. 2012;40:37–46.
6. Giza CC, Hovda DA. The neurometabolic cascade of concussion. J Athl Train. 2001;36:228.
7. Maugans TA, Farley C, Altaye M, Leach J, Cecil KM. Pediatric sports-related concussion produces cerebral blood flow alterations. Pediatrics. 2012;129:28–37.
8. Teel EF, Ray WJ, Geronimo AM, Slobounov SM. Residual alterations of brain electrical activity in clinically asymptomatic concussed individuals: an EEG study. Clin Neurophysiol. 2014;125:703–7.
9. Broglio SP, Macciocchi SN, Ferrara MS. Neurocognitive performance of concussed athletes when symptom free. J Athl Train. 2007;42:504–8.
10. Powers KC, Cinelli ME, Kalmar JM. Cortical hypoexcitability persists beyond the symptomatic phase of a concussion. Brain Inj. 2014;28:465–71.
11. Howell D, Osternig L, van Donkelaar P, Mayr U, Chou L-S. Effects of concussion on attention and executive function in adolescents. Med Sci Sports Exerc. 2013;45:1030–7.
12. Howell DR, Osternig LR, Chou L-S. Dual-task effect on gait balance control in adolescents with concussion. Arch Phys Med Rehabil. 2013;94:1513–20.
13. Guskiewicz KM, Weaver NL, Padua DA, Garrett WE. Epidemiology of concussion in collegiate and high school football players. Am J Sports Med. 2000;28:643–50.
14. Nordström A, Nordström P, Ekstrand J. Sports-related concussion increases the risk of subsequent injury by about 50% in elite male football players. Br J Sports Med. 2014;48:1447–50.
15. Rosenthal JA, Foraker RE, Collins CL, Comstock RD. National high school athlete concussion rates from 2005-2006 to 2011-2012. Am J Sports Med. 2014;42(7):1710–5.
16. Bakhos LL, Lockhart GR, Myers R, Linakis JG. Emergency department visits for concussion in young child athletes. Pediatrics. 2010;126:e550–6.
17. Doolan AW, Day DD, Maerlender AC, Goforth M, Brolinson PG. A review of return to play issues and sports-related concussion. Ann Biomed Eng. 2012;40:106–13.
18. Meehan WP, Taylor AM, Proctor M. The pediatric athlete: younger athletes with sport-related concussion. Clin Sports Med. 2011;30:133–44.
19. Guskiewicz KM, Valovich McLeod TC. Pediatric sports-related concussion. PM R. 2011;3:353–64.
20. Zemper ED. Two-year prospective study of relative risk of a second cerebral concussion. Am J Phys Med Rehabil. 2003;82:653–9.
21. Vagnozzi R, Signoretti S, Cristofori L, Alessandrini F, Floris R, Isgrò E, et al. Assessment of metabolic brain damage and recovery following mild traumatic brain injury: a multicentre, proton magnetic resonance spectroscopic study in concussed patients. Brain. 2010;133:3232–42.
22. Yuen TJ, Browne KD, Iwata A, Smith DH. Sodium channelopathy induced by mild axonal trauma worsens outcome after a repeat injury. J Neurosci Res. 2009;87:3620–5.
23. Cantu RC. Second-impact syndrome. Clin Sports Med. 1998;17:37–44.
24. Meehan 3rd WP, Mannix RC, O'Brien MJ, Collins MW. The prevalence of undiagnosed concussions in athletes. Clin J Sport Med. 2013;23:339–42.
25. McCrea M, Hammeke T, Olsen G, Leo P, Guskiewicz K. Unreported concussion in high school football players: implications for prevention. Clin J Sport Med. 2004;14:13.

26. Register-Mihalik JK, Guskiewicz KM, McLeod TCV, Linnan LA, Mueller FO, Marshall SW. Knowledge, attitude, and concussion-reporting behaviors among high school athletes: a preliminary study. J Athl Train. 2013;48:645–53.
27. Mihalik JP, Blackburn JT, Greenwald RM, Cantu RC, Marshall SW, Guskiewicz KM. Collision type and player anticipation affect head impact severity among youth ice hockey players. Pediatrics. 2010;125:e1394–401.
28. Van Kampen DA, Lovell MR, Pardini JE, Collins MW, Fu FH. The "value added" of neurocognitive testing after sports-related concussion. Am J Sports Med. 2006;34:1630–5.
29. Collins CL, Fletcher EN, Fields SK, Kluchurosky L, Rohrkemper MK, Comstock RD, et al. Neck strength: a protective factor reducing risk for concussion in high school sports. J Prim Prev. 2014;35:309–19.
30. Mansell J, Tierney RT, Sitler MR, Swanik KA, Stearne D. Resistance training and head-neck segment dynamic stabilization in male and female collegiate soccer players. J Athl Train. 2005;40:310–9.
31. Lisman P, Signorile JF, Del Rossi G, Asfour S, Eltoukhy M, Stambolian D, et al. Investigation of the effects of cervical strength training on neck strength, EMG, and head kinematics during a football tackle. Int J Sports Sci Eng. 2012;6:131–40.
32. Schmidt JD, Guskiewicz KM, Blackburn JT, Mihalik JP, Siegmund GP, Marshall SW. The influence of cervical muscle characteristics on head impact biomechanics in football. Am J Sports Med. 2014;42(9):2056–66.
33. Rowson S, Duma SM, Greenwald RM, Beckwith JG, Chu JJ, Guskiewicz KM, et al. Can helmet design reduce the risk of concussion in football? J Neurosurg. 2014;120:919–22.
34. McIntosh AS, Andersen TE, Bahr R, Greenwald R, Kleiven S, Turner M, et al. Sports helmets now and in the future. Br J Sports Med. 2011;45:1258–65.
35. Daneshvar DH, Baugh CM, Nowinski CJ, McKee AC, Stern RA, Cantu RC. Helmets and mouth guards: the role of personal equipment in preventing sport-related concussions. Clin Sports Med. 2011;30:145–63, x.
36. Cross KM, Serenelli C. Training and equipment to prevent athletic head and neck injuries. Clin Sports Med. 2003;22:639–67.
37. McIntosh AS, McCrory P. Preventing head and neck injury. Br J Sports Med. 2005;39:314–8.
38. Cusimano MD, Nastis S, Zuccaro L. Effectiveness of interventions to reduce aggression and injuries among ice hockey players: a systematic review. Can Med Assoc J. 2013;185:E57–69.
39. Roberts W, Brust J, Leonard B, Hebert BJ. Fair-play rules and injury reduction in ice hockey. Arch Pediatr Adolesc Med. 1996;150:140–5.
40. Boden BP, Tacchetti RL, Cantu RC, Knowles SB, Mueller FO. Catastrophic head injuries in high school and college football players. Am J Sports Med. 2007;35:1075–81.
41. Saunders RL, Harbaugh RE. The second impact in catastrophic contact-sports head trauma. JAMA. 1984;252:538–9.
42. Cantu RC, Gean AD. Second-impact syndrome and a small subdural hematoma: an uncommon catastrophic result of repetitive head injury with a characteristic imaging appearance. J Neurotrauma. 2010;27:1557–64.
43. Thomas M, Haas TS, Doerer JJ, Hodges JS, Aicher BO, Garberich RF, et al. Epidemiology of sudden death in young, competitive athletes due to blunt trauma. Pediatrics. 2011;128:e1–8.
44. Tomei KL, Doe C, Prestigiacomo CJ, Gandhi CD. Comparative analysis of state-level concussion legislation and review of current practices in concussion. Neurosurg Focus. 2012;33(E11):1–9.
45. Gibson TB, Herring SA, Kutcher JS, Broglio SP. Analyzing the effect of state legislation on health care utilization for children with concussion. JAMA Pediatr. 2015;169:163–8.
46. Boden BP. Direct catastrophic injury in sports. J Am Acad Orthop Surg. 2005;13:445–54.
47. Cantu RC, Mueller FO. The prevention of catastrophic head and spine injuries in high school and college sports. Br J Sports Med. 2009;43:981–6.
48. Zemper ED. Catastrophic injuries among young athletes. Br J Sports Med. 2010;44:13–20.
49. Banerjee R, Palumbo M, Fadale P. Catastrophic cervical spine injuries in the collision sport athlete, part 1: epidemiology, functional anatomy, and diagnosis. Am J Sports Med. 2004;32: 1077–87.

50. Bailes J, Petschauer M, Guskiewicz K, Marano G. Management of cervical spine injuries in athletes. J Athl Train. 2007;42:126–34.
51. Torg JS, Vegso JJ, O'Neill MJ, Sennett B. The epidemiologic, pathologic, biomechanical, and cinematographic analysis of football-induced cervical spine trauma. Am J Sports Med. 1990;18:50–7.
52. Torg JS, Sennett B, Pavlov H, Leventhal MR, Glasgow SG. Spear tackler's spine. An entity precluding participation in tackle football and collision activities that expose the cervical spine to axial energy inputs. Am J Sports Med. 1993;21:640–9.
53. Cantu RC, Mueller FO. Catastrophic spine injuries in American football, 1977-2001. Neurosurgery. 2003;53:358–62; discussion 362–3.
54. Cantu RC, Li YM, Abdulhamid M, Chin LS. Return to play after cervical spine injury in sports. Curr Sports Med Rep. 2013;12:14–7.
55. Torg JS, Guille JT, Jaffe S. Injuries to the cervical spine in American football players. J Bone Joint Surg Am. 2002;84-A:112–22.
56. Boden BP, Tacchetti RL, Cantu RC, Knowles SB, Mueller FO. Catastrophic cervical spine injuries in high school and college football players. Am J Sports Med. 2006;34:1223–32.
57. Markey KL, Di Benedetto M, Curl WW. Upper trunk brachial plexopathy. The stinger syndrome. Am J Sports Med. 1993;21:650–5.
58. Chao S, Pacella MJ, Torg JS. The pathomechanics, pathophysiology and prevention of cervical spinal cord and brachial plexus injuries in athletics. Sports Med. 2010;40:59–75.
59. Stuber K. Cervical collars and braces in athletic brachial plexus injury and excessive cervical motion prevention: a review of the literature. J Can Chiropr Assoc. 2005;49:216–22.
60. Gorden JA, Straub SJ, Swanik CB, Swanik KA. Effects of football collars on cervical hyperextension and lateral flexion. J Athl Train. 2003;38:209–15.

2 Protective Equipment

Emilie Dolan and Peter Kriz

Introduction

Injuries involving the head and neck represent a significant proportion of sports-related trauma incurred by youth athletes. Approximately 6.5 % of over 2.6 million children ≤ 19 years treated for sport and recreation-related injuries in an emergency department setting between 2001 and 2009 had sustained traumatic brain injuries or concussions [1]. In this chapter, we will review the history of protective equipment; evidence supporting the utilization of head, face, and neck protective gear in contact/collision sports; the role protective equipment plays in injury reduction; attitudes among players, medical staff, and coaches toward the use of protective equipment; issues pertaining to enforcement and mandated use of protective gear; advertising and marketing claims regarding protective equipment; and future directions and research regarding head and neck protective equipment.

History of Protective Equipment and Evidence of Effectiveness

Helmets and Headgear

Protective headgear initially was designed for combat due to the vulnerability of the head in wartime operations. With the advent of sophisticated weapons and twentieth-century manufacturing technological advances, mass production of standard-issue head protection became available for soldiers. Significant morbidity and mortality in American football sparked the adoption of modern head protection

E. Dolan, BS • P. Kriz, MD (✉)
Rhode Island Hospital, Providence, RI, USA
e-mail: emiliedolan1@gmail.com; peter_kriz@brown.edu

M. O'Brien, W.P. Meehan III (eds.), *Head and Neck Injuries in Young Athletes*, Contemporary Pediatric and Adolescent Sports Medicine,
DOI 10.1007/978-3-319-23549-3_2

in sport. The first documented use of a leather football helmet occurred during the 1893 Army-Navy game. In 1905, 18 deaths and 129 serious injuries occurred in American football, prompting President Theodore Roosevelt to call a conference with representatives of several Ivy League schools, resulting in the formation of the Intercollegiate Athletic Association, the predecessor to the National Collegiate Athletic Association (NCAA) [2, 3]. Helmet technology continued to evolve in the early twentieth century, with leather padding gradually being replaced by metal and plastic components. However, leather helmets continued to be developed and utilized routinely in American football through the 1940s. Mandatory helmet use in American football did not occur until 1939 in the NCAA and 1943 in the National Football League (NFL). Unfortunately, serious head injuries including intracranial hemorrhages and skull fractures remained prevalent in American football throughout the mid-twentieth century, prompting rule changes, coaching changes, and, ultimately, the formation of the National Operating Committee on Standards for Athletic Equipment (NOCSAE) in 1969, which ultimately implemented the first football helmet safety standards in 1973 [4, 5].

American Football

Since the development of modern-day sports concussion assessment and management guidelines [6–8], few studies regarding helmet effectiveness in reducing head injury in American football have been published. Studies conducted prior to the Prague/Zurich era tended to underreport concussive injuries, reported only the most severe concussive injuries, and relied on coach and certified athletic trainer (ATC) diagnosis [4, 9, 10]. Collins et al. performed a prospective cohort study during the 2002–2004 seasons comparing concussion rates and recovery times for 2141 high school football players. Nearly half the sample wore newer helmet technology (Riddell Revolution), and the remainder used traditional helmet designs from various manufacturers. Over the course of the study, the concussion rate of the Revolution helmet group was 5.3 % compared to 7.6 % in the traditional helmet group ($p<0.03$) [11]. However, this study was limited by lack of randomization of helmets among study participants, mean chronologic age discrepancies among study groups, and variability in age of the helmets, as the Revolution helmets were brand new while traditional helmets were reconditioned. Additionally, impact exposure was not accounted for.

Rowson et al. performed a retrospective analysis of head impact data collected from 1833 Division I collegiate football players between 2005 and 2010 utilizing helmet-mounted accelerometers, in an effort to determine whether helmet design reduces the incidence of concussion. Concussion rates were compared between two helmet models: the Riddell VSR4 and the Riddell Revolution. The Revolution helmet had a greater offset and 40 % thicker foam than the VSR4 helmet. The number of head impacts each player experienced were controlled for. ATCs or team physicians diagnosed 64 concussions by from a total of 1,281,444 recorded head impacts. Players wearing the Revolution helmets had a 53.9 % reduction in concussion risk compared to players wearing the VSR4 helmet. When each player's exposure to head impact was controlled for, a statistically significant difference was found between concussion rates for players wearing VSR4 and Revolution helmets ($\chi^2=4.7, p=0.04$). Players wearing VSR4 helmets had a per-impact concussion rate more than twice as high as players wearing Revolution helmets (8.4 vs. 3.9 concussions per 100,000 head impacts, respectively). Additionally, players wearing VSR helmets experienced higher acceleration impacts more frequently, regardless of the position they played. The authors concluded that differences in the ability to reduce concussion risk between helmet models in American football indeed exist [12]. Limitations of this study included lack of randomization of helmets among study participants and widespread underreporting of concussion in Division I college football during the study period.

McGuine et al. performed a prospective cohort study of 2081 high school football players during the 2012 and 2013 seasons to determine whether the type of protective equipment and player characteristics affect the incidence of sports-related concussion (SRC). There were 211 SRCs sustained by 206 players (9 % of included athletes), for an incidence of 1.6 SRCs per 1000 athletic-exposures. No difference in incidence of SRC for players wearing Riddell, Schutt, or Zenith helmets was identified. Additionally, helmet age and recondition status did not affect the incidence of SRC [13]. Limitations of this study included lack of randomization of helmets among study participants and lack of collection of impact exposure data.

Ice Hockey

Similar to American football, ice hockey protective headgear underwent technological advances, beginning with leather and felt construction in the 1950s and the introduction of plastic shells and foam liners in the 1970s which could absorb energy and provide a comfortable fit. In 1979, the National Hockey League (NHL) adopted head protection 11 years following a fatal head injury during NHL play [2]. Despite the widespread use of helmets at both amateur and professional levels, brain injuries remain a serious concern [14]. Recent literature has focused on the role that facial protection plays in modifying head injury risk in ice hockey and will be discussed in a later section.

Cycling

Early bicycle helmets were very rudimentary, constructed from strips of leather sewn together and reinforced with padding. Such designs were largely ineffective in reducing head injury and were replaced in the 1970s with a hard shell and expanded polystyrene (EPS) liner. Over the past several decades, this hard shell has waned in popularity and has been replaced by a thin microshell covering an EPS liner [2]. Wearing a properly fitted helmet has been shown to decrease head injuries by 63–88 % in cyclists of all ages [15]. While the debate and dispute over mandatory helmet use legislation continue, currently only two countries mandate bicycle helmet use for all cyclists: Australia and New Zealand.

Amoros et al. performed a retrospective case-control study utilizing a road trauma registry in France between 1998 and 2008. Thirteen thousand seven hundred ninety-seven cyclist injuries involving the head, face, or neck were identified. The control group consisted of cyclist injuries below the neck. Authors adjusted for age, gender, type of crash, injury severity, and crash location (road type, urban/rural). For head injury of any severity, the crude odds ratio (OR) for helmeted cyclists was estimated at 0.8 (95 % CI 0.7–0.9), whereas the crude OR for serious head injury was estimated at 0.4 (95 % CI 0.2–0.7). When adjusted for confounders, ORs were lower for both injury subgroups. Authors concluded that bicycle helmet use resulted in a decreased risk of head injury regardless of severity, with a greater decrease for risk of serious head injuries [16].

Bambach et al. performed a retrospective case-control study using linked police-reported road crash, hospital admission, and mortality data in Australia during 2001–2009. One of the primary objectives of the study was to assess the effectiveness of bicycle helmets in preventing head injuries (HIs) among cyclist crashes involving motor vehicles (CCMVs). Cases were those cyclists who sustained HIs and weren't admitted to hospital, while controls were those admitted/not admitted to hospital without HIs. A total of 6745 CCMVs were identified where helmet use was known, and the overall helmet wearing rate was 75.4 %. Of the 639 cyclists with HIs, 42.9 % sustained intracranial injury, 18.5 % sustained skull fracture, and 14.4 % sustained open wounds. Helmet use was associated with up to 74 % reduced risk of HIs in CCMVs. Cyclists not wearing a helmet had 3.9 (95 % CI 2.2–6.8) times higher odds of sustaining moderate, serious, or severe head injuries, with $p<0.0001$ for all three injury severities. Nearly 50 % of children and adolescents 19 years and younger in the study were not wearing a helmet [17].

Soccer

Headgear use in soccer is a relative newcomer to the landscape of protective equipment in contact sports. Federation International de Football Association (FIFA), the global governing body of soccer, began permitting its use in 2003. Most headgear is comprised of a thin layer of shock-absorbing foam fit between outer layers of fabric. American Society for Testing and Materials (ASTM) International set a performance standard for headgear in 2006; currently, five headgear products meet this standard [18].

Withnall et al. conducted controlled laboratory testing utilizing a human volunteer and test dummy headforms in an effort to determine whether soccer headgear had an effect on head impact responses. Impact attenuations of three commercial headgears during ball impact speeds of 6–30 m/s and in head-to-head contact with a closing speed of 2–5 m/s were measured. For ball impacts, none of the headgear provided attenuation over the full range of impact speeds. Head responses with or without headgear were not significantly different ($p>0.05$) and remained well below levels associated with mild traumatic brain injury. The authors concluded that while headgear provided a measurable benefit during head-to-head impact (both linear and rotational acceleration were reduced by nearly 33 % for all three headgear in head-to-head contacts), the headgear models tested did not provide any benefit during ball impact, likely due to the large amount of ball deformation relative to the headband thickness [19].

Delaney et al. performed a retrospective online survey of 278 Canadian youth soccer players aged 12–17 years old in an effort to assess the role of headgear on concussion symptoms. Respondents were asked how many concussions they had experienced in the prior season, as well as how many times they had experienced concussion-specific symptoms in response to a collision. 7.2 % of players reported at least one concussion, while 7.8 % reported experiencing concussion symptoms at least once in the prior season. Players self-selected on the decision to wear headgear, and those players who had suffered a previous concussion were more likely to wear headgear. Players who did not wear headgear were 2.6 times more likely to sustain a concussion compared to those players who did [20]. Limitations of this study include the lack of randomization of headgear use and recall bias as information in this retrospective study was collected from athletes at the conclusion of the season.

Facemasks and Face Shields

Ice Hockey

Variable standards are imposed at different levels of ice hockey with regard to the use of face shields. Full-face shields cover the entire face and can either be made of impact-resistant plastic or metal cages, while half-face shields or visors cover only the upper half of the face. The National Federation of State High School Associations (NFHS) and the NCAA require all players to wear full-face shields, while USA Hockey only requires the use of full-face shields until the adult level [21]. Asplund et al. found that wearing facemasks significantly reduced the occurrence of facial, ocular, and dental injuries in hockey [14]. Lemaire and Pearsall demonstrated that ice hockey helmets with full-face shields produce lower post-impact peak acceleration (10–100 g) than do helmets alone (100–130 g), consequently concluding that facial protector use may lower the incidence as well as severity of head injuries by decreasing post-impact head acceleration [22].

Reduction of facial injuries by facemasks should not be confused with evidence for the reduction of concussions in ice hockey. Injury data obtained from the NHL ($n=787$ players) during the 2001–2002 season found that players wearing half visors were not less likely to sustain concussions than those players without face shields. Visors were shown to prevent eye injuries and significantly reduce non-concussion head injuries. The data provided by the NHL is representative of the visor trends throughout North American and European hockey leagues [23]. Similarly, at the amateur level, Asplund et al. found no difference in the concussion rates between players who wear half vs. full-face shields [14]. Although there is a lack of evidence that visors and full-face shields prevent concussions, there is evidence demonstrating that the use of visors and face shields reduces the recovery time from a concussion. In a study by Benson et al., concussed hockey players wearing visors missed over twice as many practices and games compared to those wearing a full-face shield (4.1 vs. 1.7 sessions; 95 % CIs 3.5–4.7 and 1.3–2.2, respectively) [24]. Despite this, NHL players have claimed that wearing a visor shows lack of toughness, making them a prime target for the opposing team [23, 25].

Baseball/Softball

In baseball and softball, catchers are required to wear a facemask, and for good reason: a 2010 study showed that facemask wear reduced the resultant post-impact peak acceleration by 85 %, from a range of 140–180 to a range of 16–30 g. Not only did the catcher's mask reduce the peak acceleration post-impact, but it was also shown to reduce the head injury criterion number from 93–181 without a mask to 3–13 with a mask, as well as the severity index from 110–210 to 3–15 with a mask [26]. Recent discussions have focused on the idea of requiring headgear and facemasks for pitchers, who have suffered rare albeit serious injuries from receiving baseballs to the head.

Marshall et al. analyzed data from over 6.7 million player-seasons when studying the effectiveness of faceguards in youth baseball. They found that the use of faceguards reduced the risk of facial injury (adjusted rate ratio, 0.7, 95 % CI 0.4–1.0) [27].

Lacrosse

Lincoln et al. studied 507,000 high school and 649,573 collegiate lacrosse players of both genders to find the most common occurrences of head, face, and eye injuries. At the high school level, the rate of head, face, and eye injuries for girls was significantly higher than that for boys (0.5 vs. 0.4 per 1000 AEs, respectively). The same trend was found among college athletes, with women having a higher injury rate than men (0.8 vs. 0.4 per 1000 AEs, respectively). Of these injuries, boys and men were more likely to sustain concussions (73 % for boys, 85 % for men vs. 40 % for girls and 41 % for women), while girls and women presented higher rates of face injuries. The majority of concussions for men were the result of direct contact with another player, whereas female concussions were usually due to stick, ball, or ground contact [28]. It remains unclear, from such striking evidence, why helmets and protective gear are required for men's but not women's lacrosse. As in all contact sports, there is a concern that players who wear more protective equipment will play more aggressively and possibly incur injury more frequently. However, studies of the implementation of additional protective equipment in ice hockey and field hockey do not support such claims [29, 30].

Protective Eyewear

Sports are responsible for a third of eye injuries in the United States that lead to blindness [31]. Recent studies reviewing data from the National Electronic Injury Surveillance System reveal that 208,517 sports-related eye injuries were treated in US emergency departments between 2001 and 2009. Data from the National Eye Trauma System show that sports account for 13 % of all penetrating ocular injuries. While eye injury trends declined from 2001 to 2005, recent data show increasing injury rates from 2007 to 2009 [32, 33]. Despite policy and position statements that strongly recommend certified protective eyewear from organizations including the American Academy of Ophthalmology and the American Academy of Pediatrics [34], few youth sports organizations mandate protective eyewear, and few studies have been published which demonstrate the effectiveness of protective eyewear in reducing eye injuries.

Lincoln et al. performed a prospective cohort study involving American female high school lacrosse players during the 2000–2009 seasons, comparing eye injury rates before and after implementation of a protective eyewear mandate during the 2004 season. The study population included 9430 player-seasons over the study period. ATCs recorded all injury and athletic exposure data. Eye injury rates were reduced from 0.1 injuries per 1000 AEs in 2000–2003 to 0.02 injuries per 1000 AEs in 2004–2009. Injuries to the eyelid, eyebrow, eye orbit, and eye globe were virtually eliminated after mandated use of eyewear, with the exception of injuries that occurred when standard eyewear was not being worn [35].

Kriz et al. performed a prospective cohort study involving American female high school field hockey players during two seasons of play immediately before (fall 2009 and fall 2010) and immediately after (fall 2011 and fall 2012) a national mandate for protective eyewear in girls' field hockey was exercised by the National Federation of High School Associations. Eye injury incidence rates were compared between players competing in US states that mandated protective eyewear (MPE), players competing in states with no protective eyewear mandate (no MPE), and the postmandate group. Players from 16 of the 19 states that sanctioned high school field hockey at the time of the study were represented. Four hundred fifteen eye/orbital, head, and facial injuries were recorded during 624,803 AEs. The incidence of eye/orbital injuries was significantly higher in states without MPE (0.080 injuries per 1000 AEs) than in states with MPE (before the 2011/2012 mandate) and the postmandate group (0.025 injuries per 1000 AEs) (odds ratio 3.20, 95 % CI 1.47–6.99, $p = 0.003$). There was no significant difference in concussion rates for the two groups (odds ratio 0.77, 95 % CI 0.58–1.02, $p = 0.068$), challenging a perception in contact/collision sports that increased protective equipment yields increased injury rates [30]. After the 2011/2012 MPE, severe eye/orbital injuries (time loss > 21 days) were reduced by 67 %, and severe/medical disqualification head/face injuries were reduced by 70 %. Limitations of this study included lack of randomization as enrollment in MPE and non-MPE groups was predetermined by individual state interscholastic league mandates.

Mouthguards

The first sport to require mouthguards was professional boxing in the 1920s. Decades later, in 1962, mouthguards became mandatory in high school football. Currently, both the NFHS and the NCAA require the use of mouthguards in football, ice hockey, field hockey, and lacrosse [36]. When properly fitted, mouthguards can greatly reduce the severity of dental and maxillofacial injuries [21]. In a 2007 study by Knapik et al., athletes who did not wear mouthguards were 1.6–1.9 times more likely to receive an oral-facial injury than those wearing mouthguards [36].

There are three main types of mouthguards: stock, boil-and-bite, and custom made. Stock mouthguards are ready to wear, while boil-and-bite mouthguards must first be heated and then can be molded to the teeth while cooling. Custom mouthguards must be made by a dental professional and offer the best fit [21].

There has been great debate as to the effectiveness of mouthguards in preventing concussions. It has been postulated that mouthguards may be able to absorb some of the shock that would otherwise reach the brain [36]. Studies of hits to the underside of the jaw of a mechanical skull have demonstrated that mouthguards reduce deformations and fractures to the jaw by 54.7 % and significantly decrease the acceleration of the head by 18.5 % [21]. In a number of other impact studies, it has been shown that mouthguards do reduce the injury to teeth and dampen impact forces [36]. However, due to ethical concerns, these studies were not done on live humans, putting into question the ability to generalize the results to athletes.

In other studies, comparisons were made between concussion occurrences in athletes who wear mouthguards vs. those who do not [37–39]. In all three studies, no significant difference was found between those who used mouthguards and those who did not. There also is no evidence that custom-fit mouthguards provide superior protection compared to stock and boil-and-bite models.

Despite the lack of clear evidence as to the effectiveness of mouthguards in the prevention of concussions, the NFHS remains steadfast that mouthguards are necessary for safe participation in sports. The NFHS has determined that prior to the use of mouthguards and facemasks, over 50 % of football injuries were oral-facial. That number has been reduced to 1 % with the use of mouthguards [40].

Neck Straps

Neck guards are most commonly seen in ice hockey, yet they are not a required piece of equipment in most hockey programs. In 2008, following the neck laceration of an NHL player, Stuart et al. conducted a retrospective Internet-based survey and follow-up of 328,821 registered USA Hockey players, inquiring about personal experience with a neck laceration during hockey or their witnessing of such an injury. Of 26,589 responses received, only 485 (1.8 %) had sustained a neck laceration. In more than one quarter (27 %) of the incidents, the player was wearing a neck guard [41]. The survey had a number of limitations, including a response rate of only 5.8 %. Nevertheless, USA Hockey's position statement continues to recommend the use of neck guards by all hockey players.

Loyd et al. evaluated the effectiveness of different neck guards against skate lacerations. They reviewed 46 samples of 14 different types of neck guards with both low force and high force tests at differing skate orientations (45° and 90°). The authors found that neck lacerations were more likely to occur when the skate blade was angled at 45° compared with 90°. They also concluded that neck guards containing Spectra® fibers were the most resistant to lacerations [42].

Football Collars

Football collars are commonly employed in American football to reduce the incidence of burners and stingers by limiting extremes of cervical motion. However, their use and purported effectiveness are based largely on empiric data [43–45].

Up to 65 % of collegiate players experience a burner during their careers with recurrence rates approaching 85 % [46], resulting in widespread implementation of preventive strategies that includes neck and shoulder conditioning, learning proper blocking and tackling technique, and utilization of protective equipment. Gorden et al. conducted a laboratory study to evaluate the effectiveness of 3 football collars in reducing cervical range of motion in 15 Division I collegiate football players. Cervical hyperextension and lateral flexion (both active and passive) were measured with video analysis. All three collars reduced hyperextension when compared to helmet and shoulder pads alone ($p<0.05$). Additionally, the Cowboy collar was superior to a traditional foam neck roll in reducing hyperextension ($p<0.05$). No collar reduced passive lateral flexion when compared to helmet and shoulder pads alone; however, the foam neck roll permitted significantly less active lateral flexion than the other collars ($p<0.01$). From these results, the authors concluded that (1) cervical hyperextension could be controlled in a laboratory setting using various cervical collars and (2) cervical lateral flexion could not be controlled by any of the cervical collars tested, and foam collars may reduce active lateral flexion while providing no additional protection during cervical loading [45]. Study limitations included testing in a laboratory setting rather than during live, full contact play. Additionally, as football collars collectively appear to reduce active motion without an accompanying reduction in passive motion, clinicians and athletic trainers should question the use of any piece of protective equipment which limits function without providing protective benefits.

Attitudes of Players, Medical Staff, and Coaches Toward Protective Equipment Use

In a number of contact and collision sports, certain protective equipment including mouthguards, protective eyewear, face shields/visors, and athletic cups for genital protection is recommended but not mandatory. In certain sports or levels of participation, such protective equipment is mandatory, but compliance is low due to suboptimal enforcement. Factors that can affect utilization in these circumstances can include discomfort; interference with vision, breathing, speech, or running/movement; poor esthetics; peer perceptions; lack of instruction/advice on usage; and lack of education regarding injuries associated with disuse. Oftentimes, indifferent attitudes of players, parents, and/or coaching staffs can contribute to suboptimal compliance with various sports protective equipment. In other circumstances, sport tradition or culture can dictate utilization. For instance, American football players tend to demonstrate high compliance with mouthguard use but rarely choose to wear athletic cups [47]. Conversely, male ice hockey players demonstrate poor compliance with proper mouthguard use but demonstrate high compliance with athletic cup use.

Raaii et al. conducted a cross-sectional survey of 180 Canadian travel hockey players aged 9–12 years who participated in leagues allowing bodychecking and mandating mouthguard use, in an effort to determine if youth hockey players engage in proper mouthguard wear. A 12-question written questionnaire ascertained what types of mouthguards were worn, whether mouthguards were worn at all, worn properly, and reasons for noncompliance. Sixty-eight percent of players reported "always" wearing mouthguards, but only 31.7 % wore them properly during games and 51.1 % during practice. Custom mouthguards were most likely to be worn properly, followed by boil-and-bite and stock-type guards. Younger players wore mouthguards more consistently than older players ($p<0.01$). Incidentally, many mouthguards were noted to be worn out from chewing, which significantly altered their protective function [48].

Hawn et al. performed a survey of 104 NCAA ATCs who covered men's varsity ice hockey to determine enforcement patterns and athlete compliance with a rule requiring mouthguard wearing during the collegiate season. Key questions inquired about attitudes of coaching and medical staff toward mouthguard use, enforcement of mouthguard use, percentage of players wearing mouthguards in competition, and estimated number of penalties incurred secondary to mouthguard violations. The overall response rate was 82 % (104/127 programs). ATCs reported 63 % of athletes consistently wore mouthguards in competition, with significantly higher compliance at the Division II/III level compared to Division I (82 % vs. 65 %, respectively). Twenty-six percent of ATCs reported that neither the ATC nor the coach enforced mouthguard wear, despite 93 % of ATCs reporting they believed mouthguards play a role in injury prevention. Overall, only 19 mouthguard violation penalties (14/19 in Division III) were reported during the 1997 season [49].

Loopholes

Despite the existence of mandates pertaining to protective equipment in youth sports, circumstances exist in youth sports which circumvent universal compliance with these protective mandates. In the United States, the NFHS enacted a mandate regarding protective eyewear in field hockey, effective with the 2011–2012 season [50]. However, enforcement of this mandate is only applicable to public high school and interscholastic leagues that sanction field hockey. High school-age players participating in private/independent schools and leagues, as well as club teams, showcases, tournaments, and instructional camps do not have to comply with this mandate, and subsequently protective eyewear is not required for play but can be worn on a voluntary basis. The NCAA and USA Field Hockey, the governing body of field hockey in the USA, allow but do not require protective eyewear [51, 52].

Advertising/Marketing

As the focus on sports-related concussion has recently expanded to include prevention, sporting goods manufacturers have been aggressively marketing helmets, headgear, and mouthguards to youth sport participants and their parents, often with advertising campaigns that include performance test results conducted by the manufacturer. Consequently, these campaigns have been misleading to the general population as the advertising appears scientific and convincing. In 2010, Cascade Sports marketed the

M11 hockey helmet, which was endorsed by a former professional ice hockey player. The National Advertising Division of the Council of Better Business Bureaus inquired into the manufacturer's claims and ultimately recommended that Cascade Sports modify or discontinue certain advertising campaigns, after Cascade claimed the M11 helmet provided "maximum protection" and reduced the risk of concussions [53]. In 2012, the Federal Trade Commission reached a settlement with Brain-Pad, Inc., prohibiting the company from claiming that its mouthguards can reduce risk of concussions [54]. In 2014, the US Senate Committee on Commerce, Science, and Transportation passed the Youth Sports Concussions Act (S. 1014), which increased potential penalties for using false injury prevention claims to sell youth sports equipment [55].

Future Research and Direction

Current evidence pertaining to the effectiveness of protective equipment in youth sports is limited by study design, study setting, study population, standardization of reporting, sample size/power constraints, bias and confounding, ethical considerations (e.g., control group in helmeted collision sports), and expense, as longitudinal studies are costly in time and resources. Future research pertaining to youth sport protective equipment—specifically mouthguards, headgear/helmets, facial protection, and neck protection—should ideally: be prospective; be performed in natural experimental sport settings; utilize pediatric/adolescent populations; include adequate sample sizes/be sufficiently powered; utilize validated injury surveillance systems and standardized measurements, definitions (e.g., of injury and exposure), and reporting; and utilize multivariate analyses which adjust for covariates [56].

Conclusion

Protective equipment use in contact/collision sports has undergone substantial technological advancement over the past half century, resulting in significant reduction of morbidity and mortality in athletes participating in these activities. However, as more youth play competitive sports and engage in sport-specific training including strength and conditioning programs, they can resultantly generate high-magnitude impacts—forces previously thought to be achieved only by college and professional athletes. There is a collective effort by youth sports organizations, medical, safety, and scientific communities to reduce injury risk in young athletes, specifically injuries to the head and neck. Contact and collision sports have inherent safety risks that will remain despite protective equipment advances and rule modifications. Current literature demonstrates a lack of evidence regarding the role that protective equipment plays in injury reduction of youth athletes. There is a need for well-designed, prospective studies enrolling pediatric and adolescent participants utilizing standardized, validated data collection and clinical assessment tools to ultimately provide research that can guide the medical, scientific, and youth sport organization communities in establishing protective equipment regulations that ultimately make contact and collision sports safer for their participants.

References

1. Trojian TH, Mohamed N. Demystifying preventive equipment in the competitive athlete. Curr Sports Med Rep. 2012;11(6):304–8.
2. Hoshizaki TB, Brien SE. The science and design of head protection in sport. Neurosurgery. 2004;55(4):956–66; discussion 66–7.
3. Roper WW. Football today and tomorrow. New York: Duffield and Co.; 1927.
4. Daneshvar DH, Baugh CM, Nowinski CJ, et al. Helmets and mouth guards: the role of personal equipment in preventing sport-related concussions. Clin Sports Med. 2011;30(1):145–63, x.
5. Bennett T. The NFL's official encyclopedic history of professional football. 2nd ed. New York: Macmillan; 1977.
6. McCrory P, Johnston K, Meeuwisse W, et al. Summary and agreement statement of the 2nd international conference on concussion in sport, Prague 2004. Br J Sports Med. 2005;39(4):196–204.
7. McCrory P, Meeuwisse W, Johnston K, et al. Consensus statement on concussion in sport: the 3rd international conference on concussion in sport held in Zurich, November 2008. Br J Sports Med. 2009;43 Suppl 1:i76–90.
8. McCrory P, Meeuwisse WH, Aubry M, et al. Consensus statement on concussion in sport: the 4th international conference on concussion in sport held in Zurich, November 2012. Br J Sports Med. 2013;47(5):250–8.
9. Covassin T, Elbin 3rd R, Stiller-Ostrowski JL. Current sport-related concussion teaching and clinical practices of sports medicine professionals. J Athl Train. 2009;44(4):400–4.
10. Notebaert AJ, Guskiewicz KM. Current trends in athletic training practice for concussion assessment and management. J Athl Train. 2005;40(4):320–5.
11. Collins M, Lovell MR, Iverson GL, et al. Examining concussion rates and return to play in high school football players wearing newer helmet technology: a three-year prospective cohort study. Neurosurgery. 2006;58(2):275–86; discussion 86.
12. Rowson S, Duma SM, Greenwald RM, et al. Can helmet design reduce the risk of concussion in football? J Neurosurg. 2014;120(4):919–22.
13. McGuine TA, Hetzel S, McCrea M, et al. Protective equipment and player characteristics associated with the incidence of sport-related concussion in high school football players: a multifactorial prospective study. Am J Sports Med. 2014;42(10):2470–8. pii: 0363546514541926.
14. Asplund C, Bettcher S, Borchers J. Facial protection and head injuries in ice hockey: a systematic review. Br J Sports Med. 2009;43(13):993–9.
15. Goudie R, Page JL. Canadian Academy of Sport and Exercise Medicine position statement: mandatory use of bicycle helmets. Clin J Sport Med. 2013;23(6):417–8.
16. Amoros E, Chiron M, Martin JL, et al. Bicycle helmet wearing and the risk of head, face, and neck injury: a French case-control study based on a road trauma registry. Inj Prev. 2012; 18(1):27–32.
17. Bambach MR, Mitchell RJ, Grzebieta RH, et al. The effectiveness of helmets in bicycle collisions with motor vehicles: a case-control study. Accid Anal Prev. 2013;53:78–88.
18. National Federation of State High School Associations. Soccer headgear and ATSM product performance. http://www.nfhs.org/sports-resource-content/soccer-headgear-and-astm-product-performance/. Accessed 31 Aug 2014.
19. Withnall C, Shewchenko N, Wonnacott M, et al. Effectiveness of headgear in football. Br J Sports Med. 2005;39 Suppl 1:i40–8; discussion i8.
20. Delaney JS, Al-Kashmiri A, Drummond R, et al. The effect of protective headgear on head injuries and concussions in adolescent football (soccer) players. Br J Sports Med. 2008;42(2):110–5; discussion 5.
21. Protection and prevention strategies. In: Graham R, Rivara FP, Ford MA, Spicer CM, editors. Sports-related concussions in youth: improving the science, changing the culture. Washington,

DC: Institute of Medicine of the National Academies, The National Academies Press; 2013. http://www.iom.edu/Reports/2013/Sports-Related-Concussions-in-Youth-Improving-the-Science-Changing-the-Culture.aspx. Accessed 31 Aug 2014.
22. Lemair M, Pearsall DJ. Evaluation of impact attenuation of facial protectors in ice hockey helmets. Sports Eng. 2007;10(2):65–74.
23. Stevens ST, Lassonde M, de Beaumont L, et al. The effect of visors on head and facial injury in National Hockey League players. J Sci Med Sport. 2006;9(3):238–42.
24. Benson BW, Rose MS, Meeuwisse WH. The impact of face shield use on concussions in ice hockey: a multivariate analysis. Br J Sports Med. 2002;36(1):27–32.
25. Stuart MJ, Smith AM, Malo-Ortiguera SA, et al. A comparison of facial protection and the incidence of head, neck, and facial injuries in Junior A hockey players. A function of individual playing time. Am J Sports Med. 2002;30(1):39–44.
26. Shain KS, Madigan ML, Rowson S, et al. Analysis of the ability of catcher's masks to attenuate head accelerations on impact with a baseball. Clin J Sport Med. 2010;20(6):422–7.
27. Marshall SW, Mueller FO, Kirby DP, et al. Evaluation of safety balls and faceguards for prevention of injuries in youth baseball. JAMA. 2003;289(5):568–74.
28. Lincoln AE, Hinton RY, Almquist JL, et al. Head, face, and eye injuries in scholastic and collegiate lacrosse: a 4-year prospective study. Am J Sports Med. 2007;35(2):207–15.
29. Hagel B, Meeuwisse W. Risk compensation: a "side effect" of sport injury prevention? Clin J Sport Med. 2004;14(4):193–6.
30. Kriz PK, Comstock RD, Zurakowski D, et al. Eye protection and risk of eye injuries in high school field hockey. Pediatrics. 2015;136(3):521–527.
31. U.S. Consumer Product Safety Commission. Sports and recreational eye injuries. Washington, DC: U.S. Consumer Product Safety Commission; 2000.
32. Cass SP. Ocular injuries in sports. Curr Sports Med Rep. 2012;11(1):11–5.
33. Kim T, Nunes AP, Mello MJ, et al. Incidence of sports-related eye injuries in the United States: 2001-2009. Graefes Arch Clin Exp Ophthalmol. 2011;249(11):1743–4.
34. American Academy of Pediatrics Committee on Sports Medicine and Fitness. Protective eyewear for young athletes. Pediatrics. 2004;113(3 Pt 1):619–22.
35. Lincoln AE, Caswell SV, Almquist JL, et al. Effectiveness of the women's lacrosse protective eyewear mandate in the reduction of eye injuries. Am J Sports Med. 2012;40(3):611–4.
36. Knapik JJ, Marshall SW, Lee RB, et al. Mouthguards in sport activities: history, physical properties and injury prevention effectiveness. Sports Med. 2007;37(2):117–44.
37. Benson BW, Hamilton GM, Meeuwisse WH, et al. Is protective equipment useful in preventing concussion? A systematic review of the literature. Br J Sports Med. 2009;43 Suppl 1:i56–67.
38. Labella CR, Smith BW, Sigurdsson A. Effect of mouthguards on dental injuries and concussions in college basketball. Med Sci Sports Exerc. 2002;34(1):41–4.
39. Wisniewski JF, Guskiewicz K, Trope M, et al. Incidence of cerebral concussions associated with type of mouthguard used in college football. Dent Traumatol. 2004;20(3):143–9.
40. National Federation of State High School Associations. Position statement and recommendations for mouthguard use in sports. http://www.nfhs.org/sports-resource-content/position-statement-and-recommendations-for-mouthguard-use-in-sports/. Accessed 31 Aug 2014.
41. Stuart MJ, Link AA, Smith AM, et al. Skate blade neck lacerations: a survey and case follow-up. Clin J Sport Med. 2009;19(6):494–7.
42. Loyd AM, Berglund L, Twardowski CP, et al. The most cut-resistant neck guard for preventing lacerations to the neck. Clin J Sport Med. 2015;25(3):254–9.
43. Di Benedetto M, Markey K. Electrodiagnostic localization of traumatic upper trunk brachial plexopathy. Arch Phys Med Rehabil. 1984;65(1):15–7.
44. Markey KL, Di Benedetto M, Curl WW. Upper trunk brachial plexopathy. The stinger syndrome. Am J Sports Med. 1993;21(5):650–5.
45. Gorden JA, Straub SJ, Swanik CB, et al. Effects of football collars on cervical hyperextension and lateral flexion. J Athl Train. 2003;38(3):209–15.
46. Sallis RE, Jones K, Knopp W. Burners: offensive strategy for an underreported injury. Phys Sportsmed. 1992;20(11):47–55.

47. Borden S. Helmet? Check. Shoulder pads? Check. Cup? No thanks. http://www.nytimes.com/2012/12/09/sports/football/helmet-check-shoulder-pads-check-cup-no-thanks.html?_r=0. Accessed 31 Aug 2014.
48. Raaii F, Vaidya N, Vaidya K, et al. Patterns of mouthguard utilization among atom and pee wee minor ice hockey players: a pilot study. Clin J Sport Med. 2011;21(4):320–4.
49. Hawn KL, Visser MF, Sexton PJ. Enforcement of mouthguard use and athlete compliance in National Collegiate Athletic Association men's collegiate ice hockey competition. J Athl Train. 2002;37(2):204–8.
50. National Federation of State High School Associations. NFHS field hockey rules committee—eyewear ruling. https://nfhs-fieldhockey.arbitersports.com/Groups/105408/Library/files/Field%20Hockey%20Eyewear%20Press%20Release.pdf . Accessed 31 Aug 2014.
51. National Collegiate Athletic Association. NCAA field hockey rule modifications 2014. http://www.ncaa.org/sites/default/files/2014_NCAA_Field_Hockey_Rules_Modifications_072214.pdf. Accessed 31 Aug 2014.
52. USA Field Hockey. Approved FIH and USA field hockey protective eyewear. http://www.teamusa.org/USA-Field-Hockey/Features/2011/April/22/Approved-FIH-and-USA-Field-Hockey-protective-eyewear.aspx. Accessed 31 Aug 2014.
53. Boucicaut JR. Press release concerning Cascade M11 concussion claims. http://modsquad-hockey.com/forums/index.php/topic/53357-press-release-concerning-cascade-m11-concussion-claims/. Accessed 31 Aug 2014.
54. Federal Trade Commission. FTC approves final order settling charges against marketer Brain-Pad, Inc. for allegedly deceptive claims that its mouthguards can reduce risk of concussions. http://www.ftc.gov/news-events/press-releases/2012/11/ftc-approves-final-order-settling-charges-against-marketer-brain. Accessed 31 Aug 2014.
55. U.S. Senate Committee on Commerce, Science, and Transportation. Commerce Committee passes youth sports concussions bill. http://www.commerce.senate.gov/public/index.cfm?p=PressReleases&ContentRecord_id=bf3be696-553f-41d0-93a3-e95136cc1fbd&ContentType_id=77eb43da-aa94-497d-a73f-5c951ff72372&Group_id=1d6521ef-f1d5-407b-a471-1ae71d0935b3. Accessed 31 Aug 2014.
56. Benson BW, McIntosh AS, Maddocks D, et al. What are the most effective risk-reduction strategies in sport concussion? Br J Sports Med. 2013;47(5):321–6.

Sideline Response and Transport

3

Lisa M.G. Vopat

Introduction

Although catastrophic head and neck injuries are rare in youth sports, these injuries are serious, causing permanent neurological deficits or death. Traumatic brain injury is the leading cause of death in youth athletes that sustain direct injury [1]. Twenty-one percent of all traumatic brain injuries among children and adolescents are the result of sports and recreational activities [2]. An estimated 7.6 % of all cervical spinal cord injuries sustained by adults are related to sports, of which 86 % resulted in tetraplegia [3]. The proportion of cervical spine fractures sustained by children that is related to sports is nearly 1 in 4 [4]. The school sports with the highest risk for catastrophic injury are ice hockey, American football, gymnastics, wrestling, cheerleading, and lacrosse [1]. Since many more youths play football than the other sports combined, American football is the sport with the highest absolute number of head and spine injuries [1].

On-field emergencies can occur during any physical activity and at any level of participation [5], but due to the low incidence of catastrophic events, athletic program personnel may develop a false sense of security over time [5]. Less than 20 % of the two to four million youth athlete coaches in the United States have received any formal training in injury prevention or first aid [6, 7]. Therefore, proper education, training, and preparation are critical to emergency management of the youth athlete.

Sideline physicians along with athletic trainers and coaches need be prepared with an organized approach to acutely evaluate and manage these injuries. Paradoxically, a seemingly minor head trauma can result in a developing intracranial bleed, while a

L.M.G. Vopat, MD (✉)
Orthopedics/Division of Sports Medicine, Boston Children's Hospital,
319 Longwood Ave, Boston, MA 02115, USA
e-mail: lisa.vopat@childrens.harvard.edu

M. O'Brien, W.P. Meehan III (eds.), *Head and Neck Injuries in Young Athletes*,
Contemporary Pediatric and Adolescent Sports Medicine,
DOI 10.1007/978-3-319-23549-3_3

more violent head trauma with loss of consciousness may only result in a mild concussion. Injuries can vary in severity, and differentiating these injuries can be difficult even for highly trained physicians. Early recognition of spinal cord injury is vital due to the risk of neurologic deterioration during initial management of the injury and the need for rapid intervention. In this chapter, we will review an organized approach for initial assessment and stabilization of the pediatric athlete with a suspected head or neck injury. We will review guidelines for safe transport with immobilization and discuss sideline and emergency preparedness.

Primary Survey and Stabilization

When a head or neck injury is suspected, the athlete should be assessed quickly and efficiently to identify life-threatening conditions. This can be achieved by following the ABCD sequence of trauma care:

Airway maintenance with cervical spine protection
Breathing and ventilation
Circulation
Disability and neurologic status

This initial assessment typically begins by asking the athlete two simple questions: "*What is your name?*" and "*Can you describe what happened?*" An appropriate response indicates that the athlete can speak clearly (no major airway compromise), they can generate adequate air to allow speech (breathing is not compromised), and they are alert enough to describe what happened (no major decrease in level of consciousness). Inability to respond or an inappropriate response warrants further assessment and prompt management [8].

Head and neck injuries often occur simultaneously. An athlete suspected of having a head or neck injury should not be moved and should be managed as though they have a spinal injury until the primary assessment is complete. During the initial survey, the presence of any or all of the following warrants use of spinal precautions: unconscious or altered level of consciousness, bilateral neurologic findings or complaints, significant cervical spine pain with or without palpation, and obvious spinal deformity [9].

Airway Maintenance with Cervical Spine Protection

Ensuring a patent airway while protecting the cervical spine is the highest priority in caring for an injured athlete. Similar to adults, the pediatric cervical spine is protected using in-line immobilization. Having one person manually hold the cervical position while maintaining the airway is recommended during the initial assessment until a more permanent means of immobilization can be obtained [10]. If the athlete is restless or combative, a second person should hold distal portions of the body for complete immobilization. Younger children (especially athletes 8 years of age or younger) have a disproportionately larger cranium and occiput compared to their midface and torso [8]. This imbalance results in excessive passive flexion of the neck and an anterior buckling of the posterior pharynx that leads to airway occlusion when in the supine position [8, 10]. The plane of the midface should be parallel to the spine in a neutral position [8]. Placement of padding underneath the child's torso will keep the athlete's midface parallel to the spine while maintaining neutral alignment of the spinal column [8, 10, 11].

The airway should be evaluated simultaneously with manual in-line cervical spine stabilization. Airway occlusion can occur due to the relatively large soft tissues of the oropharynx (tongue and tonsils) falling posterior to obstruct the more anterior airway. A jaw-thrust maneuver (using the index fingers to push the angle of the mandible upward) pulls these tissues forward to assist in ensuring a patent airway while maintaining spinal protection [8, 10] (Fig. 3.1).

Protective equipment such as helmet and shoulder pads can make safe airway management more challenging; however, an athlete wearing such protective equipment should have their gear left in place, if it is possible to do so while still performing resuscitation, in order to minimize risk of further injury from undue cervical spine motion [12]. If the facemask, however, interferes with access to the airway, it should be removed. The tool and technique used to remove the facemask should be fast and easy to use and most importantly create the least head and neck motion. A combined-tool approach is recommended to avoid chance of failure. For football helmets, a screwdriver or cordless screwdriver can be used in the first attempt, followed by the use of a backup cutting tool to cut away any remaining loop straps if necessary. More recently developed helmets have quick-release mechanisms triggered by

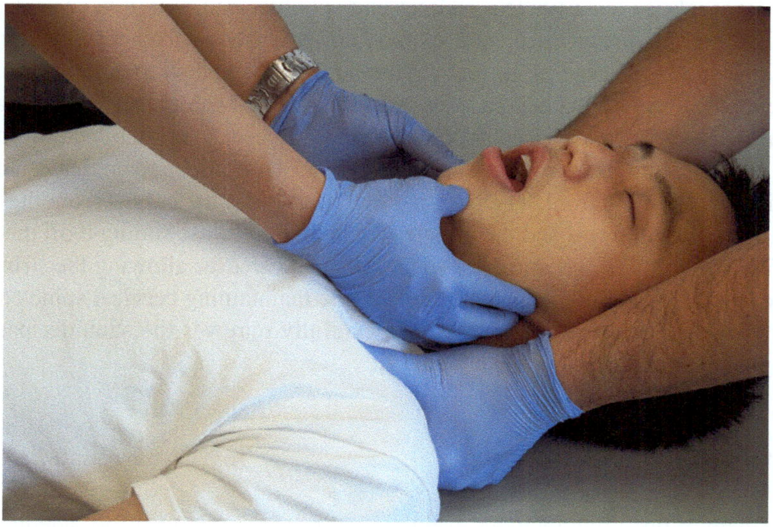

Fig. 3.1 Manual in-line cervical spine stabilization with jaw-thrust maneuver. Image provided by Anthony Luke, M.D.

depressing a button. Regardless of the type of helmet, the goal is the same; remove the facemask in the most efficient manner without causing further harm [9].

The helmet and shoulder pads should not be removed unless the airway is unable to be accessed by other means. This should follow an “all or none” principal whereby the helmets and shoulder pads are either both removed or both left in place. Removal of the helmet alone results in hyperextension of the athletes’ cervical spine, while removal of only the shoulder pads alone leads to neck flexion and inability to maintain neutral cervical spine stabilization.

Similar to adults, pediatric athletes ages 8 and older should ideally have their equipment left in place [13]. While athletes 8 years and older may have residual skeletal disproportion until maturity is reached, no modification of alignment is necessary. No statistically significant difference in cervical spine angulation has been found for this age group when comparing the fully equipped athletes to those without equipment. Therefore, adult guidelines following the “all or none” equipment principle apply to the older child or adolescent athlete [13]. If equipment is properly fitted, leaving the helmet and shoulder pads strapped in place will minimize motion and angulation of the cervical spine, thus decreasing the risk of further injury [14]. For younger athletes (age 8 years old and younger), the emphasis on performing the necessary modifications to maintain neutral alignment is the same, although no formal guidelines on equipment have been established.

In certain situations, it may be necessary to remove an athlete’s protective equipment. An athlete’s equipment should be removed if: the helmet and chin strap do not hold the head securely to allow for complete immobilization; the airway and ventilation cannot be controlled despite removal of the facemask; the facemask is unable to be successfully removed; the helmet prevents proper neutral alignment for cervical spine immobilization; or the equipment is interfering with needed access to the chest, neck, or head [9, 15]. Helmet and shoulder pad design is variable, and therefore, the sideline medical team should familiarize themselves with their team’s particular model. In general, to remove the helmet, the chinstrap is removed from the helmet followed by cheek pad removal. Helmet air bladders should be drained with a needle or blade to loosen fit of the helmet. Cervical spine stabilization should be transferred from the person at the athlete’s head to another person that can apply stabilization from the front. The person at the head grabs the helmet from the sides pulling the sides outward and then rotates the helmet up while sliding it off the head [9]. The athlete’s jersey is slit along the midline and sleeves allowing the strings or buckles on the front of the pads to be cut. While maintaining cervical spine control from the front, the rescuer from the head carefully removes the shoulder pads by sliding them out from under the athlete [9].

Breathing

Assessment of breathing includes evaluation of respiratory rate, effort, adequacy of air excursion, and the presence or absence of cyanosis to ensure adequate oxygenation and ventilation [16]. Airway patency does not ensure adequate ventilation.

Hypoxia is the most common cause of cardiac arrest in a child and is of significant concern especially in a head injured athlete [10]. Younger athletes (ages 4–5) have faster respiratory rates at 22–34 breaths per minute, while adolescents have rates similar to adults (12–18 breaths per minute) [16]. Children also have small tidal volumes so chest wall rise may be subtle, but should be readily seen when the chest clothing is uncovered [10, 16]. Breath sounds should be assessed for symmetry. Transient respiratory arrest and hypoxia are common with severe brain injury [8]. Bag-valve-mask ventilation should be initiated if breathing is inadequate and equipment is available. Bag-valve-mask ventilation is much easier in children than adults due to smaller size and more compliant physiology, but regardless of age it is always essential to ensure a proper seal around the mouth. Care should be taken to avoid overventilation. In cases of traumatic brain injury, hyperventilation can be detrimental by worsening cerebral ischemia [10].

Circulation

Rapid assessment of hemodynamic status can be achieved by evaluating skin color, pulse, and level of consciousness. Pink skin and normal capillary refill, especially in the face and extremities, are suggestive of adequate perfusion. However, skin assessment can be affected by ambient temperature and is not always reliable. Pulse should be assessed for quality, rate, and regularity [8, 10]. In addition to several other etiologies (e.g., traumatic brain injury or metabolic dysregulation), reduced central and cerebral perfusion may be a cause of an altered level of consciousness.

Vital signs are less sensitive for identification of shock in children than in adults [10]. Children have increased physiologic reserve that allows for maintenance of perfusion even in the presence of shock [8, 10]. The presentation of a child in early shock can be subtle; thus, a high index of suspicion is warranted. Tachycardia is the earliest finding of circulatory compromise in children and therefore mandates closer attention and evaluation [10]. Slowing of the heart rate below normal is also a concerning sign, which may indicate neurogenic shock in an athlete with cervical spinal cord injury [8].

Disability and Neurologic Status

A focused neurologic evaluation quickly establishes the athlete's level of consciousness, pupillary response, and focal neurologic deficit. The goal during the primary survey is to assess the *general* level of injury until there is more time for an in-depth evaluation. The most rapid assessment can be performed using the Alert-Voice-Painful-Unresponsive (AVPU) mnemonic. Those athletes that are not fully alert and only respond to voice, pain, or not at all should be presumed to have a head injury [10, 16]. These athletes have an unreliable neurologic exam and therefore should have full spinal precautions. Subsequent steps should include checking the size and reactivity of the pupils followed by gross assessment for movement and sensation in each extremity. Unequal or poorly reactive pupils can indicate brain injury. Abnormal posturing (involuntary flexion or extension of the arms and legs) also signifies severe brain injury and poorer outcomes. Any evidence of loss of sensation, paralysis, or weakness of the extremities suggests spinal cord injury [8, 10].

The Glasgow Coma Scale is a simple, objective, and reproducible clinical measure of level of consciousness and neurologic status. This 15-point system estimates the severity of brain injury by evaluating eye opening, verbal response, and best motor response (Table 3.1) to different stimuli. A GCS score less than 8 is concerning for severe brain injury or coma; a score of 9–12 is moderate, while a score of 13–15 is the classification for possible minor injury. The AVPU mnemonic is preferred during the primary assessment; therefore, determination of the athlete's GCS can be deferred until there is time for more in-depth evaluation [10].

Identifying Head or Neck Injury

At completion of the primary survey, the presence of any or all of the following necessitates use of spinal precautions: unconscious or altered level of consciousness, bilateral neurologic findings or complaints, significant cervical spine pain with or without palpation, and obvious spinal deformity [9]. Intoxication and a distracting injury such as a long bone fracture are other criteria that should prompt cervical spine immobilization [8–10]. Any abnormality identified during the ABCD sequence should have resuscitation measures initiated to immediately improve the

Table 3.1 Glasgow Coma Scale

Assessment		Scale
Eye opening (E)	Spontaneous	4
	To speech	3
	To pain	2
	None	1
Verbal response (V)	Oriented	5
	Confused	4
	Inappropriate words	3
	Incomprehensible sounds	2
	None	1
Best motor response (M)	Obeys commands	6
	Localizes pain	5
	Flexion withdrawal to pain	4
	Abnormal flexion (decorticate)	3
	Extension (decerebrate)	2
	None (flaccid)	1

GCS Score = E + V + M

Best possible score 15; worst possible score 3

condition [8]. The athlete should be prepared for immediate transport to an emergency department.

Conscious, neurologically intact athletes without concern for cervical spine injury can be assisted to a sitting position. If stable in a sitting position, the athlete can be helped to stand and then be walked off the field for further evaluation [17].

Immobilization and Transport

For the athlete with a suspected cervical spine injury, once the primary survey is complete, and all emergent issues have been addressed, manual stabilization of the head and neck is transferred to mechanical stabilization using an external device. A rigid cervical collar is applied to athletes without equipment to maintain cervical spine immobilization. In the equipment-laden athlete, a cervical collar can be difficult to apply due to lack of space between the helmet and shoulder pads, and attempts to do so may cause undue cervical motion. If the helmet and shoulder pads maintain neutral alignment, fit properly, and can be secured in place, then a rigid cervical collar does not need to be applied. The rescuer at the head should maintain neutral alignment, which should be continued despite external stabilization devices while the athlete is being secured for transport [9, 15].

Full spinal immobilization via a long spine board is used to transport the athlete to an emergency department. Either the log-roll or lift-and-slide technique is used to place the athlete on a spine board. In either technique, the head and trunk must be moved as a unit. The log-roll technique involves multiple rescuers with one at the head, two or three kneeling on one side of the trunk, and another on the opposite side with the spine board. With the athlete's arms at their side or crossed over their body, the rescuer at the head commands the team to roll the athlete onto their side toward the kneeling rescuers. The spine board is positioned at a 45° angle beneath the athlete. On command the rescuers lower the athlete onto the spine board. This technique can be used for the supine athlete as well an athlete found in lying on their side [9, 15].

If the athlete is found in the prone position, the log-roll technique can also be used with a few modifications (Figs. 3.2 and 3.3). The rescuer at the head is going to stabilize the cervical spine beginning with their arms crossed so that they will uncross when the athlete is rolled. Rescuers kneeling on the side of the athlete roll the athlete onto their side. Another rescuer slides the spine board underneath the athlete so that athlete is rolled into a supine position on the board [9, 15].

The lift-and-slide technique is an alternative to the log roll (Figs. 3.4, 3.5, and 3.6). This technique also requires multiple personnel to simply lift the athlete up on command to allow for spine board placement. This technique may be easier for athletes with equipment but can only be used for the supine athlete. While a variety of techniques exist, rescuers should use the technique with which they are most comfortable and one that will produce the least amount of spinal movement [9].

Once on the spine board, the head and the body need to be secured for transport. The body should be secured before the head to minimize cervical movement.

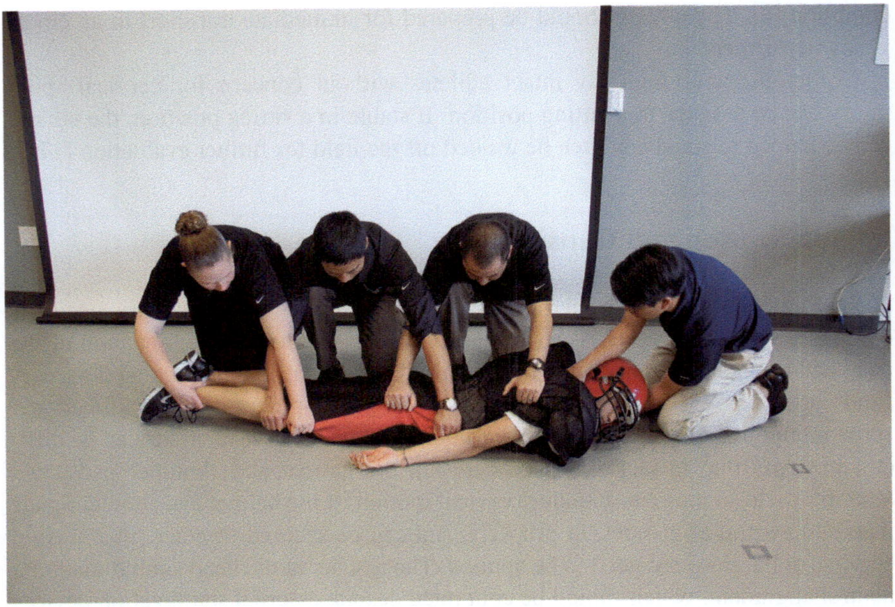

Fig. 3.2 Log-roll technique with manual in-line cervical spine stabilization for an athlete found in the prone position. Image provided by Anthony Luke, M.D.

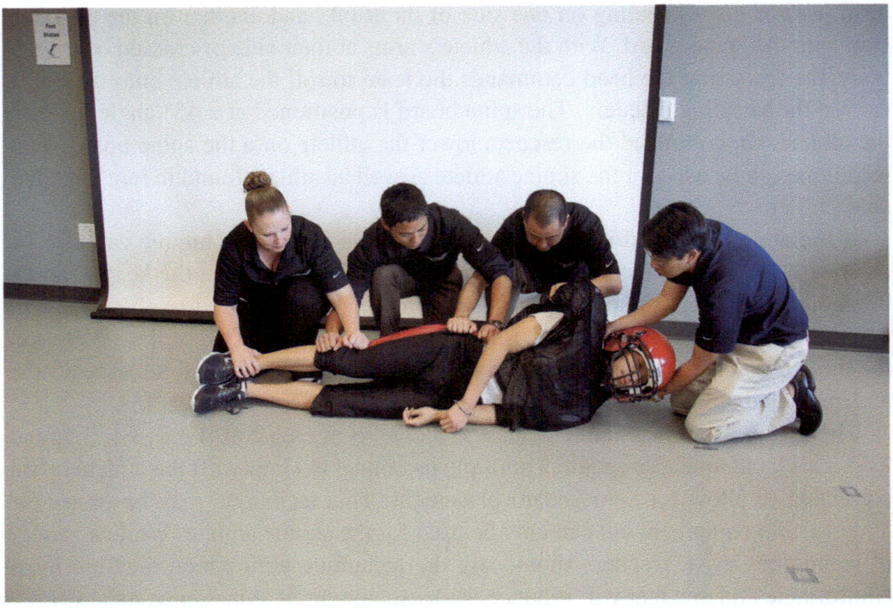

Fig. 3.3 Log-roll technique with manual in-line cervical spine stabilization for an athlete found in the prone position. Image provided by Anthony Luke, M.D.

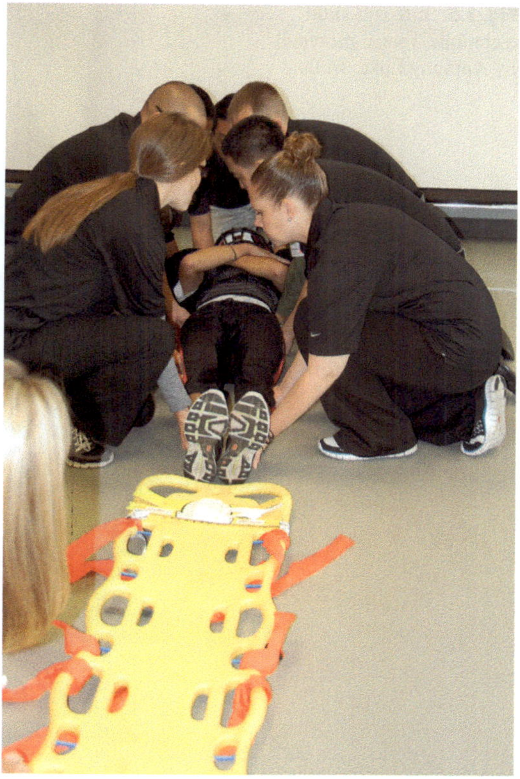

Fig. 3.4 Lift-and-slide technique. Image provided by Anthony Luke, M.D.

A variety of strapping options exist including the traditional three-strap technique (chest, pelvis, and thighs). Proper strapping should minimize or eliminate sliding in any direction. The head is the last part secured to the spine board. This can be achieved with a variety of head immobilization devices including helmet blocks, foam blocks, and towel rolls. The head is then further secured to the board with tape or straps. The tape or strap should have two points of contact at the chin and the forehead [9]. With the head and body in full immobilization, and with airway and circulation secured, the athlete is ready for transport.

Emergency Planning and Sideline Preparedness

An organized response plan is critical to the emergency management of an athlete with a suspected head or cervical spine injury. While the incidence of catastrophic injury is low, these events are unpredictable and easily complicated by heightened emotions and a chaotic atmosphere. A well-designed and rehearsed emergency action plan is practical and establishes a coordinated response to allow for a rapid and effective care of the athlete.

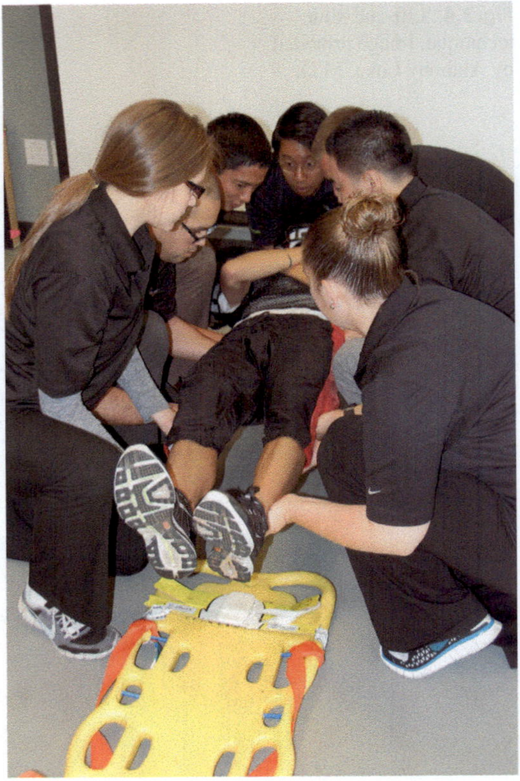

Fig. 3.5 Lift-and-slide technique. Image provided by Anthony Luke, M.D.

The Emergency Action Plan is a written plan that identifies the proper personnel needed to carry out the plan, including but not limited to physicians, athletic trainers, coaches, and officials in conjunction with local emergency medical service personnel. Sideline personnel should be trained in automatic external defibrillation, cardiopulmonary resuscitation, and first aid. Proper equipment including an automatic external defibrillator, spine board, cervical collar, facemask removal kit, and ventilation supplies should be readily available especially for contact and collision sports [5]. It is the responsibility of the sideline personnel to ensure they know the location and working conditions of this type of essential equipment before the start of a contest. A system of communication, the mode of transportation, and the location of the emergency facility should be predetermined. The plan should be flexible in order to adapt to any athletic situation and should be rehearsed and revised on a regular basis [5, 14, 15].

While schools and events have adopted these recommendations, there is room for improvement. A national survey of athletic trainers reported that 70 % of schools in the United States have a written emergency plan and 54 % have activated their emergency action plan in response to a life-threatening sport-related emergency within the past school year. Only a quarter of these schools, however, practiced their plan [18]. Of these athletic trainers, 20 % had no CPR training and only 61 % had an available AED. While many pediatric and adolescent athletes participate in

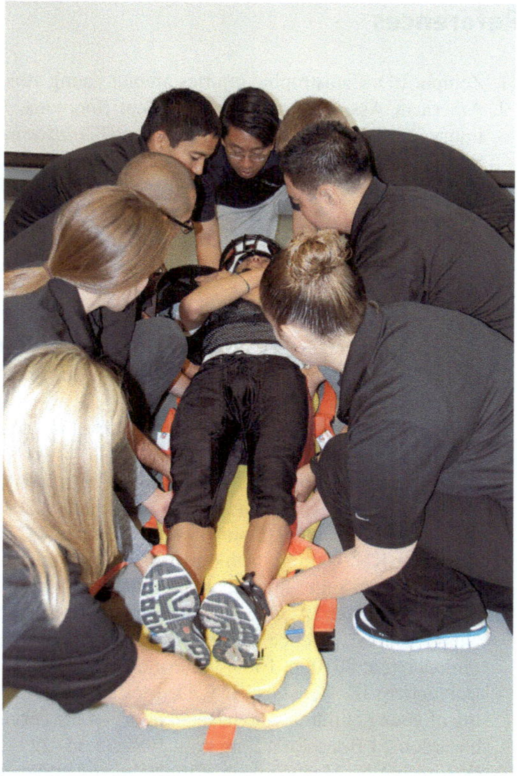

Fig. 3.6 Lift-and-slide technique. Image provided by Anthony Luke, M.D.

interscholastic sports with access to athletic training services and sports medicine personnel, participants in independent sports leagues may not have such resources. A coach may be the only person to initiate life-saving resuscitation. The 2008 National Coaching Report indicates that only 29 % of states require formal CPR training for coaches [19]. Therefore, better promotion of proper education, training, and preparation is critical to emergency management of the youth athlete.

Conclusion

On-field management of an athlete with a head or neck injury should follow an organized approach as part of a well-designed emergency protocol. Athletes, coaches, trainers, physicians, and other health-care providers should be familiar with the ABCD sequence of assessment to identify potential head and neck injury and initiate stabilizing treatment. Rescuers should use extreme caution and have a low threshold for spinal immobilization of any athlete suspected of a cervical spine injury. Knowledge and familiarity with protective equipment will assist in safe care, packaging, and transport of the injured athlete. Proper education of all individuals involved in the care of the athlete will optimize successful emergency management and promote safety for the athlete.

References

1. Zemper ED. Catastrophic injuries among young athletes. Br J Sports Med. 2010;44:13–20.
2. American Association of Neurological Surgeons. Patient information: sports-related head injury. 2010. http://www.aans.org/Patient%20Information/Conditions%20and%20Treatments/Sports-Related%20Head%20Injury.aspx. Accessed 22 Aug 2014.
3. American Association of Neurological Surgeons. Patient information: sports-related neck injury. 2010. http://www.aans.org/Patient%20Information/Conditions%20and%20Treatments/Sports-Related%20Neck%20Injury.aspx. Accessed 22 Aug 2014.
4. Meehan III WP, Mannix R. A substantial proportion of life-threatening injuries are sport-related. Pediatr Emerg Care. 2013;29:624–7.
5. Andersen JC, Courson RW, Kleiner DM, McLoda TA. National Athletic Trainers' Association position statement: emergency planning in athletics. J Athl Train. 2002;37:99–104.
6. Merkel DL, Molony JT. Medical sports injuries in the youth athlete: emergency management. Int J Sports Phys Ther. 2012;7:242–51.
7. DeWitt TL, Unruh SA, Seshadri S. The level of medical services and secondary school-aged athletes. J Athl Train. 2012;47:91–5.
8. American College of Surgeons. Advanced trauma life support (ATLS) student course manual. 9th ed. Chicago: American College of Surgeons; 2012. Print.
9. Swartz EE, Boden BP, Courson RW, Decoster LC, Horodyski M, Norkus SA, Rehberg RS, Waninger KN. National Athletic Trainers' association position statement: acute management of the cervical spine-injured athlete. J Athl Train. 2009;44:306–31.
10. Place RC, Mayer TA. General approach to pediatric trauma. In: Wolfson AB, editor. Harwood-Nuss' clinical practice of emergency medicine. 5th ed. Lippincott Williams & Wilkins: Philadelphia; 2010. p. 1089–96. Print.
11. Herzenberg JE, Hensinger RN, Dedrick DK, Phillips WA. Emergency transport and positioning of young children who have an injury of the cervical spine: the standard backboard may be hazardous. J Bone Joint Surg Am. 1989;71:15–22.
12. Waninger KN. Management of the helmeted athlete with suspected cervical spine injury. Am J Sports Med. 2004;32:1331–50.
13. Treme GT, Diduch DR, Hart J, et al. Cervical spine alignment in the youth football athlete. Am J Sports Med. 2008;36:1582–6.
14. Kleiner D, Almquist J, Bailes J, et al. Prehospital care of the spine-injured athlete: a document from the inter-association task force for appropriate care of the spine-injured athlete. 2001. http://www.nata.org/sites/default/files/PreHospitalCare4SpineInjuredAthlete.pdf. Accessed 22 Aug 2014.
15. Walters R. Management of the critically injured athlete: packaging of head and cervical spine injuries. South Med J. 2004;97:843–6.
16. American Heart Association. Pediatric advanced life support (PALS) provider manual. Dallas: American Heart Association; 2006. Print.
17. Miele VJ, Norwig JA, Bailes JE. Sideline and ringside evaluation for brain and spinal injuries. Neurosurg Focus. 2006;21:E8.
18. Olympia RP, Dixon T, Brady J, et al. Emergency planning in school-based athletics. Pediatr Emerg Care. 2007;23:703–8.
19. National Association for Sport and Physical Education. National coaching report 2008. Reston, VA. http://www.shapeamerica.org/publications/resources/teachingtools/coachtoolbox/loader.cfm?csModule=security/getfile&pageid=8390. Accessed 22 Aug 2014.

Contusions, Abrasions, and Lacerations of the Head and Neck in Young Athletes

4

Andrew F. Miller and Andrea Stracciolini

Introduction

The injury rate of abrasions, lacerations, and contusions in youth sports is relatively high in comparison to more severe sports injuries [1–3]. The challenge with these types of injuries often lies with the assessment. Determining whether or not an injury is minor, such as a superficial contusion or abrasion/laceration, versus major in nature, requiring more advanced medical treatment, can be very difficult. This is especially true when dealing with young athletes, who may be less cooperative with the physical examination or may not be able to describe their symptoms as well as adults.

Young athletes in all sports have many opportunities to sustain an abrasion, laceration, or contusion, especially when participating in sports that involve a significant amount of contact and/or collision. Contusions are a leading cause of youth sports injuries and are often minor in severity, without taking the athlete away from the game [1, 4]. On the other hand, more severe contusions can cause deep tissue damage and can lead to complications that may keep the athlete out of sports for months.

A.F. Miller, MD
Division of Emergency Medicine, Department of Medicine, Boston Children's Hospital, Harvard Medical School, Boston, MA,, USA

A. Stracciolini, MD (✉)
Division of Sports Medicine, Department of Orthopaedics, Boston Children's Hospital, Boston, MA, USA

Division of Emergency Medicine, Department of Medicine, Boston Children's Hospital, Boston, MA, USA

Harvard Medical School, Boston, MA, USA
e-mail: Andrea.Stracciolini@childrens.harvard.edu

M. O'Brien, W.P. Meehan III (eds.), *Head and Neck Injuries in Young Athletes*, Contemporary Pediatric and Adolescent Sports Medicine,
DOI 10.1007/978-3-319-23549-3_4

Definitions

- *Contusion*—an injury that occurs when a direct blow or repeated blows from a blunt object strike part of the body, crushing underlying muscle fibers and connective tissue without breaking the skin. A contusion can result from falling or jamming the body against a hard surface.
- *Abrasion*—an injury that occurs to the skin when it is rubbed or scraped against another surface. Abrasions tend to involve the superficial epidermis, but can be deeper, involving the dermis and adipose tissue.
- *Laceration*—an injury resulting from a cut or tear in the skin, caused by blunt or shearing forces or sharp objects making forceful contact with the skin. Lacerations can involve a range of depth, from the epidermis to the muscle and fascial layers.
- *Minor injury*—an injury that can be expected to heal with minimal medical intervention.
- *Major injury*—an injury that requires advanced medical attention and intervention.

Head and neck injuries are common body locations for youth sports injuries [2, 3]. Children participating in sports incur head and neck contusions, abrasions, and lacerations that vary greatly in severity and nature. The injury ranges from minor injuries to the muscle and other soft tissue structures to more severe injuries, including intracranial contusions of the brain. Differentiating minor injuries from more severe injuries can be difficult. Injury severity may not immediately be apparent, even to highly trained and experienced personnel attending to young athletes. Longitudinal reassessment to identify the athlete who has sustained an injury that is more severe, and subject to clinical deterioration, is required in many cases. This chapter focuses on contusions, abrasions, and lacerations of the head and neck in sports participation by young athletes.

A discussion of the epidemiology of head and neck contusions in sports participation by youths is difficult at the outset. The diagnosis of "contusion" often serves as a nonspecific diagnosis "proxy" when a more accurate diagnosis is lacking or has not yet been determined. Also, contusions occur often in sports [5], are minor in nature, and generally have a good outcome requiring minimal treatment. These factors make it likely that most of these injuries go unreported. Contusions, as a definitive diagnosis, have been shown in some studies to be the most frequent type of injury sustained by children playing baseball [6, 7]. Finally, epidemiology studies specific to head and neck injuries in sports in children are also lacking. In a study evaluating injuries sustained during organized community sports participation in children aging 7–13 years, Radelet et al. found that almost 54 % of the injuries were "bruises," and, when combined with lacerations and abrasions, over two-thirds of the total injuries fell into this category [6]. The authors note that the coaches had difficulty recording minor bruises and abrasions, which speaks to the difficulty of obtaining accurate epidemiological data for these categories of injuries.

Abrasions and lacerations are a continuum of injury to the skin, ranging from minor, more superficial injuries to deeper injuries, extending to the muscle or fascial layers. Abrasions are caused by sheer forces to the skin and are often caused by the skin sliding across turf during sports participation. Abrasions can be broken up into categories, including superficial and deep. Superficial abrasions cause a removal of the epidermis and do not cause injury to underlying structures. Deep abrasions may entail removal of all skin layers, up to and including the subcutaneous fat, and potentially are associated with significant damage to underlying structures [8]. Most lacerations are a result of direct sheering forces from sharp objects. Other lacerations are caused by compressive forces (i.e., a blunt compressive force to the head resulting in a stellate laceration from an external force hitting the underlying skull) [9]. Lacerations are a very common type of injury. Nearly 12 million wounds are treated annually in the emergency department; approximately 7 million of those are lacerations [10, 11]. As stated, the true epidemiology of these injuries is unknown, although most experts agree that they are common in sports and likely underreported due to their frequent minor nature [8].

Pathophysiology

Any injury to soft tissue may cause bleeding and tissue destruction. This activates humoral and cellular mechanisms to stop bleeding and to resist infection. The sequential healing processes starting immediately after trauma can be divided into three phases: the exudative or inflammatory phase, the proliferative phase, and the reparative phase.

In the initial inflammatory phase, there is a massively increased interaction between the leukocytes and the injured microvascular endothelium. The importance of oxygen in wound healing should be emphasized. Fibroblast and leukocyte functions are depressed by hypoxia [12]. Furthermore, the number of bacteria killed by leukocytes in vitro increases as local oxygen tension is raised [13]. Soft tissue injuries in hypoxic areas heal poorly. Ischemic, desiccated tissue cannot be adequately perfused and thus is exceedingly accessible to infection [14]. The infiltrating granulocytes and macrophages, with their capacity to resist infection and to engulf cell debris and bacteria (physiological wound debridement), play a key role in the inflammatory response of traumatized tissue and therefore have a decisive effect on the subsequent reparative processes [15]. However, extensive debridement with removal of all necrotic tissue is a crucial component of preventing infection because these cells have only limited capacity for phagocytosis.

After successful occlusion of the vessels, the proliferative phase begins, followed by a smooth transition to the reparative phase. Stimulated by the mitogenic growth factors, fibroblasts, followed by endothelial cells, migrate into the area of the wound and proliferate there. Fibrosis and scarring following this process can take up to 12 months to establish the highest level of strength.

All wounds that extend beyond the dermis have the potential for scar formation [16]. Wounds heal either by primary or secondary intention. Primary intention refers to wounds being closed by approximation of the wound edges with a form of primary closure. Secondary intention implies that the wound edges are not approximated and therefore heals from the deepest portion of the wound to the most superficial. The former is typically the preferred option and creates the least amount of scarring. The latter method of healing is appropriate in conditions when wound contamination is severe and the wound occurred more than 6–12 h from the time of repair (24 h if on a cosmetically important region such as the face) and in cases of human or animal bite wounds due to the high risk of infection. Another example of a wound that should be allowed to heal by secondary intention is a wound that was closed primarily and then became secondarily infected.

Head Contusions, Abrasions, and Lacerations in Youth Sports

Ear

The ear is uniquely subject to trauma due in part to the unique external position on the head and the protuberant nature of the organ. Traumatic perichondral contusions to the ear in the sport of wrestling are common and are related to the frequent friction or shearing type of injury inherent to the sport of wrestling. The cosmetic result of this injury is often referred to as "cauliflower ear." Traumatic auricular hematoma is most often seen in wrestlers who do not wear headgear or wear improperly fitting headgear [17]. The resultant hematoma disrupts the normal blood supply to the underlying cartilage, causing necrosis, fibrosis, and disfigurement of the auricle.

Auricular hematoma management is typically performed within 7 days [18]. Brickman et al. found that aspiration and drainage procedure with angio-catheter drain placement for the management of auricular hematomas within 3 weeks of onset was successful in allowing athletes to return to activity with minimal downtime and achieved excellent results [17].

Wounds sustained to the external ear can be challenging based on the architecture of the ear itself and the fact that there is only a thin layer of skin overlying the cartilaginous structure. The perichondrium provides nutrients and oxygen to the cartilage and, if disrupted, may lead to necrosis and damage to the cartilage. In contrast, the superficial skin covering to the ear has a great blood supply which allows for good healing and a lower risk of infection [19].

Treatment of superficial lacerations to the ear on the sidelines is reasonable if the wounds are clean and do not involve the perichondrium or underlying cartilage. This should be done with great care, so as to not inflict injury to the cartilage when suturing the wound. It is imperative to completely close the wound to ensure that there is no cartilage exposed and to minimize the risk of infection to the cartilage (chondritis). If the perichondrium is affected, subspecialty consultation with plastic surgery, or ear–nose–throat (ENT) surgery, is recommended. Likewise, large avulsion injuries or amputations of the ear should be evaluated and treated by a plastic or ENT surgeon. If no subspecialty care is available, optimal closure of the cartilage is achieved with a minimal amount of 5–0 absorbable sutures to approximate the edges [19].

Nose

The treatment of nasal injuries can be challenging to clinicians due to the functional and cosmetic importance of the nose. Because of the prominent location of the nose on the face, it is very susceptible to injuries during youth sports participation [20]. The nose is a centerpiece to the face and small amounts of malalignment can be very aesthetically displeasing. A recent survey of nasal injuries occurring during sports participation of children and adults reported that 33 % of the diagnoses were contusions and basketball and baseball were the leading cause of nasal injuries (26 % and 22 %, respectively) [21]. Like the ear, the nose has a cartilaginous structure and is dependent on the perichondrium for its metabolic demands. The nose has an added inner mucosal layer as well.

Trauma to the nose can result in the formation of a septal hematoma that requires drainage. Inserting an 18-gauge needle into the hematoma for drainage is appropriate. Alternatively, an incision may be made. Nasal packing should be inserted after drainage, and prophylactic antibiotics must be prescribed. In the majority of cases of athletes with nasal contusions, return to sport can occur immediately after comprehensive evaluation [21]. After injury, a patient may choose to wear a splint, shield, or other types of protective device when resuming his or her sport or activity. This protective gear may decrease the chance of reinjury, including nasal fracture [22].

Nasal lacerations that simply involve the superficial skin require simple closure with 6–0 suture. Full-thickness nasal lacerations through the outer skin, cartilaginous structure, and inner mucosa are much more serious and challenging to treat. This type of injury requires a three-layer repair, starting with the inner mucosa, preferably using absorbable sutures. This portion of the repair can be particularly difficult due to, in particular, the small space and poor light availability. The next step is repair of the cartilaginous structure, with a minimum number of 5–0 absorbable sutures required to approximate the edges. In some circumstances, the cartilage may be approximated with simple sutures, placed only in the skin. This likely holds true if there are no defects to the cartilage, and the edges can be well approximated with only external skin sutures. The last step is closure of the superficial skin with a typical skin suture repair. This type of full-thickness repair to the nose often requires subspecialist consultation, such as a plastic surgeon or ENT surgeon, due to the technical challenges and aesthetic requirements [23].

Eye

Contusions to the eyes are also common in sports participation, with one hospital-based study reporting sports injuries being responsible for 60 % of the traumatic hyphemas [24]. Certain sports played by youth may be more susceptible to injuries to the head, specifically the face and eyes. A good example of this is girls' lacrosse which has a relatively high rate of injuries to this region, likely related to the nature of the sport involving multiple players, fast running, swinging sticks, and high-speed projectiles [25, 26]. The use of protective eyewear in women's lacrosse is associated with a reduction in the number of eye injuries and no associated change in overall injury rates [27]. Although rare, pediatric golf injuries can be devastating to the eye, visual system, and periocular adnexa (i.e., eyelids, muscles, conjunctiva, lacrimal apparatus) [28]. Blunt force can cause such injuries as retinal tear and detachment, choroidal rupture, vitreous hemorrhage, commotio retinae, retinal hemorrhage, hyphema, traumatic iritis, and subconjunctival hemorrhage.

Wounds involving the eye, and surrounding structures, can be potentially serious. Specifically, wounds to the lower medial eyelid (due to concerns for lacrimal duct injury), the levator palpebrae muscle, medial canthal ligament, and the eyelid margin necessitate ophthalmologic referral. All lacerations to the globe require emergent ophthalmologic referral due to the risk of permanent visual disturbance and complete loss of the eye. Other injuries to the eye, such as corneal abrasion, are typically less concerning and can be treated by the emergency medical provider.

Scalp

Scalp lacerations can be challenging to repair due to the presence of multiple layers of subcutaneous structures and hair (see Fig. 4.1). Stapling scalp wounds and hair apposition techniques with tissue adhesive have been shown to be equivalent to suturing, with respect to wound healing outcome [29, 30]. Because stapling is more cost-effective and time efficient, it has become the preferred method of closure [31]. The galea aponeurotica (muscular layer), if involved, must be closed in addition to the superficial layer. Galea closure can be achieved with deep absorbable sutures [32].

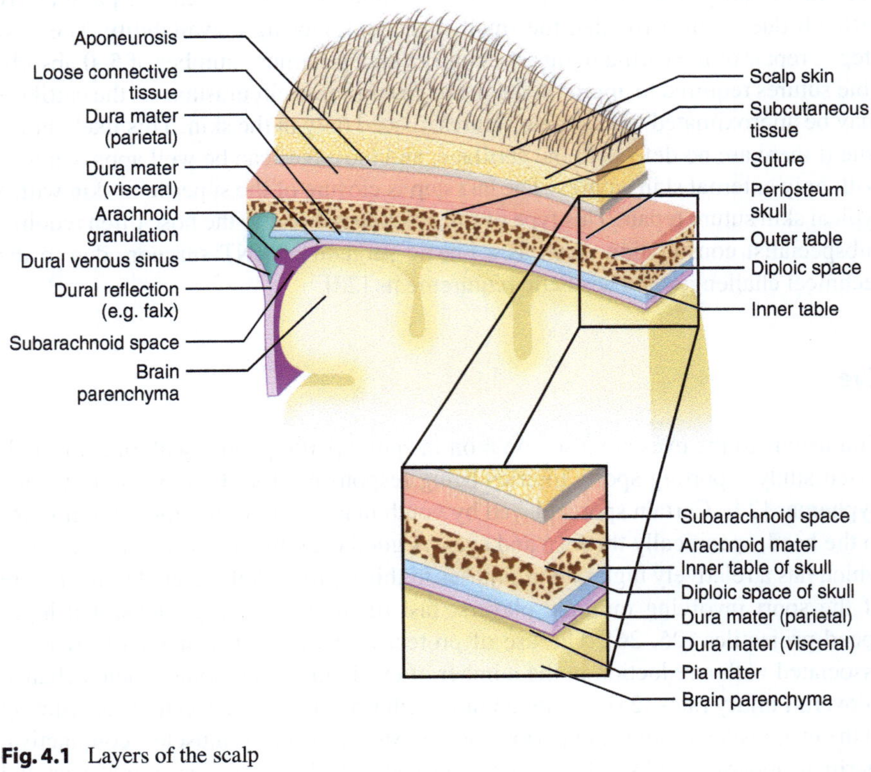

Fig. 4.1 Layers of the scalp

Mouth

Mouth injuries are still prevalent in youth sports, despite many sports requiring helmets and/or mouthguards [33]. Intraoral lacerations commonly occur from injury caused by biting of the buccal mucosa. These wounds require evaluation for depth and involvement of the underlying structures. Tongue lacerations typically occur after a fall when the tongue is bitten by the athlete's teeth. Lacerations that affect the lip should be evaluated for involvement of the vermilion border. Small intraoral lacerations heal without intervention [23]. However, if they are greater than 2–3 cm in length, or have a large flap, these wounds are best closed with 5–0 Vicryl suture [34].

The tongue can be difficult to repair simply because it is a difficult area to access. If there is a large laceration involving the free edge of the tongue, or if there is persistent bleeding, the tongue should probably be repaired. When repairing these lacerations, simple interrupted 4–0 absorbable sutures (e.g., chromic gut) with full-thickness bites are recommended [34]. Tongue lacerations can be difficult to repair due to the patients' inability to tolerate the procedure and concerns surrounding airway compromise. Sedation may be used when deemed necessary. In situations where the patient's airway is tenuous, surgical consultation, with repair under general anesthesia, may be warranted [35].

The vermilion border is the area of the lip where the dry mucosa meets the skin of the face. Strict attention to alignment of this border is of great aesthetic importance, so that there is no discontinuity of the lip. A 1-mm discordance can be aesthetically displeasing [36]. Repair of the vermilion border is best achieved using 6–0 nonabsorbable sutures placed in a simple interrupted fashion to first align the edges; repair of the rest of the laceration can follow in standard fashion. Specific care should be taken to maintain the architecture of the lip when using local infiltration of anesthesia. Regional blocks should be used, such as infraorbital and mental nerve blocks, for anesthesia to the upper and lower lip, respectively [37].

Face Lacerations

Careful consideration for the deeper structures of the face when exploring and examining facial lacerations is important. The central portion of the cheek contains the parotid gland and the facial nerve. Notable caution should be taken with injuries close to the tragus of the ear, where the bulk of the parotid gland is located and the facial nerve branches are larger. Other locations to note include outlets of the V1, V2, and V3 branches of the trigeminal nerve—the supraorbital, infraorbital, and mental foramen of the skull, respectively. Wounds that involve ligation of nerves, injury to the parotid gland or Stenson's duct, or large lacerations that penetrate the oral cavity often necessitate subspecialty surgical consultation.

Neck Contusions, Abrasions, and Lacerations in Youth Sports

Penetrating neck injuries in the pediatric population are rare and are associated with a mortality risk of approximately 10 % [38]. No sports-related mechanisms have been reported in large retrospective reviews in the literature [38, 39]. However, there are case reports of lacerations to the neck in ice hockey from the ice skate blades, leading to significant injuries [40]. A database study reported neck lacerations in football and hockey, but no injuries in soccer [41]. The anatomy of the very young pediatric patient provides relatively good inherent protection to the neck unless the neck is in an extended position [42]. This is secondary to a relatively large head and mandible in relation to the neck. This anatomic protection is less likely in young athletes, as head and neck proportions begin to change quickly, approaching adult proportions when the child is approximately school-age or older.

The spectrum of injury to the neck is broad, spanning from superficial contusions, lacerations, or abrasions to more serious injury to deeper structures. The neck harbors many vital structures including the trachea and relatively superficial large blood vessels. The neck is anatomically broken up into three vertical zones and two anterior and posterior zones.

Zone I—area from the thoracic inlet extending to the cricoid cartilage
Zone II—area from the cricoid cartilage extending to the angle of the mandible
Zone III—area above the angle of the mandible to the base of the skull
Anterior Zone—area anterior to the palpable transverse processes of the cervical spine
Posterior Zone—area posterior to the palpable transverse processes of the cervical spine

These zones are very important to the description and management of penetrating neck injuries.

Zone I

Zone I of the neck includes the area from the thoracic inlet to the cricoid cartilage (see Fig. 4.2). This zone is less protected by the jaw but proportionately smaller in size, as compared to the other zones of the neck. The structures in this region tend to be much deeper which increases the level of protection.

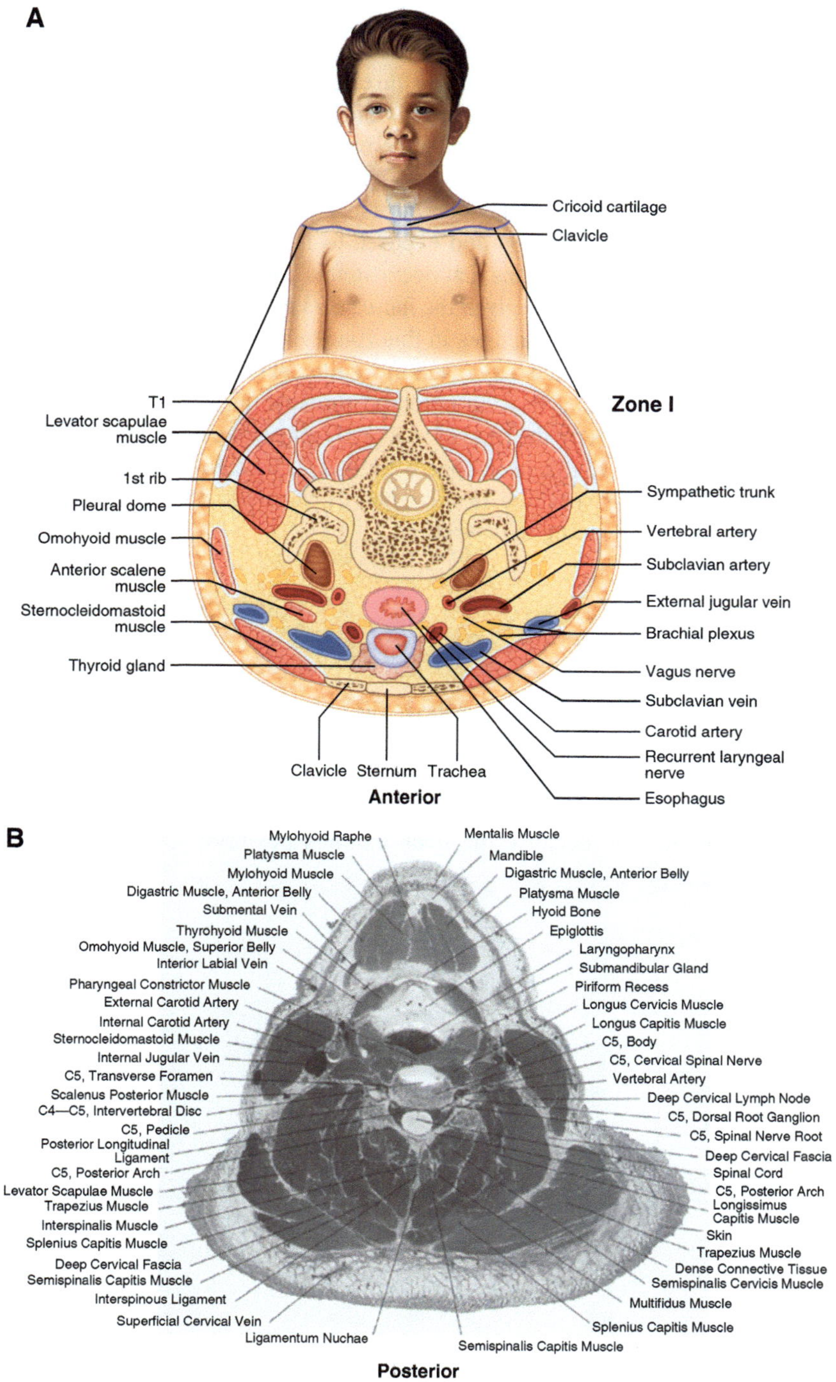

Fig. 4.2 Zone I Anatomy of the neck

Zone II

Zone II of the neck includes the area above the cricoid cartilage and below the angle of the mandible (see Fig. 4.3). Vital structures, such as the major vessels of the neck, traverse this zone very superficially, when compared to the other zones [38]. This zone has the protection of the mandible draping over this region inferiorly, which is more pronounced in younger-aged children versus adolescents. As a result this zone is in the most vulnerable position and exposed to injury, when the neck is in an extended position [42]. Contusions that occur in this zone of the neck are the most likely to cause significant injury given the increased vulnerability to vital structures that this region affords. The structures in this zone will most likely sustain injuries including tracheal injury, which may result in significant subcutaneous emphysema, a large deep hematoma that has the potential to cause airway compromise, and laryngeal injury associated to the triad of stridor, dyspnea, and hemoptysis. Vascular injury from a contusion to this neck zone is unlikely. The carotid artery is the most likely involved vascular structure in this zone of the neck; the most concerning would be intimal tears leading to dissections.

Zone III

Zone III of the neck includes the area above the angle of the mandible and extends to the base of the skull (see Fig. 4.4). This area of the neck is well protected from injury by the bony mandible and its relatively small exposed surface. This neck zone should be considered with penetrating injuries that occur in the submaxillary region of the face because the neck extends posterior to the face in this region.

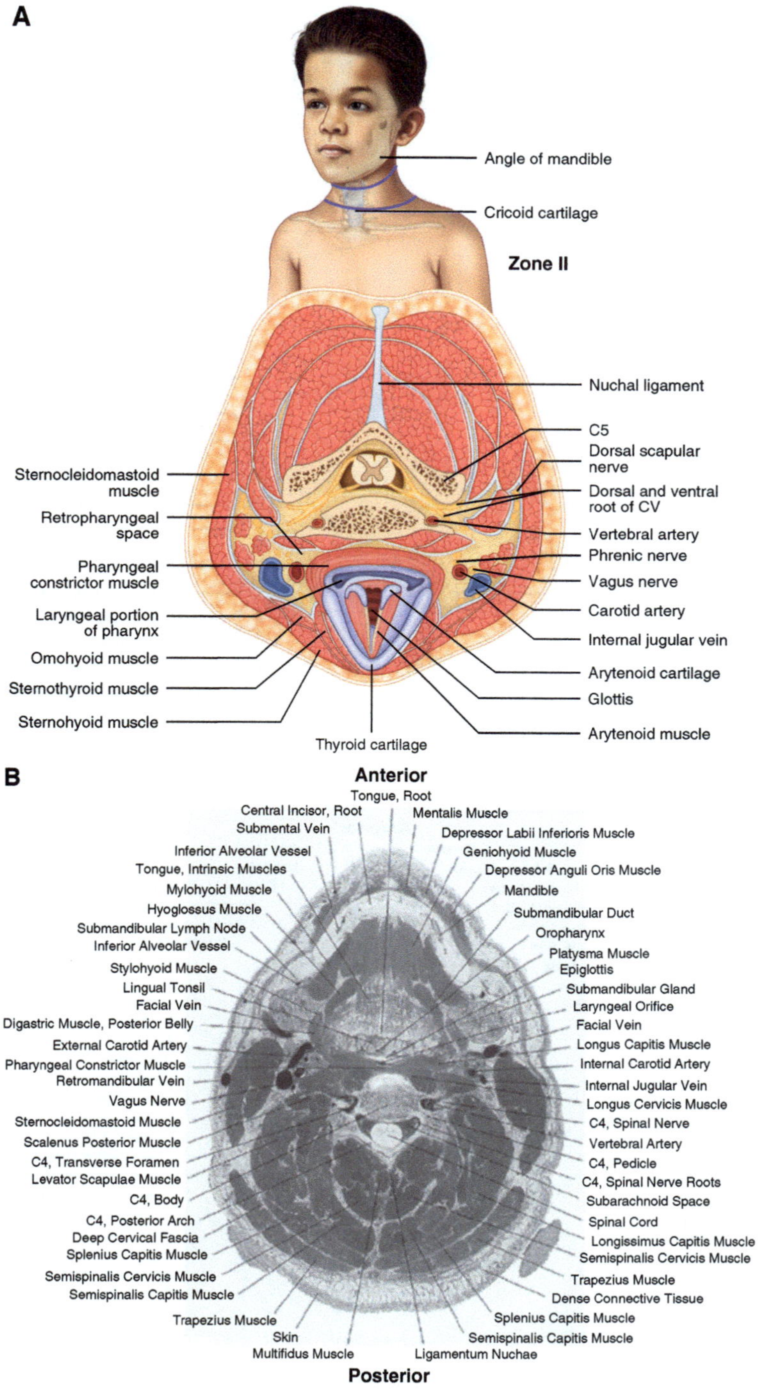

Fig. 4.3 Zone II Anatomy of the neck

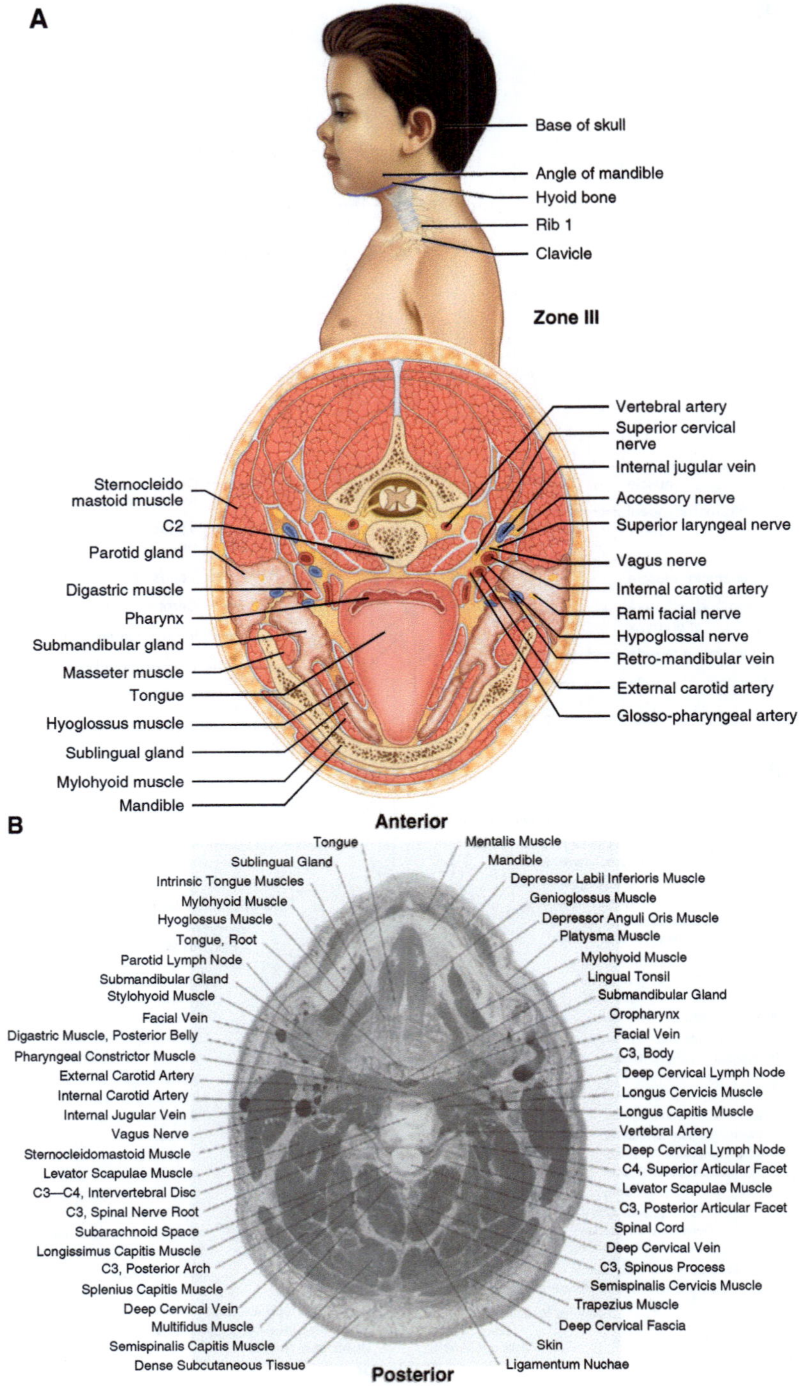

Fig. 4.4 Zone III Anatomy of the neck

Anterior/Posterior

The anterior aspect of the neck contains the most important structures, while the posterior aspect contains mainly bony and muscular structures. However, it can be difficult to determine if the wound extends deeper into the opposite zone, especially in penetrating trauma. The superficial aspect to the neck is remarkable for the platysma muscle, which has its origin in the superior fascia of the pectoralis major and deltoid. It inserts on the mandible and portions of the inferior face [43]. As a result, it spans the majority of the zones of the neck, sparing the most superior portion of zone III. Lacerations to the platysma require sutured repair of the muscle belly itself to maintain its structural integrity.

Clinical Evaluation and Management of Head and Neck Contusions, Abrasions, and Lacerations in Youth Sports

History

Many young athletes are involved in events that lead to contusion, abrasion, or laceration of the head and neck. A thorough history regarding the injury is critical in assisting the healthcare provider assess the need for clinical management. The condition of the wound after injury is determined by the following factors:

- Type of insult and area of contact (blunt, penetrating, pointed, sharp, crush, etc.)
- Degree of force applied
- Direction of force (vertical or tangential)
- Area of body affected (to determine possibility of underlying structures being affected)
- Timing of the injury
- Contamination of the abrasion or laceration (sterile surgical wound, degree of dirt, foreign bodies, etc.)
- Environment in which it occurred
- General physical condition of the patient (age, associated illness, immune response, etc.)
- Tetanus status (if the skin barrier is broken)

Contusions cause swelling and pain and limit joint range of motion near the injury. Torn blood vessels and deep bleeding beneath the soft tissue are responsible for the discoloration of the skin. The injured muscle or tissue may feel weak and stiff. Sometimes a pool of blood collects within damaged tissue, forming a hematoma. The most common sites of soft tissue bruising in children are the head and lower legs [44]. The location of the bruise requires clinical examination for deeper structural injury. In severe cases, swelling and bleeding beneath the skin may be significant. If tissue damage is extensive, suspicion should be heightened for a fracture, dislocated joint, sprain, torn muscle, or other injuries. The extent of the bruising is not a good indication of the amount of force sustained. Commonly there is impressive bruising and few, if any, other clinical signs [44]. If bruising is extensive, has an atypical pattern, and occurs in the absence of trauma or involves only minor trauma, the child may have an underlying preexisting condition or coagulopathy [44].

Examples of abrasions and lacerations to the head and neck in youth sports include abrasions from friction of the helmet strap or a hard surface. Many of the lacerations in the region of the head and neck occur with blunt traumatic force over a bony prominence causing the skin to open. Examples in youth sports with no helmets include a head-to-head collision while attempting a header in soccer or an elbow strike to the cheekbone during a basketball game. In helmeted sports, a significant collision in football may cause the chin strap to lacerate the chin. Other examples of sports causing trauma from sharp objects include ice hockey and lacrosse whereby a skate blade or stick may get caught underneath the helmet in the region of the neck causing injury.

Physical Examination

A comprehensive physical examination, including a detailed neurologic examination, is important to determine the exact location and extent of injury and the need for emergent medical care. If there is a change in mental status or a focal neurologic deficit, further urgent evaluation with advanced diagnostics, including MRI or CT, may be warranted.

Contusions are more difficult to assess accurately given that deeper structures can be damaged without an open wound to view the extent of the injury. It is important to know the underlying anatomy and to separate out deeper pathology from more superficial benign injury. Head contusion physical examination is dependent on the location of the contusion and the mechanism of injury. For example, if the mechanism of injury suggests a major injury (e.g., a high-speed or forceful collision/tackle or a fall from a height of ≥ 2 m), assessment of the child athlete should begin with a primary survey, including evaluation of airway, breathing, circulation, and conscious state, including a Glasgow Coma Score (GCS). The secondary survey should focus on assessing the location and size of the contusion, areas of ecchymosis, and tenderness or presence of bony step-offs on palpation. Prompt immobilization of the neck and spine is warranted with any concern for neck injury.

The evaluation of lacerations and abrasions is different given the ability to assess structures below within the extent of the wound. A complete physical examination when the skin is broken should include the following steps:

- Assess for vascular damage and control bleeding if necessary
- Determine the depth of the wound
- Explore the wound for foreign bodies and material
- Evaluate for any damage to major nerves
- Assess for tendon injury
- Evaluate the bony structures in the region of the wound

Medical Management

Prior to any treatment, a basic assessment needs to be made either on the field of play or on the sideline depending on the severity of the situation. Initial assessment of the airway, breathing, and circulation (ABC) is crucial in all sports injuries. This is especially important in head and neck injuries because this area is densely packed with structures essential to all of these basic functions. An evaluation of the GCS is also helpful to determine the mental status of an individual who has just sustained a traumatic injury. Finally, when assessing the neck, it is vital to finish the initial evaluation with an assessment of cervical spine stability to ensure proper immobilization when necessary. It is important to make cervical spine stability assessment an integral part of all sports injury management so that life-threatening injuries are not missed.

The decision to treat a young injured athlete on the sideline versus in the emergency department (ED) treatment can be difficult in many cases. The decision many times is obvious; however, in some situations, it is not immediately obvious that referral is required, for example, an athlete who sustains a deep laceration through the ear that penetrates the cartilage. The treating provider must recognize the risk for necrosis and infection, if the wound is not cleaned and closed with a layered sutured repair.

On-Field Treatment

On-field treatment for most injuries should begin with pain, bleeding, and inflammation control using the RICE formula:

- *Rest.* Protect the injured area from further harm by stopping play. Provide protective devices as needed (i.e., crutches, sling).
- *Ice.* Apply ice wrapped in a clean cloth. (Remove ice after 20 min.)
- *Compression.* Lightly wrap the injured area in a soft bandage or ace wrap.
- *Elevation.* Raise it to a level above the heart.

Most athletes with contusions get better quickly with simple treatment measures. The use of nonsteroidal anti-inflammatory drugs (NSAIDs), such as ibuprofen, or other medications for pain relief usually is all that is required for most injuries. It is important to correctly instruct patients with regard to frequent use of ice in the acute phase for pain control and to help control swelling and bleeding. It is important to avoid heat during this phase, as it promotes vasodilatation and can worsen the bleeding. Also, it is important to advise against massage of the injured area. Providing specific instructions regarding elevation above the level of the heart is very important in the acute phase of injury to minimize swelling. For athletes, encouraging cross-training or relative rest while encouraging exercise of the uninjured parts of the body to maintain an overall level of fitness is an important component of the instructions to the injured athlete.

Irrigation of all lacerations is the most useful intervention to avoid infection by reducing bacterial load of the wound and contaminants prior to closure [45]. The proper way to perform wound irrigation is with high pressure using a 60-mL syringe with a

16–18-gauge angio-catheter or splash guard [46]. Although normal saline solution was the commonly used solution in the past due to isotonicity and availability, tap water has now been proven to be equally efficacious and should be used in its place [47].

Wound Repair

Local infiltration of medications such as lidocaine, or other available local anesthetics, should be used to provide a field block to the wound prior to suture or staple closure. Lidocaine, epinephrine, and tetracaine (LET) mixture can be used as a sole treatment in certain scenarios or as an adjunct to local infiltration. Regional anesthesia can be used for certain areas of the face.

Steri-Strips—used for superficial wounds that are not under a large amount of tension.

Skin adhesive—used for superficial wounds that are not under a large amount of tension. It can be a great needleless alternative to sutures; however, this type of closure may have an increased risk of infection due to the completely occlusive closure of the wound.

Staples—reserved for wounds on the scalp, as stapled closure can be performed quickly and does not require shaving of the scalp.

Sutures—a sutured repair is used with any wound that requires closure that is not a candidate for any of the aforementioned methods of closure. There are two general types of closure, a single-layer repair or multiple-layer closure. Single-layer repair, meaning a single layer of sutures at the skin surface, is used when a wound requires closure, but is relatively well approximated, and minimal suture tension is required at the wound edges. A multiple-layer repair is required when a wound is gaping and deep, thus requiring subcutaneous sutures to be placed to help approximate the edges and allow for ease of closure at the skin surface.

Post-wound Care

The initial wound dressing should be nonocclusive and remain on the wound for the first 24–48 h, to allow for epithelialization and reduce the risk of infection [48]. Applying topical antibiotic ointment may help the wound epithelialize more quickly, as well as decrease the risk of infection [49, 50].

Suture duration is one of the most important factors in preventing aesthetically displeasing scar formation or residual "train tracks" [51]. Suture removal timing for sutures placed in the neck, face, and scalp is 3–4 days, 5 days, and 5 days, respectively [52].

Tetanus Prophylaxis

Tetanus prophylaxis should be considered for all wound management [53]. Prophylaxis, if needed, may require administration of tetanus immune globulin (TIG) in addition to vaccination with DTap, Tdap, or Td, depending on the athletes' vaccination history and degree of wound contamination. The use of certain vaccine types is dependent upon patient age and vaccination status. DTaP is given to injured athletes less than 7 years old. Tdap and Td are used when athletes are older than 7 years. Tdap is preferred to Td when the athletes are under immunized or they have not previously received Tdap.

For clean and minor wounds, three vaccines are required if the young athlete has not previously received three doses of tetanus vaccine or it has been greater than 10 years since the last tetanus-containing vaccine. "Dirty" wounds are considered wounds that are contaminated with soil, dirt, or saliva or wounds that are puncture, avulsion, or crush injuries. These wound types require the appropriate vaccine and TIG, if the athlete has not previously received three doses of tetanus vaccine. If the athlete has received three doses of tetanus vaccine and it has been greater than 5 years since their last tetanus vaccine, then appropriate tetanus vaccine is required for adequate prophylaxis [53].

Antibiotic Prophylaxis

The routine use of antibiotics in laceration prophylaxis has been shown to be ineffective and is not recommended [54]. Antibiotics should be reserved for complicated and contaminated lacerations including bites, exposed tendons, heavily soiled wounds, or a specific mechanism or environmental exposure. Antibiotics are useful only in cases of human bites, as in the case of head-to-head collision [55]. Antibiotic choice for most lacerations should cover for *Staphylococcus* and *Streptococcus* species of skin flora with a first-generation cephalosporin. Human bites require more broad-spectrum coverage for human oral flora species of *Eikenella* (e.g., amoxicillin–clavulanate) [51].

Emergency Department Treatment

The clinical management of pediatric head and neck wounds has not been researched extensively, and studies guiding care are lacking at this time. Standard radiographs to detect a possible radiopaque foreign body in wounds are recommended, specifically when the foreign object is glass [56]. Ultrasound evaluation of the wound may serve as an alternate imaging modality when radiographs fail to detect the foreign body [57].

Decisions regarding the clinical investigation for structural damage to the neck largely depend upon the injured zones of the neck. The goals for advanced diagnostics are to ensure that airway, vascular, or esophageal damage has not occurred. The use of CT angiogram, as compared to surgical exploration for deep vessel injury to the neck, is largely determined case by case, depending upon clinical suspicion.

Conclusions

Contusions, abrasions, and lacerations to the head and neck are very common in youth sports, with most of these wounds being benign in nature and healing with no significant long-term adverse effects. Many are treated on the field or in training rooms, by coaches, athletic trainers, or parents. However, the head and neck regions of the body harbor many vital structures that can result in severe life-threatening injury, and concern regarding poor aesthetic outcome is warranted in many cases.

Diligent evaluation by a skilled and experienced provider is often needed to ensure that there are no injuries to deeper structures and to monitor the young athlete over time for any worsening of the clinical status. Optimizing cosmetic outcomes is often very important when treating wounds to the head and neck in athletes, necessitating specialist evaluation and treatment, in some selected cases. Although life-threatening contusions or lacerations are rare, it is important that all of these injuries are approached in a systematic fashion and that the appropriate levels of care are called into play when necessary.

References

1. Lislevand M, Andersen TE, Junge A, Dvorak J, Steffen K. Injury surveillance during a 2-day national female youth football tournament in Kenya. Br J Sports Med. 2014;48(11):924–8.
2. Howard AF, Costich JF, Mattacola CG, Slavova S, Bush HM, Scutchfield FD. A statewide assessment of youth sports- and recreation-related injuries using emergency department administrative records. J Adolesc Health. 2014;55(5):627–32.
3. Loder RT, Feinberg JR. Orthopaedic injuries in children with nonaccidental trauma: demographics and incidence from the 2000 kids' inpatient database. J Pediatr Orthop. 2007;27(4):421–6.
4. Faude O, Rossler R, Junge A. Football injuries in children and adolescent players: are there clues for prevention? Sports Med. 2013;43(9):819–37.
5. Junge A, Dvorak J. Injury surveillance in the World Football Tournaments 1998-2012. Br J Sports Med. 2013;47(12):782–8.
6. Radelet MA, Lephart SM, Rubinstein EN, Myers JB. Survey of the injury rate for children in community sports. Pediatrics. 2002;110(3):e28.
7. American Academy of Pediatrics. Risk of injury from baseball and softball in children. Pediatrics. 2001;107(4):782–4.
8. Foster DT, Rowedder LJ, Reese SK. Management of sports-induced skin wounds. J Athl Train. 1995;30(2):135–40.
9. Edlich RF, Rodeheaver GT, Morgan RF, Berman DE, Thacker JG. Principles of emergency wound management. Ann Emerg Med. 1988;17(12):1284–302.
10. Singer AJ, Dagum AB. Current management of acute cutaneous wounds. N Engl J Med. 2008;359(10):1037–46.
11. Nawar EW, Niska RW, Xu J. National Hospital Ambulatory Medical Care Survey: 2005 emergency department summary. Adv Data. 2007;(386):1–32.
12. Hunt TK, Hopf HW. Wound healing and wound infection. What surgeons and anesthesiologists can do. Surg Clin North Am. 1997;77(3):587–606.
13. Hohn DC, MacKay RD, Halliday B, Hunt TK. Effect of O2 tension on microbicidal function of leukocytes in wounds and in vitro. Surg Forum. 1976;27(62):18–20.
14. Oestern HJ, Tscherne H. Pathophysiology and classification of soft tissue injuries associated with fractures. In: Tscherne H, Gotzen L, editors. Fractures with soft tissue injuries. Berlin: Springer-Verlag; 1984. p. 1–9.
15. Cromack DT, Porras-Reyes B, Mustoe TA. Current concepts in wound healing: growth factor and macrophage interaction. J Trauma. 1990;30(12 Suppl):S129–33.
16. Fleisher GR, Ludwig S. Textbook of pediatric emergency medicine (Chapter 106, Minor trauma—lacerations). 6th ed. Philadelphia: Lippincott Williams & Wilkins; 2010.
17. Brickman K, Adams DZ, Akpunonu P, Adams SS, Zohn SF, Guinness M. Acute management of auricular hematoma: a novel approach and retrospective review. Clin J Sport Med. 2013;23(4):321–3.
18. Cassaday K, Vazquez G, Wright JM. Ear problems and injuries in athletes. Curr Sports Med Rep. 2014;13(1):22–6.

19. Eagles K, Fralich L, Stevenson JH. Ear trauma. Clin Sports Med. 2013;32(2):303–16.
20. Perkins SW, Dayan SH, Sklarew EC, Hamilton M, Bussell GS. The incidence of sports-related facial trauma in children. Ear Nose Throat J. 2000;79(8):632–4, 636, 638.
21. Cannon CR, Cannon R, Young K, Replogle W, Stringer S, Gasson E. Characteristics of nasal injuries incurred during sports activities: analysis of 91 patients. Ear Nose Throat J. 2011;90(8):E8–12.
22. Morita R, Shimada K, Kawakami S. Facial protection masks after fracture treatment of the nasal bone to prevent re-injury in contact sports. J Craniofac Surg. 2007;18(1):143–5.
23. Brown DJ, Jaffe JE, Henson JK. Advanced laceration management. Emerg Med Clin North Am. 2007;25(1):83–99.
24. Schein OD, Hibberd PL, Shingleton BJ, et al. The spectrum and burden of ocular injury. Ophthalmology. 1988;95(3):300–5.
25. Webster DA, Bayliss GV, Spadaro JA. Head and face injuries in scholastic women's lacrosse with and without eyewear. Med Sci Sports Exerc. 1999;31(7):938–41.
26. Xiang J, Collins CL, Liu D, McKenzie LB, Comstock RD. lacrosse injuries among high school boys and girls in the united states: academic years 2008-2009 through 2011-2012. Am J Sports Med. 2014;42(9):2082–8.
27. Lincoln AE, Caswell SV, Almquist JL, et al. Effectiveness of the women's lacrosse protective eyewear mandate in the reduction of eye injuries. Am J Sports Med. 2012;40(3):611–4.
28. Pujalte GGA. Eye Injuries in Sports. Athletic Therapy Today. September 2010;15(5):14–18.
29. Hock MO, Ooi SB, Saw SM, Lim SH. A randomized controlled trial comparing the hair apposition technique with tissue glue to standard suturing in scalp lacerations (HAT study). Ann Emerg Med. 2002;40(1):19–26.
30. Khan AN, Dayan PS, Miller S, Rosen M, Rubin DH. Cosmetic outcome of scalp wound closure with staples in the pediatric emergency department: a prospective, randomized trial. Pediatr Emerg Care. 2002;18(3):171–3.
31. Kanegaye JT, Vance CW, Chan L, Schonfeld N. Comparison of skin stapling devices and standard sutures for pediatric scalp lacerations: a randomized study of cost and time benefits. J Pediatr. 1997;130(5):808–13.
32. Semer N. Facial lacerations in practical plastic surgery for nonsurgeons (Chapter 16), vol. 16. Philadelphia: Hanley & Belfus, Inc.; 2001.
33. Kaplan Y, Myklebust G, Nyska M, Palmanovich E, Victor J, Witvrouw E. Injuries can be prevented in contact flag football! Knee Surg Sports Traumatol Arthrosc. 2014.
34. Armstrong BD. Lacerations of the mouth. Emerg Med Clin North Am. 2000;18(3):471–80, vi.
35. Buntic RF, Buncke HJ. Successful replantation of an amputated tongue. Plast Reconstr Surg. 1998;101(6):1604–7.
36. Lammers RL. Principles of wound management. In: Roberts JR, Hedges JR, Chanmugam AS, et al., editors. Clinical procedures in emergency medicine. 4th ed. Philadelphia: WB Saunders Co; 2004. p. 623–54.
37. Zide BM, Swift R. How to block and tackle the face. Plast Reconstr Surg. 1998;101(3):840–51.
38. Abujamra L, Joseph MM. Penetrating neck injuries in children: a retrospective review. Pediatr Emerg Care. 2003;19(5):308–13.
39. Cooper A, Barlow B, Niemirska M, Gandhi R. Fifteen years' experience with penetrating trauma to the head and neck in children. J Pediatr Surg. 1987;22(1):24–7.
40. Bisson LJ, Sanders SM, Noor S, Curl R, McCormack R. Common carotid artery laceration in a professional hockey player: a case report. Am J Sports Med. 2009;37(11):2249–51.
41. Delaney JS, Al-Kashmiri A. Neck injuries presenting to emergency departments in the United States from 1990 to 1999 for ice hockey, soccer, and American football. Br J Sports Med. 2005;39(4):e21.
42. Fleisher GR, Ludwig S. Textbook of pediatric emergency medicine (Neck trauma, Chapter 115). 6th ed. Philadelphia: Lippincott Williams & Wilkins; 2010.
43. Netter F. Atlas of human anatomy (Head and neck, Chapter 1). 4th ed. Philadelphia: Saunders; 2006.

44. Young SJ, Barnett PL, Oakley EA. 10. Bruising, abrasions and lacerations: minor injuries in children I. Med J Aust. 2005;182(11):588–92.
45. Stevenson TR, Thacker JG, Rodeheaver GT, Bacchetta C, Edgerton MT, Edlich RF. Cleansing the traumatic wound by high pressure syringe irrigation. JACEP. 1976;5(1):17–21.
46. Singer AJ, Hollander JE, Subramanian S, Malhotra AK, Villez PA. Pressure dynamics of various irrigation techniques commonly used in the emergency department. Ann Emerg Med. 1994;24(1):36–40.
47. Valente JH, Forti RJ, Freundlich LF, Zandieh SO, Crain EF. Wound irrigation in children: saline solution or tap water? Ann Emerg Med. 2003;41(5):609–16.
48. Schauerhamer RA, Edlich RF, Panek P, Thul J, Prusak M, Wangensteen OH. Studies in the management of the contaminated wound. VII. Susceptibility of surgical wounds to postoperative surface contamination. Am J Surg. 1971;122(1):74–7.
49. Hinman CD, Maibach H. Effect of air exposure and occlusion on experimental human skin wounds. Nature. 1963;200:377–8.
50. Dire DJ, Coppola M, Dwyer DA, Lorette JJ, Karr JL. Prospective evaluation of topical antibiotics for preventing infections in uncomplicated soft-tissue wounds repaired in the ED. Acad Emerg Med. 1995;2(1):4–10.
51. Singer AJ, Hollander JE, Quinn JV. Evaluation and management of traumatic lacerations. N Engl J Med. 1997;337(16):1142–8.
52. Fleisher GR, Ludwig S. Textbook of pediatric emergency medicine (Chapter 106, Minor trauma—lacerations). 6th ed. Philadelphia: Lippincott Williams & Wilkins; 2010.
53. American Academy of Pediatrics Committee on Infectious Diseases. Tetanus. In: Pickering LK, editor. Red book. 29th ed. Elk Grove Villiage, IL: American Academy of Pediatrics; 2012.
54. Cummings P, Del Beccaro MA. Antibiotics to prevent infection of simple wounds: a meta-analysis of randomized studies. Am J Emerg Med. 1995;13(4):396–400.
55. Medeiros I, Saconato H. Antibiotic prophylaxis for mammalian bites. Cochrane Database Sys Rev. 2001;(2):CD001738.
56. Orlinsky M, Bright AA. The utility of routine x-rays in all glass-caused wounds. Am J Emerg Med. 2006;24(2):233–6.
57. Hill R, Conron R, Greissinger P, Heller M. Ultrasound for the detection of foreign bodies in human tissue. Ann Emerg Med. 1997;29(3):353–6.

Concussions

5

Michael O'Brien and Purnima Bansal

Definition and Epidemiology

Mild traumatic brain injury and concussion are a growing source of concern in today's sports environment. There is increased emphasis on diagnosing and managing concussions at all levels of athletic endeavor. The reasons for this are multifactorial and include advances in medical science and technology, as well as interest generated by high-profile cases and lawsuits in professional football.

It is natural that the concern about mild traumatic brain injury and concussion should extend to the pediatric and adolescent sports milieu. With major implications on young athletes relative to their sports participation, school performance, and future health, there is a desire for a clear understanding of current evaluation and management principles among athletes, parents, coaches, and clinicians.

Approximately 3.8 million sports-related traumatic brain injuries occur every year [1–5], and approximately 13–15 % of all sports-related injuries sustained by high school athletes are concussions [1–3]. Injury rates vary by sport and gender with the highest rates seen in boys playing collision sports such as American football, ice hockey, and lacrosse [1, 3]. Among girls, soccer, lacrosse, and field hockey have the highest incidences of concussion [1, 3].

There has been a dramatic increase in the diagnosis of concussion among pediatric and adolescent athletes in outpatient and emergency department settings [6–8] and approximately one-quarter to one-half of these injuries are sustained during sports or recreational activities. Primary care clinicians and athletic trainers manage

M. O'Brien, MD (✉)
Division of Sports Medicine, Childrens Hospital Boston, Boston, MA, USA
e-mail: michael.obrien@childrens.harvard.edu

P. Bansal, MD
Jennie Stuart Medical Center, Hopkinsville, KY

M. O'Brien, W.P. Meehan III (eds.), *Head and Neck Injuries in Young Athletes*,
Contemporary Pediatric and Adolescent Sports Medicine,
DOI 10.1007/978-3-319-23549-3_5

the majority of these patients, with approximately 10 % of cases managed by specialists such as sports medicine physicians, neurosurgeons, or neurologists [1].

The consensus statement from the 4th International Conference on Concussion in Sport, held in Zurich in 2012, defines concussion as a complex pathophysiological process affecting the brain with several common features [4]. A concussion may be caused by a direct blow to the head or impact elsewhere to the body with an impulsive force transmitted to the head. It typically results in the rapid onset of short-lived impairment in neurologic function that may be manifested by several different types of symptoms. Concussion symptoms may be present immediately after a collision but may also take minutes to hours to develop. Recovery is typically spontaneous, though it may be prolonged in certain cases. Loss of consciousness is not a requirement to make the diagnosis, and lack of loss of consciousness does not predict recovery rate and cannot be used to justify a more rapid return to play (RTP).

Pathophysiology

Rotational acceleration of the brain is hypothesized to cause a shear strain of the underlying neural elements and a subsequent cascade of effects [9]. Current theory is that there is neuronal depolarization, local lactic acid accumulation, and decreased cerebral blood flow in the days to weeks following a concussion. The decreased blood flow correlates to decreased glucose delivery, precisely at a time when the injured brain cells are demanding more fuel for recovery. This supply/demand mismatch likely creates the varied symptoms of concussion. While shear strain likely produces a microscopic structural disruption, in most concussions current neuroimaging such as standard MRI and CT scans typically does not show any gross abnormality. Neuroimaging is not necessarily part of standard concussion evaluation and management, and indications for imaging are discussed below.

The signs and symptoms of concussion are varied, but the most common symptoms are described in Table 5.1 [2, 4]. Headache is the most commonly reported

Table 5.1 Table of concussion symptoms

Symptoms of concussion	
Headache	"Don't feel right"
Pressure in head	Difficulty concentrating
Neck pain	Difficulty remembering
Nausea or vomiting	Fatigue or low energy
Dizziness	Confusion
Blurred vision	Drowsiness
Balance problems	Trouble falling asleep
Sensitivity to light	More emotional
Sensitivity to noise	Irritability
Feeling slowed down	Sadness
Felling like "in a fog"	Nervous or anxious

symptom, followed by dizziness, difficulty concentrating, confusion, and visual changes such as sensitivity to light. If a patient experiences these symptoms in the minutes to hours after a collision, then concussion must be suspected. The athlete should be removed from sports or activities where further injury might occur until a qualified clinician has done a thorough evaluation.

In the past, severity of concussion was graded either numerically (grade 1, 2, or 3) or as mild, moderate, or severe. These grading systems were largely based upon the presence and duration of loss of consciousness with pre-prescribed times out of sports. However, the general consensus is to no longer use these types of grading scales, primarily because evidence now suggests that a brief loss of consciousness in association with concussion does not predict clinical course or long-term cognitive impairment [4–6]. In addition, it has become clear that duration of symptoms until full recovery and the timing for return to sports will be different for each athlete. An individualized treatment plan is necessary for each injury, and return to contact sports is restricted at least until there is a confirmation of full resolution of symptoms, full academic and exercise tolerance, and an estimation of full cognitive recovery [4, 10].

During initial evaluation, if the athlete has a loss of consciousness or there is any concern for potential concomitant cervical spine injury, then the principles of traumatology must be followed. Airway, breathing, and circulation must take priority. Athletes with possible cervical spine injury, including those with neck pain or neurologic symptoms (e.g., paresthesias, numbness, paralysis), should undergo cervical spine immobilization until spine injury is excluded clinically or radiographically. CT scan is considered to exclude serious intracranial injuries (e.g., epidural hematoma, subdural hematoma, parenchymal hemorrhage, or cerebral contusion) in athletes with posttraumatic seizure activity, loss of consciousness for longer than a minute, signs of skull fracture, persistent alteration in mental status, or focal neurologic abnormality [4, 10]. Patients with headache, vomiting, or a questionable loss of consciousness should have monitoring for the first several hours following the injury. Worsening of symptoms may warrant imaging, although this may be avoided if patients show improvement during observation. Because CT scan is often readily available and the results are rapid as well as sensitive for evaluating potential fractures or intracranial hemorrhages, it is the test of choice in the acute setting. However, it delivers a relatively large dose of ionizing radiation, so the decision as to if and when it should be used must be made carefully.

Recognizing and diagnosing concussion often begin with a subjective symptom survey, though other sideline tools are employed as well. These tools include a careful cervical spine and neurologic exam, along with balance and cognitive assessments. The 4th International Conference on Concussion in Sport produced the SCAT3 (and the Child SCAT 3). This evaluation tool includes simple methods for the sideline assessment of balance (the modified Balance Error Scoring System, or BESS) and cognitive function (the Standardized Assessment of Concussion, or SAC) [4]. Both the BESS and the SCAT 3 tests are best used when there are healthy, baseline scores that the athlete has completed before the injury for comparison is available, but they can still be useful in the absence of a baseline. Researchers have shown that compared with baseline, a 3.5-point drop in SCAT-2 score had 96 % sensitivity and 81 % specificity in detecting concussion. When examined to exclude baseline scores, a cutoff value of 74.5 was associated with 83 % sensitivity and 91 % specificity in predicting concussion versus controls [11]. "Normal" performance on sideline assessment tools does not necessarily rule out a concussion, and it should be recognized that symptoms may evolve over minutes to hours after a collision. If the athlete has new onset of concussion-like symptoms after a collision, then removal from the contest may be appropriate, even if sideline tests are normal. Particularly in younger athletes, the medical community as a whole has made a commitment to sit a player out if there is any doubt about their concussion status.

Management

Clinical management is based upon observational studies and clinical experience that have culminated in consensus guidelines. The majority of evidence is based on athletes over age 12, but the principals of management are the same for all ages [1, 4, 5, 10, 12–16].

Once the diagnosis of concussion is made, the top two priorities are to avoid additional injury and minimize the impact on the athlete's academic life. If concussion is suspected, the athlete should be immediately removed from the contest with no plans to RTP the same day. This is a departure from previous management principles that were held years ago, where athletes who reported no symptoms after 15 or 30 min may be allowed to return to their sport. Athletes should also refrain from other activities that have a potential for injury, such as skateboarding, skiing, or climbing until a qualified licensed clinician confirms their full recovery [4, 5, 7].

Factors for emergency department (ED) assessment or for neuroimaging are discussed earlier in this chapter. If the patient is stable and the exam is reassuring, the patient may be allowed to recover at home if a responsible adult is available to transport and supervise them.

Cognitive and physical rest are the primary interventions [4, 12–17]. Frequent waking throughout the night is no longer part of current medical recommendations. However, if the patient's status worsens throughout the night (e.g., recurrent vomiting, lethargy, worsening confusion), then urgent evaluation at an ED equipped with neuroimaging capabilities is warranted.

A treatment plan that ensures effective communication between athletic trainers, coaches, medical personnel, and parents should be in place before the start of the season to ensure effective handoff and monitoring of injured athletes.

The amount of rest required is different for each individual patient. But removal from high-risk activities is essential because during recovery, athletes suffering from concussions may be particularly vulnerable to worsening symptoms, additional concussions, or potential catastrophic outcomes, such as second impact syndrome if repeated injury occurs. Animal models and human observational studies suggest that these additional injuries may occur even with relatively low-energy collisions [10, 18–23].

Additionally, it is difficult to know how much cognitive rest is optimal. Care is taken to optimize recovery, but avoid unnecessary interruptions in the academic school year. Overdoing cognitive rest and academic restrictions can significantly affect a student athlete's future school plans, increase the stress of trying to make up a large volume of school work (which by itself may increase symptoms), and can create unnecessary social isolation [24].

Although observational, studies suggest that athletes suffering from concussions who engage in very high levels of cognitive and physical activity have longer recovery times than those who engaged in low to moderate levels of activity [25, 26], those same studies suggest that low levels of activity are not harmful. The recommendation for physical rest is primarily based upon expert consensus and observational studies that suggest physical rest is associated with fewer concussion symptoms, a shorter duration of symptoms, and a lower risk of repeat concussion [10, 14, 19].

Physical Rest

During the prescribed physical rest, activities that significantly increase heart rate and blood pressure should be avoided, such as running, weight lifting, or pushups. The athlete should perform activities of daily living, and basic exercise such as stretching and walking can be encouraged. It should be noted that young, motivated student athletes often feel better when they can be proactive in their recovery. Continuous passive waiting can be frustrating and uncomfortable. In particular, patients who remain home from school, with instructions to do nothing but rest, and refrain from their typical exercise patterns, often have disruption to their normal homeostasis. For instance, a pattern of sleeping during the day and insomnia at night will, by itself, quickly contribute to daytime fatigue, irritability, trouble concentrating, and several other symptoms that are being monitored on the post-concussion symptom survey. Simple and safe suggestions such as dedicated time for daily stretching and walking can give the athlete an opportunity to be more proactive and perhaps stave off some degree of physical deconditioning.

Physical rest should be prescribed until there is resolution of symptoms back to the patient's personal pre-injury baseline, normalization of balance, and recovery of cognitive function. Cognitive assessments may be made with tools such as the SCAT 3 [4] or with computerized neuropsychological testing, but at the very least, the patient should demonstrate the ability to attend full days of school and perform normal study habits without return of symptoms.

In the minority of athletes with prolonged symptoms beyond 14 days after injury, a light, sub-symptom threshold level of aerobic exercise (e.g., light stationary bicycling for 10–15 min trials) may be introduced. This light to moderate exercise challenge can often be well tolerated and may improve symptoms [27], provide a psychological boost, and potentially help mitigate the effects of physical deconditioning.

Cognitive Rest

Although there is evidence that high levels of cognitive challenge may exacerbate symptoms and perhaps even prolong recovery [17], a priority is given to attempts at academic work for several reasons. The implications of several weeks or (rarely) months of missed school work, while waiting for all symptoms to resolve, can threaten the success of a student athlete's semester or school year. In addition, there is no current evidence that cognitive demand, even at high intensity, would contribute to long-term or structural brain damage. This is an obvious difference from the concerns that exist for a return to contact sports before full symptom recovery. For these reasons, patients may attempt a return to school even before complete symptom resolution. In fact, if symptoms are resolved by the next day after injury, the patient may be able to continue with school uninterrupted. However, if significant symptoms persist, then staying home from school with full cognitive rest for 3–5 days, followed by potential temporary academic adjustments, should be considered. For these patients, often they will attempt half days of school with minimal cognitive participation for the first 2–3 days back to school if necessary. It has been suggested that a return to school should occur when the student can tolerate the length of a typical school period (30–45 min) of uninterrupted reading [28].

During cognitive rest, the athlete may engage in light mental activities, such as watching limited amounts of television and family interaction, if symptoms are not exacerbated [28, 29]. Social visits and trips should be limited in an effort to minimize opportunities for symptom exacerbation. Extended texting, video gaming, movie theaters, exposure to loud music, or computer use should be avoided [10].

Academic adjustments may include limited course load, shortened classes or school day, increased rest time, aids for learning (e.g., class notes or supplemental tutoring), or postponement of high-stakes testing [28, 30]. Other adjustments may be offered based on the most prominent symptoms [28]. Strategies to avoid symptom exacerbation are suggested as well, including optimization of sleep patterns, nutrition, and hydration status for the athlete. Frequent breaks from prolonged reading including potential visits to a quiet dark location like the nurse's office may be necessary. For athletes who suffer prolonged recoveries, plans to make up incomplete work may include assignments during scheduled school breaks or summer vacation [23, 31–33].

Prolonged Recovery

Most young athletes will recover readily from sports-related concussions in a matter of days to weeks [1–4, 33, 34]. Over 90 % of high school athletes who sustain a sports-related concussion will be symptom-free and cleared for play within 1 month of injury [1, 2, 10]. Some athletes, however, will take several months to recover from their concussions.

A minority of patients will have prolonged post-concussion symptoms lasting more than 3–4 weeks, and a multidisciplinary approach is warranted that includes treatment by a physician with concussion management expertise, physical therapist, neuropsychologists, and, in selected patients, behavioral management by a psychologist or psychiatrist [30]. Although it appears that initial symptom load (i.e., more severe or numerous initial signs or symptoms) seems to be one of the only reliable predictors of prolonged recovery [12, 35], other features have been debated as contributing factors. These include premorbid conditions such as prior concussion, multiple collisions before concussion was recognized and treatment was initiated, preexisting headache history, learning disability, or psychiatric disorder (e.g., depression) [10, 33, 36].

Symptom Management and Prolonged Recovery

While acetaminophen or nonsteroidal anti-inflammatory medications (NSAIDs) are reasonable adjuncts to physical and cognitive rest during the first few days after injury, they may be ineffective. Although uncommon, rebound headaches after frequent and prolonged use can complicate treatment and recovery [13, 31, 37, 38].

Headache is the most common symptom of concussion and is the most common complaint in patients with prolonged recovery [2]. For patients who have a preexisting migraine history, they may have increased incidence of migraines after injury. In these cases, the patient may use their typical migraine abortive therapy.

There are no medications that are specifically approved by the FDA for the treatment of concussions. There are a handful of prescription medications that are employed in off-label use in the setting of persistent recovery, when there is a heavy symptom burden and when there is interruption of activities of daily living, such as school tolerance [13]. Discussions about the specific indications, dosing, and side effects of these medications are beyond the scope of this chapter. The use of pharmaceuticals should only be considered by a clinician with specific knowledge and experience with concussion management and with extensive knowledge of the potential side effects or contraindications for these medications.

Non-medication interventions can be considered for all patients and in particular for patients that are experiencing prolonged recovery. If there exists cervical muscle pain and tension, or myofascial strains and trigger points, then massage or physical therapy may be helpful. Acupuncture has been suggested for relief of headaches and represents a relatively noninvasive measure that does not carry the same potential for side effects as prescription medications.

Insomnia is a frequent complaint, particularly if athletes are not exercising as they typically do, or who may be sleeping extensively during the day during a period of cognitive rest. Lack of quality nighttime sleep can, by itself, create or exacerbate several symptoms on the post-concussion symptom survey, including fatigue, irritability, headache, trouble concentrating, or even anxiety. If sleep hygiene has not resulted in improved sleep, then a trial of melatonin (up to 3 mg in older children and 5 mg in adolescents) may be considered [13, 39]. This over-the-counter supplement has very little side effects or toxicity and may be effective in initiating sleep. Benzodiazepines should be avoided in patients with concussion because of daytime sleepiness and memory impairment, which hampers the assessment of recovery [13].

Vertigo and balance impairment following concussion typically resolve with physical and cognitive rest, but, for patients with prolonged symptoms, observational studies have suggested that vestibular rehabilitation by a trained physical therapist may have benefit [10, 40, 41]. Dizziness, visual acuity impairment, or exacerbation of symptoms (particularly headache or eye pain) with reading or with exposure to movement in the visual periphery (e.g., while riding in a car, or with walking in a crowded shopping mall) may indicate a need for formal ophthalmology evaluation.

Neuropsychological Testing

As symptoms resolve, academics are tolerated, and return to higher levels of exercise and potential RTP is contemplated, cognitive recovery should be assessed. It should be noted that cognitive recovery may lag behind physical symptom resolution and that every athlete will perform differently on neuropsychological testing. For these reasons, validated tools like the SCAT 3 or more formal computerized neuropsychological tests are typically employed before an athlete returns to contact sports. These tests can typically be completed within 30 min and are best used with a pre-injury, healthy baseline for comparison [1, 2, 35]. In patients with prolonged symptoms, medical symptom validity testing may need to be considered to ensure that symptoms are being exaggerated [42].

As athletes recover and remain symptom-free, they should complete a course of noncontact exercise challenges of gradually increasing intensity [4, 12, 16]. The graded RTP protocol advances through the following rehabilitation stages: light aerobic exercise, more intensive training, sports-specific exercises, noncontact participation, full practice, and ultimately game play as shown in Table 5.2 [4].

Athletes should remain symptom-free during and after exertion at a given activity level before progressing to the next level and remain at each stage for no less than 24 h before advancing to the next level. Therefore, a minimum of 5 days should pass before consideration of full return to competition [10, 12]. If symptoms return at any level, the athlete should rest until the symptoms resolve and then attempt the protocol again beginning at previous level of symptom-free exertion.

Athletes younger than 13 years of age and those at higher risk (e.g., longer duration of symptoms, higher numbers of previous concussions, or returning to higher-risk sports) typically engage in a longer symptom-free waiting period at each stage on their way to RTP [10]. For young athletes with prolonged recovery or with a prior history of concussions, a week of success at each level of noncontact exercise challenge may be advocated. Some clinicians have suggested an arbitrary requirement of equal number of symptom-free weeks as there were symptomatic weeks during recovery before return to contact practice and play is considered.

Thus, the plan for RTP after a concussion should be individualized, gradual, and progressive. This progression permits the athlete to restore confidence, sharpen

Table 5.2 Graduated return to play protocol

Rehabilitation stage	Functional exercise at each stage of rehabilitation	Objective of each stage
1. No activity	Symptom limited physical and cognitive rest	Recovery
2. Light aerobic exercise	Walking, swimming, or stationary cycling keeping intensity, 70 % maximum permitted heart rate	Increase HR
	No resistance training	
3. Sports-specific exercise	Skating drills in ice hockey, running drills in soccer	Add movement
	No head impact activities	
4. Noncontact training drills	Progression to more complex training drills, e.g., passing drills in football and ice hockey	Exercise, coordination, and cognitive load
	May start progressive resistance training	
5. Full-contact practice	Following medical clearance participate in normal training activities	Restore confidence and assess functional skills by coaching staff
6. Return to play	Normal game play	

Source: From: McCrory P, Meeuwisse W, Aubry M, et al. Consensus statement on concussion in sport—the 4th International Conference on Concussion in Sport held in Zurich, November 2012. Clin J Sport Med 2013; 23:89

skills, and simulate sports-specific activity in a controlled setting before entering competitive play. A licensed clinical provider should make the final decision for RTP with experience in the evaluation and management of sports-related concussions. The presenting features of a concussion cannot easily predict the prognosis for RTP. Full RTP exercise progression may take days, weeks, or months although most athletes will be cleared to play within 1 month [1, 2, 4, 10, 12, 16].

Retirement

Some of the most complicated and difficult questions that arise in the management of concussions surround the issue of withdrawal or retirement from contact sports. Decisions regarding retirement from certain sports should be done in conjunction with an experienced clinician and may require ancillary testing, such as neuroimaging or formal neuropsychological testing. Retirement from contact sports is considered when there are multiple concussion over the course of an athletic career, increased recovery times for successive injuries, or a pattern of decreased threshold for repeat concussions, especially when associated with persistent prolonged symptoms [10, 43, 44].

In summary, the medical community has adopted a lower threshold for withdrawing athletes from competition if a concussion is suspected and more formalized conditions to define complete recovery. Loss of consciousness is not a sine qua non for concussion, and the lack of loss consciousness should not be a factor in more rapid return to sports. Injured athletes are no longer permitted to return to competition on the same day as a suspected injury, and formal evaluation with a trained clinician is required before attempted RTP. Before complete recovery and RTP, the athlete should be expected to have complete resolution of concussion symptoms, normalized balance and physical exam, demonstrate academic tolerance or cognitive recovery, and should tolerate exercise in a graded, noncontact stepwise fashion. Neuroimaging and referral to a concussion specialist should be considered in patients with prolonged recovery, persistent or worsening symptoms, or in patients where prolonged abstinence or retirement from contact sports is being considered.

References

1. Meehan 3rd WP, d'Hemecourt P, Collins CL, Comstock RD. Assessment and management of sport-related concussions in United States high schools. Am J Sports Med [Internet]. 2011;39(11):2304–10. http://www.ncbi.nlm.nih.gov/pubmed/21969181
2. Meehan 3rd WP, d'Hemecourt P, Comstock RD. High school concussions in the 2008-2009 academic year: mechanism, symptoms, and management. Am J Sports Med [Internet]. 2010;38(12):2405–9. 2010/08/19 ed. http://www.ncbi.nlm.nih.gov/pubmed/20716683
3. Marar M, McIlvain NM, Fields SK, Comstock RD. Epidemiology of concussions among United States high school athletes in 20 sports. Am J Sports Med. 2012;40(4):747–55.
4. McCrory P, Meeuwisse WH, Aubry M, Cantu B, Dvorak J, Echemendia RJ, et al. Consensus statement on concussion in sport: the 4th international conference on concussion in sport held in Zurich, November 2012. J Am Coll Surg [Internet]. 2013;216(5):e55–71. 2013/04/16 ed. http://www.ncbi.nlm.nih.gov/pubmed/23582174
5. Gómez JE, Hergenroeder AC. New guidelines for management of concussion in sport: special concern for youth. J Adolesc Health. 2013;53(3):311–3.
6. Bakhos LL, Lockhart GR, Myers R, Linakis JG. Emergency department visits for concussion in young child athletes. Pediatrics. 2010;126(3):e550–6.
7. Mannix R, O'Brien MJ, Meehan WP. The epidemiology of outpatient visits for minor head injury: 2005 to 2009. Neurosurgery. 2013;73(1):129–34.
8. Rosenthal JA, Foraker RE, Collins CL, Comstock RD. National high school athlete concussion rates from 2005-2006 to 2011-2012. Am J Sports Med [Internet]. 2014;42(7):1710–5. http://www.ncbi.nlm.nih.gov/pubmed/24739186
9. Giza CC, Hovda DA. The neurometabolic cascade of concussion. J Athl Train. 2001;36(3):228–35.
10. Meehan 3rd WP, O'Brien MJ. Sports-related concussion in children and adolescents: manifestations and diagnosis. In: Hergenroeder AC, Bachur RB, Wiley JF, editors. Up to date. Waltham, MA: U to Date. Accessed Dec 2014.
11. Putukian M, Echemendia R, Dettwiler-Danspeckgruber A, Duliba T, Bruce J, Furtado JL, et al. Prospective clinical assessment using sideline concussion assessment tool-2 testing in the evaluation of sport-related concussion in college athletes. Clin J Sport Med [Internet]. 2015;25(1):36–42. http://www.ncbi.nlm.nih.gov/pubmed/24915173
12. Halstead ME, Walter KD. American Academy of Pediatrics. Clinical report—sport-related concussion in children and adolescents. Pediatrics. 2010;126(3):597–615.
13. Meehan 3rd WP. Medical therapies for concussion. Clin Sport Med [Internet]. 2011;30(1):115–24, ix. 2010/11/16 ed. http://www.ncbi.nlm.nih.gov/pubmed/21074086
14. Concussion, recognition, diagnosis, and management. In: Graham R, Rivara FP, Ford MA, Mason Spicer C, editors. Sports-related concussions in youth: improving the science, changing the culture. Washington, DC: Institute of Medicine of the National Academies, The National Academies Press; 2013. Accessed 6 Nov 2013.

15. Putukian M. The acute symptoms of sport-related concussion: diagnosis and on-field management. Clin Sports Med. 2011;30(1):49–61.
16. Harmon KG, Drezner JA, Gammons M, Guskiewicz KM, Halstead M, Herring SA, et al. American Medical Society for sports medicine position statement: concussion in sport. Br J Sports Med [Internet]. 2013;47(1):15–26. http://www.ncbi.nlm.nih.gov/pubmed/23243113
17. Brown NJ, Mannix RC, O'Brien MJ, Gostine D, Collins MW, Meehan 3rd WP. Effect of cognitive activity level on duration of post-concussion symptoms. Pediatrics [Internet]. 2014;133(2):e299–304. 2014/01/08 ed. http://www.ncbi.nlm.nih.gov/pubmed/24394679
18. Boden BP, Tacchetti RL, Cantu RC, Knowles SB, Mueller FO. Catastrophic head injuries in high school and college football players. Am J Sports Med. 2007;35(7):1075–81.
19. Meehan 3rd WP, Zhang J, Mannix R, Whalen MJ. Increasing recovery time between injuries improves cognitive outcome after repetitive mild concussive brain injuries in mice. Neurosurgery [Internet]. 2012;71(4):885–91. 2012/06/30 ed. http://www.ncbi.nlm.nih.gov/pubmed/22743360
20. Longhi L, Saatman KE, Fujimoto S, Raghupathi R, Meaney DF, Davis J, et al. Temporal window of vulnerability to repetitive experimental concussive brain injury. Neurosurgery [Internet]. 2005;56(2):364–74. 2005/01/27 ed. http://www.ncbi.nlm.nih.gov/pubmed/15670384
21. Vagnozzi R, Tavazzi B, Signoretti S, Amorini AM, Belli A, Cimatti M, et al. Temporal window of metabolic brain vulnerability to concussions: mitochondrial-related impairment—part I. Neurosurgery. 2007;61(2):379.
22. Laurer HL, Bareyre FM, Lee VM, Trojanowski JQ, Longhi L, Hoover R, et al. Mild head injury increasing the brain's vulnerability to a second concussive impact. J Neurosurg. 2001;95(5):859–70.
23. Saunders RL, Harbaugh RE. The second impact in catastrophic contact-sports head trauma. JAMA [Internet]. 1984;252(4):538–9. 1984/07/27 ed. http://www.ncbi.nlm.nih.gov/pubmed/6737652
24. Thomas DG, Apps JN, Hoffmann RG, McCrea M, Hammeke T. Benefits of strict rest after acute concussion: a randomized controlled trial. Pediatrics. 2015;135(2):213–23.
25. Zuckerbraun NS, Atabaki S, Collins MW, Thomas D, Gioia GA. Use of modified acute concussion evaluation tools in the emergency department. Pediatrics [Internet]. 2014;133(4):635–42. http://www.ncbi.nlm.nih.gov/pubmed/24616361
26. Majerske CW, Mihalik JP, Ren D, Collins MW, Reddy CC, Lovell MR, et al. Concussion in sports: postconcussive activity levels, symptoms, and neurocognitive performance. J Athl Train. 2008;43(3):265–74.
27. Leddy JJ, Kozlowski K, Donnelly JP, Pendergast DR, Epstein LH, Willer B. A preliminary study of subsymptom threshold exercise training for refractory post-concussion syndrome. Clin J Sport Med. 2010;20(1):21–7.
28. Halstead ME, McAvoy K, Devore CD, Carl R, Lee M, Logan K. Returning to learning following a concussion. Pediatrics [Internet]. 2013;132(5):948–57. http://www.ncbi.nlm.nih.gov/pubmed/24163302
29. Sady MD, Vaughan CG, Gioia GA. School and the concussed youth: recommendations for concussion education and management. Phys Med Rehabil Clin N Am. 2011;22(4):701–19.
30. Makdissi M, Cantu RC, Johnston KM, McCrory P, Meeuwisse WH. The difficult concussion patient: what is the best approach to investigation and management of persistent (>10 days) postconcussive symptoms? Br J Sports Med. 2013;47(5):308–13.
31. McGrath N. Supporting the student-athlete's return to the classroom after a sport-related concussion. J Athl Train. 2010;45(5):492–8.
32. Master CL, Gioia GA, Leddy JJ, Grady MF. Importance of "return-to-learn" in pediatric and adolescent concussion. Pediatr Ann. 2012;41(9):1–6.
33. Guskiewicz KM, McCrea M, Marshall SW, Cantu RC, Randolph C, Barr W, et al. Cumulative effects associated with recurrent concussion in collegiate football players: the NCAA Concussion Study. JAMA [Internet]. 2003;290(19):2549–55. 2003/11/20 ed. http://www.ncbi.nlm.nih.gov/pubmed/14625331

34. Kerr ZY, Collins CL, Mihalik JP, Marshall SW, Guskiewicz KM, Comstock RD. Impact locations and concussion outcomes in high school football player-to-player collisions. Pediatrics [Internet]. 2014;134(3):489–96. http://www.ncbi.nlm.nih.gov/pubmed/25113292
35. Meehan 3rd WP, d'Hemecourt P, Collins CL, Taylor AM, Comstock RD. Computerized neurocognitive testing for the management of sport-related concussions. Pediatrics. 2012;129(1):38–44.
36. Collins MW, Grindel SH, Lovell MR, Dede DE, Moser DJ, Phalin BR, et al. Relationship between concussion and neuropsychological performance in college football players. JAMA [Internet]. 1999;282(10):964–70. 1999/09/15 ed. http://www.ncbi.nlm.nih.gov/pubmed/10485682
37. Leddy JJ, Sandhu H, Sodhi V, Baker JG, Willer B. Rehabilitation of concussion and post-concussion syndrome. Sports Health. 2012;4(2):147–54.
38. Zafonte RD, Mann NR, Fichtenberg NL. Sleep disturbance in traumatic brain injury: pharmacologic options. NeuroRehabilitation. 1996;7(3):189–95.
39. Owens JA. Pharmacotherapy of pediatric insomnia. J Am Acad Child Adolesc Psychiatry. 2009;48(2):99–107.
40. Gurley JM, Hujsak BD, Kelly JL. Vestibular rehabilitation following mild traumatic brain injury. NeuroRehabilitation. 2013;32(3):519–28.
41. Alsalaheen BA, Mucha A, Morris LO, Whitney SL, Furman JM, Camiolo-Reddy CE, et al. Vestibular rehabilitation for dizziness and balance disorders after concussion. J Neurol Phys Ther. 2010;34(2):87–93.
42. Kirkwood MW, Peterson RL, Connery AK, Baker DA, Grubenhoff JA. Postconcussive symptom exaggeration after pediatric mild traumatic brain injury. Pediatrics [Internet]. 2014;133(4):643–50. http://www.ncbi.nlm.nih.gov/pubmed/24616360
43. Sedney CL, Orphanos J, Bailes JE. When to consider retiring an athlete after sports-related concussion. Clin Sports Med. 2011;30(1):189–200.
44. Protection and prevention strategies. In: Graham R, Rivara FP, Ford MA, Mason Spicer C, editors. Sports-related concussions in youth: improving the science, changing the culture. Washington, DC: Institute of Medicine of the National Academies, The National Academies Press; 2013. Accessed 18 Nov 2013.

Cumulative Effects of Concussion/ Chronic Traumatic Encephalopathy

6

Alex M. Taylor and Laura S. Blackwell

Introduction

To reduce the risk of worse outcomes and prevent longer-term sequelae of concussion, there has been a concerted effort by experts in the field to develop management guidelines, particularly for younger individuals in which symptoms of injury have a direct bearing on academic and social progress. Most guidelines focus on safely returning athletes to play and have clearly defined criteria for medical clearance. While these guidelines are intended to modify the risk of re-injury, many young athletes will go on to sustain a subsequent concussion. The purpose of this chapter is to review the chronic or later to develop cognitive, physical, and emotional sequelae that are potentially associated with repetitive concussion.

Developmental Considerations

Sport-related concussion (SRC) is a common occurrence in young athletes, accounting for 8.9 % of all high school injuries and 5.9 % of all collegiate injuries [1]. Acute symptoms in children are similar to those described in adult populations, including somatic, cognitive, emotional, and sleep-related difficulties [2–6]. However, conclusions based on adults do not necessarily generalize to younger children. The

A.M. Taylor, PsyD (✉)
Department of Neurology, Boston Children's Hospital, BCH 3124, 300 Longwood Ave, Boston, MA 02115, USA

Brain Injury Center, Boston Children's Hospital, Boston, MA, USA
e-mail: alex.taylor@childrens.harvard.edu

L.S. Blackwell, PhD
Center for Neuropsychology, Boston Children's Hospital, Boston, MA, USA
e-mail: laura.blackwell@childrens.harvard.edu

M. O'Brien, W.P. Meehan III (eds.), *Head and Neck Injuries in Young Athletes*, Contemporary Pediatric and Adolescent Sports Medicine,
DOI 10.1007/978-3-319-23549-3_6

biomechanics and pathophysiological response to trauma, as well as the risk of repeat injury may be age related.

Anatomical and mechanical properties of the body and brain differ between developing and mature individuals. With regard to mechanics, it is accepted that concussion occurs when linear and/or rotational forces are applied to the head, neck, face, or body such that an impulsive force is imparted to the brain [7]. While rotational forces are thought to be more instrumental in SRC than linear [8], both are subject to neck strength. This was examined in Collins and colleague's 2014 [9] study of 6704 high school athletes, which found that smaller neck circumference, smaller mean neck to head circumference, and weaker mean overall neck strength were associated with incidence of concussion. By extension, children or adolescents may be at greater risk of injury by nature of their still developing musculature.

Ongoing brain development also distinguishes the risk and response to injury in young and mature athletes. Brain water content, cerebral blood volume, myelination, skull geometry, and suture elasticity are related to maturation. A combination of these developmental factors may place children at increased risk for more widespread and prolonged cerebral swelling following head injury. Youths are also vulnerable to greater metabolic sensitivities compared to similarly injured adults. These differences are seen in experimental models of concussion that report a longer temporal window of vulnerability following trauma in younger animals and suggest that the brain may be particularly sensitive to additional injury during the acute recovery phase [10–14].

Although research examining the longer-term impact of pediatric concussion is limited, longitudinal studies of more severe traumatic brain injury (TBI) in younger children show that insult occurring during infancy and preschool is associated with worse outcomes compared to injury sustained in later childhood or adolescence. Undeveloped or developing skills, particularly executive control processes, are particularly vulnerable [15–18]. Moreover, contextual factors including access to care and academic demands may impact recovery in younger athletes [3, 19–21].

In sum, ongoing development that occurs throughout childhood and adolescence may play a role in recovery from concussion. This has implications for both the risk and response to injury in the younger athlete. The clinical and neuropathological effects of sustaining repeat concussion are reviewed within this context.

Acute Effects and Recovery

Research indicates that recovery from a single concussion typically occurs within 2–14 days, although younger athletes may take longer [22–27]. However, there is evidence of acute differences between individuals with a prior history of concussion and those without. First, individuals with a prior history of concussion are likely to experience more severe markers of injury with subsequent trauma, including loss of consciousness, amnesia, and confusion [28]. Similarly, repeat concussion is associated with a higher initial symptom burden following injury such that individuals with a prior history of concussion endorse more symptoms and rate them as being more severe than individuals with no history of concussion [29, 30].

Studies also demonstrate different trajectories of recovery following repeat concussion. For example, a recent investigation by Eisenberg and colleagues [30] demonstrated that children presenting to the emergency department with a prior history of concussion are more likely to report longer symptom duration than those with no prior history. Similar findings have been shown in athletic populations [31]. For example, Guskiewicz and colleagues found that college football players with a self-reported history of three or more concussions experienced longer recovery times than players with no history of concussion [32]. In addition, prolonged impairment has been found to extend beyond self-report measures of function, with some studies demonstrating more chronic deficits on objective measures of postural stability following repeat concussion [33, 34].

Neurocognitive findings in athletes with a history of concussion are variable. The effects of a single concussion typically result in short-lived deficits in executive function, speed of information processing, attention, and memory [22, 35]. However, there is evidence indicating that concussed athletes who deny subjective symptoms demonstrate worse performance on neurocognitive measures compared to uninjured controls, but better performance than their symptomatic counterparts [26]. This finding suggests that subtle deficits signifying incomplete recovery may linger beyond reported symptoms, which raises concern that the risk of re-injury is greater than previously thought. It also highlights the utility of neurocognitive testing in determining full recovery from acute symptomatology following concussion.

While several studies have shown that repeat concussion is associated with more pronounced neurocognitive deficits[24, 36–39], others do not show any difference between those with a history of concussion and uninjured controls [40–44]. These inconsistencies highlight the heterogeneity of concussion, as well as some of the methodological limitations inherent to cross-sectional analyses. In the extreme (e.g., boxing), however, repetitive trauma is associated with more consistent findings of neurocognitive impairment, with data showing a dose–response relationship [45]. Readers are referred to the section entitled “Long-Term Effects of Chronic Repetitive Concussion” for a more detailed review of prolonged exposure to repeat injury.

Risk of Repeat Injury

The most consistently reported finding in studies examining athletes with a history of concussion is increased susceptibility to additional injury [32, 36, 46–48]. In high school and college athletes, the risk of re-injury for those who report a prior history of concussion is 2–5.8 times greater than in non-injured athletes [49]. Several factors have been suggested to explain this risk, including persistent neuropathological changes, personality/behavioral factors (e.g., aggressive playing style), position, or size and strength. Of these, the number of previous concussions and time elapsed since the most recent prior concussion may be the best predictor of repeat injury

[30, 32]. Guskiewicz et al. [32], for example, found a dose–response relationship between history of concussion and new injury in their sample of 2905 college football players when controlling for division (i.e., NCAA I, II, III), position, years of participation, academic level, and body mass index. This study also indicated that the risk of repeat concussion was greatest within the first 7–10 days after an initial injury [32].

Eisenberg and colleagues' [30] recent study of patients presenting to the emergency department with concussion confirms previous findings demonstrating a dose–response effect of previous injuries. Results also suggest a temporal vulnerability to prolonged recovery with repeat injury. Specifically, subjects who had suffered a concussion within the previous year experienced prolonged symptom duration following repeat injury, whereas subjects with a history of a single concussion occurring more than a year prior to a second injury were indistinguishable from those with no history of concussion. Similar findings are well documented in animal models of concussion [50, 51]. For example, Meehan et al. [51] showed that shorter intervals (1 day) between concussive injury in mice were associated with worse performance on measures of learning and memory compared to those with longer, 1 month intervals between injury or uninjured controls. Moreover, the mice that received daily concussions demonstrated reduced functioning 1 year post injury.

At its extreme, repetitive head injury within a short period of time can have devastating effects. Although presumed to be related to an extraordinarily rare cascade of events, second impact syndrome (SIS) is characterized by catastrophic brain injury occurring when an athlete sustains a second, typically benign head trauma while still symptomatic from a previous concussion [52]. Physiologically, SIS is thought to reflect cerebrovascular congestion or a loss of cerebrovascular autoregulation, which leads to increased intracranial pressure and, ultimately, brain herniation through the foramen magnum [53, 54]. To date, most cases of SIS have been reported in children, adolescents, and young adults, suggesting that the developing brain may be more vulnerable to the effects of this condition, although this may simply reflect the larger numbers of athletes in this age group participating in collision sports. Other investigators have questioned the existence of SIS [55–57] and suggested that the syndrome reflects malignant brain edema, a rare but equally devastating effect of mild brain trauma in youths that has been documented in neurosurgical literature [58]. Despite the debate about SIS and its extremely low incidence, experts generally agree that athletes should be removed from play until all symptoms have resolved to prevent its occurrence [52, 55].

Imaging and Physiologic Studies in Repetitive Concussion

Although useful in ruling out more serious pathology, traditional neuroimaging techniques [e.g., computed tomography (CT) or magnetic resonance imaging (MRI)] are unable to detect concussion [7, 59]. However, functional imaging studies reveal differing patterns of activation in patients diagnosed with concussion compared to uninjured controls [60–63]. Of these, investigations utilizing functional MRI (fMRI) have consistently shown physiological differences following concussion that tend to correlate with self-reported symptoms. Similar findings are documented in studies involving positron emission tomography (PET) or single-photon emission computed tomography (SPECT). None of these studies has looked specifically at the effect of repeat concussion. However, in one investigation examining the acute effects of a single concussion on metabolic function with magnetic resonance spectroscopy (MRS), participants who sustained a second injury during the study period showed more prolonged metabolic dysfunction compared to those who sustained only one concussion [64]. Although speculative, a similar trajectory of prolonged hypo- or hyper-activation may exist in patients who continue to experience symptoms following repeat concussion.

Emerging brain imaging techniques capable of detecting white matter integrity have demonstrated structural injury in the absence of findings on CT or MRI studies. The most consistent findings are reported in studies utilizing diffusion tensor imaging (DTI). This technique measures directionality and regularity of white matter tracts, and it is particularly sensitive to axonal injury. Initial findings indicate that both neurocognitive test performance and self-reported symptoms are associated with DTI findings [65, 66]. Moreover, as with other studies examining repetitive concussion, current research suggests a dose–response relationship such that the extent of white matter or axonal damage may be associated with exposure to concussion [67, 68].

There is also evidence of neurophysiological dysfunction following concussion. While standard electroencephalogram (EEG) readings have shown some utility in detecting change immediately following head injury [69], long-term effects are shown less consistently. However, variants of EEG that are sensitive to cognitive and sensory processing, including evoked potentials (EP) and event-related potentials (ERP), have demonstrated a cumulative effect of multiple concussions [70–72]. Consistent with studies utilizing neurocognitive function as an outcome, there is evidence that altered brain function seen in ERP studies may extend beyond reported symptoms [71–73].

Long-Term Effects of Chronic Repetitive Concussion

Investigations involving athletes with prolonged exposure to repetitive head injury indicate a risk of significant longer-term neurobehavioral and neuropathic sequelae [74–76]. Martland [77] was the first to describe what was initially referred to as punch-drunk syndrome in his review of boxers who presented with confusion, loss of coordination, problems with speech, and upper body tremors [77]. More recently, neuroanatomical investigations of similarly injured boxers have revealed cerebral atrophy, cortical and subcortical neurofibrillary tangles (NFTs), and cellular loss in the cerebellum with some consistency [74, 78]. Not unexpectedly, these neuropathic changes are often accompanied by neurocognitive impairment, with most studies suggesting a dose–response relationship wherein the degree of impairment is associated with the number of bouts fought [45]. Extrapolating from data collected in boxers, the genetic protein apolipoprotein E (apoE) ϵ4 allele may be a risk factor for development of neurobehavioral and neuropathic impairment in those exposed to chronic repetitive trauma [79].

Within the past decade, scientific inquiry has extended beyond boxers in its effort to gain a better understanding of the cumulative effects of concussion. Much of this followed literature suggesting a greater risk of Alzheimer's dementia [76], suicidality [80], and depression [81] in retired professional football players. Methodological limitations in studies to date have prompted investigators to push for more well-controlled, prospective epidemiological studies to determine the true risk of chronic repetitive concussion [80, 82, 83]. Of particular interest to researchers and athletes is the constellation of symptoms first described in 1928 by Martland and later detected neuropathically by Corsellis in 1973, chronic traumatic encephalopathy (CTE).

As currently understood, CTE represents a progressive neurodegenerative disease associated with repetitive symptomatic and asymptomatic brain trauma. Diagnosis is based upon the presence of uniquely distributed tauopathy at postmortem neuropathological examination [75, 84–87]. As noted, while early descriptions of the disease focused on boxing, recent investigations extend to a more diverse group of individuals exposed to repetitive head impacts, most notably American football players.

Clinical Presentation: Studies documenting the clinical presentation of CTE are somewhat variable, as they rely on proxy reports of the patient's premortem behaviors. However, a pattern tends to emerge of progressive cognitive deficits, irritability, aggression, chronic headaches, slurred speech, and parkinsonism [88–90]. Within this broad cluster of neurobehavioral/cognitive symptoms, a recent investigation describes two distinct clinical presentations of CTE [91]. One subset is characterized by more prominent behavioral or mood changes whereas the other is more likely to exhibit cognitive symptoms. Age of onset between these subtypes is reported to differ such that the type involving behavior or mood changes emerges earlier than the type involving cognitive symptoms, although all forms of CTE are thought to eventually result in cognitive impairment.

It is important to note that CTE is distinct from acute or prolonged symptoms of concussion. The clinical symptoms of CTE typically do not manifest until one to two decades after retirement from contact or collision sports [87], although there are documented cases in younger athletes showing symptoms consistent with the disease [75]. Furthermore, there has not been any clear evidence showing a relationship between prolonged acute concussion symptoms and CTE [83, 92].

Following the suicide of several high-profile professional athletes, some have posited a higher risk of depression and suicidality in those with exposure to repeat concussion. There is specific concern that there may be an association with CTE; the media has reported suicide as the cause of death in six retired NFL players between 2011 and 2013 [80]. While clearly worrisome, there is little empirical support showing a direct relationship between CTE and suicidality [80, 92]. To the contrary, there is evidence that the rate of suicide is higher in the general public than in retired professional football players, where it is well established that there is a high risk of repeat head injury. In a large cohort of retired NFL players, completed suicide deaths due to "intentional self-harm" were observed in 9 per 100,000 compared to 21.8 per 100,000 in the general population [93]. In nearly all cases, the risk factors associated with suicide, including depression, substance abuse, violence, and disinhibition, make it difficult to establish a causal relationship, and this remains true for CTE [80, 82, 83].

Neuropathology: CTE is characterized by gross neuropathological findings. The hallmark features include cerebral atrophy, enlargement of the lateral and third ventricles, thinning of the corpus callosum, large cavum septum pellucidum with fenestrations, and scarring and neuronal loss of the cerebellar tonsils [74]. At a microscopic level, CTE is characterized by uniquely distributed tauopathies, including NFTs, neuropil threads (NTs), and glial tangles (GTs) [90].

Tau is an intracellular protein found primarily in neurons of the central nervous system. It functions to support and strengthen the architecture of microtubules. When defective, tau collects abnormally and causes neuronal dysfunction. Tau depositions themselves are not unique to CTE, with 1 review citing 20 different neuropathic conditions involving tauopathies [83]. However, there is a unique pattern of tau distribution in CTE that includes the entorhinal cortex, hippocampus, and neighboring cortical areas [87, 94]. Although beta-amyloid (Aβ) deposits have also been identified in cases of CTE, they are significantly less than the Aβ deposits that characterize nearly all cases of Alzheimer's disease [83]. In 2013, McKee and colleagues published a large case report on individuals with neuropathologically confirmed CTE, presenting proposed criteria for four stages of CTE pathology based on the severity of the findings [88, 95]. Validation of the reliability of this staging system for diagnosis of CTE is currently being performed.

Risk Factors: At this time, the most consistently reported risk for developing CTE is exposure. In boxing, where the goal is to induce a concussion in one's opponent, the risk of exposure to repetitive trauma (i.e., head impact) is obvious. However, literature also shows an impressive risk of head impact in other sports, as well. For example, in American football, reports suggest as many as 1400 head impacts per season for offensive lineman and 2000 for bidirectional players [96–101]. In addition to type of sport played, position and duration of involvement are closely tied to exposure [98, 102, 103]. While it is generally accepted that CTE results from repetitive injury, this is not without some debate. Some authors have suggested that the disease can result from a single impact [104]. In sports with purposeful contact, this has implications for position played and the risk of CTE. For example, data on direct measurements of head impact exposure in college football indicated that compared to other players, running backs and quarterbacks suffer hardest and most severe blows to the head, while linemen and linebackers suffer a greater number of head impacts during a game [98].

As noted, previous investigations have shown that genetic factors may be an important risk factor in the development of CTE. Studies have linked the apolipoprotein E (APOE) gene to worse cognitive functioning in athletes and prolonged recovery following a single head injury [79, 104, 105]. The APOE ϵ4 allele is the largest known genetic risk factor for sporadic AD and has been associated with Aβ, but not tau deposition in cognitively normal aging. There is suggestion that it could also be related to onset of CTE in retired athletes. Other health-related variables may also contribute to the neurodegeneration and clinical symptom spectrum associated with CTE including chronic inflammation associated with obesity, hypertension, diabetes, and heart disease [106].

Age has also been noted as a possible risk factor [87]. Previous literature has indicated that the increased plasticity of a younger brain may allow an individual to better compensate and recover after head injury [107]. However, more recent research indicates that a younger brain may be more susceptible to diffuse brain injury, which could lead to more pronounced and prolonged symptoms, particularly cognitive deficits, over time [27]. A recent study examined the relationship between exposure to repeated head impacts through tackle football prior to age 12 in former NFL players. Results indicated that those whose first impact was before age 12 performed significantly worse on measures of executive functioning, verbal memory, and reading, after controlling for total number of years of football played and age at the time of evaluation [108]. It is possible that early, repeated exposure to head injury could increase an individual's risk for neurocognitive difficulties later in life and potentially lead to CTE. Well-controlled, longitudinal research is needed in this area.

Consistent with most research examining the effects of concussion, investigations focused on CTE have mostly involved male athletes. Previous studies have indicated that females may be at higher risk for postconcussion symptoms as well as prolonged recovery times, including headaches and depression and anxiety [29, 109]. There are emerging theories and investigations about the effect of gender in concussion rates and recovery. For instance, it has been proposed that estrogen may play a role, either a harmful or protective effect, on concussion outcome [110]. With this in mind, ongoing research is needed to examine the susceptibility of females for developing this disease, as risk may be different when compared to their male counterparts.

Conclusions

Studies of athletes with a history of concussion suggest an increased risk of sustaining additional injury, worse on-field presentations with subsequent concussion, longer symptom duration, and slower recovery of neurocognitive and postural functioning. The risks extend beyond clinical findings and include alterations in brain structure and function. Based upon current literature, the effects of repeat concussion are most pronounced with shorter intervals between successive injuries. While evidence for a causal relationship between contact or collision sports and CTE is still being gathered, the finding of uniquely distributed tauopathy and neurobehavioral/cognitive impairment in some athletes is of interest and may be of particular relevance in children and adolescents where developmental factors and increased exposure to additional injury may place them at greater risk for long-term consequences. Continued research is necessary to delineate other factors contributing to the chronic effects of repetitive injury to better elucidate management considerations and prevent worse outcomes. In the interim, evidence continues to highlight the importance of an individualized approach to managing SRC.

References

1. Gessel LM, Fields SK, Collins CL, Dick RW, Comstock RD. Concussions among United States high school and collegiate athletes. J Athl Train. 2007;42:495–503. 2008/01/05 ed.
2. Carroll LJ, Cassidy JD, Peloso PM, Borg J, von Holst H, Holm L, et al. Prognosis for mild traumatic brain injury: results of the WHO Collaborating Centre Task Force on Mild Traumatic Brain Injury. J Rehabil Med. 2004:84–105. 2004/04/16 ed.
3. Kirkwood MW, Yeates KO, Wilson PE. Pediatric sport-related concussion: a review of the clinical management of an oft-neglected population. Pediatrics. 2006;117:1359–71. 2006/04/06 ed.
4. Satz P, Zaucha K, McCleary C, Light R, Asarnow R, Becker D. Mild head injury in children and adolescents: a review of studies (1970–1995). Psychol Bull. 1997;122:107–31. 1997/09/01 ed.
5. Thompson MD, Irby Jr JW. Recovery from mild head injury in pediatric populations. Semin Pediatr Neurol. 2003;10:130–9. 2003/10/24 ed.
6. Taylor HG, Dietrich A, Nuss K, Wright M, Rusin J, Bangert B, et al. Post-concussive symptoms in children with mild traumatic brain injury. Neuropsychology. 2010;24:148–59. 2010/03/17 ed.
7. McCrory P, Meeuwisse WH, Aubry M, Cantu B, Dvorák J, Echemendia RJ, et al. Consensus statement on concussion in sport: the 4th international conference on concussion in sport held in Zurich, November 2012. Br J Sports Med. 2013;47:250–8.
8. Ommaya AK, Gennarelli TA. Cerebral concussion and traumatic unconsciousness: correlation of experimental and clinical observations on blunt head injuries. Brain. 1974;97:633–54.
9. Collins CL, Fletcher EN, Fields SK, Kluchurosky L, Rohrkemper MK, Comstock RD, et al. Neck strength: a protective factor reducing risk for concussion in high school sports. J Prim Prev. 2014;35(5):309–19.
10. Lovell MR, Fazio V. Concussion management in the child and adolescent athlete. Curr Sports Med Rep. 2008;7:12–5. 2008/02/26 ed.
11. Vagnozzi R, Signoretti S, Tavazzi B, Cimatti M, Amorini AM, Donzelli S, et al. Hypothesis of the postconcussive vulnerable brain: experimental evidence of its metabolic occurrence. Neurosurgery. 2005;57:164–71. 2005/07/01 ed.
12. Vagnozzi R, Tavazzi B, Signoretti S. Temporal window of metabolic brain vulnerability to concussions: mitochondrial-related impairment—part I. Neurosurgery. 2007;61:1–10.
13. Giza CC, Hovda DA. The neurometabolic cascade of concussion. J Athl Train. 2001;36:228–35. 2003/08/26 ed.
14. Prins ML, Alexander D, Giza CC, Hovda DA. Repeated mild traumatic brain injury: mechanisms of cerebral vulnerability. J Neurotrauma. 2013;30:30–8.
15. Anderson V, Catroppa C, Morse S, Haritou F, Rosenfeld J. Functional plasticity or vulnerability after early brain injury? Pediatrics. 2005;116:1374–82. 2005/12/03 ed.
16. Ewing-Cobbs L, Prasad MR, Landry SH, Kramer L, DeLeon R. Executive functions following traumatic brain injury in young children: a preliminary analysis. Dev Neuropsychol. 2004;26:487–512. 2004/07/28 ed.
17. Ewing-Cobbs L, Barnes M, Fletcher JM, Levin HS, Swank PR, Song J. Modeling of longitudinal academic achievement scores after pediatric traumatic brain injury. Dev Neuropsychol. 2004;25:107–33. 2004/02/27 ed.

18. Ewing-Cobbs L, Prasad MR, Kramer L, Cox Jr CS, Baumgartner J, Fletcher S, et al. Late intellectual and academic outcomes following traumatic brain injury sustained during early childhood. J Neurosurg. 2006;105:287–96. 2007/03/03 ed.
19. Gioia GA, Isquith PK, Schneider JC, Vaughan CG, Vincent DT, Leaffer E, et al. Initial validation of a paediatric version of the immediate postconcussion assessment and cognitive testing (ImPACT) battery. Br J Sports Med. 2009;43:i91–105.
20. Purcell L. What are the most appropriate return-to-play guidelines for concussed child athletes? Br J Sports Med. 2009;43 Suppl 1:i51–5. 2009/05/14 ed.
21. McCrory P, Meeuwisse W, Johnston K, Dvorak J, Aubry M, Molloy M, et al. Consensus statement on concussion in sport: the 3rd international conference on concussion in sport held in Zurich, November 2008. Br J Sports Med. 2009;43 Suppl 1:i76–90. 2009/05/14 ed.
22. Belanger HG, Vanderploeg RD. The neuropsychological impact of sports-related concussion: a meta-analysis. J Int Neuropsychol Soc. 2005;11:345–57. 2005/10/08 ed.
23. Chen J-KK, Johnston KM, Collie A, McCrory P, Ptito A. A validation of the post concussion symptom scale in the assessment of complex concussion using cognitive testing and functional MRI. J Neurol Neurosurg Psychiatry. 2007;78:1231–8. 2007/03/21 ed.
24. Collins M, Grindel S. Relationship between concussion and neuropsychological performance in college football players. JAMA. 1999;282(10):964–70.
25. Erlanger D, Saliba E, Barth J, Almquist J, Webright W, Freeman J. Monitoring resolution of postconcussion symptoms in athletes: preliminary results of a web-based neuropsychological test protocol. J Athl Train. 2001;36:280–7. 2003/08/26 ed.
26. Fazio VC, Lovell MR, Pardini JE, Collins MW. The relation between post concussion symptoms and neurocognitive performance in concussed athletes. NeuroRehabilitation. 2007;22:207–16. 2007/10/06 ed.
27. Field M, Collins MW, Lovell MR, Maroon J. Does age play a role in recovery from sports-related concussion? A comparison of high school and collegiate athletes. J Pediatr. 2003;142:546–53. 2003/05/21.
28. Collins MW, Lovell MR, Iverson GLL, Cantu RCC, Maroon JCC, Field M. Cumulative effects of concussion in high school athletes. Neurosurgery. 2002;51:1175–81. 2002/10/18 ed.
29. Colvin AC, Mullen J, Lovell MR, West RV, Collins MW, Groh M. The role of concussion history and gender in recovery from soccer-related concussion. Am J Sports Med. 2009;37:1699–704. 2009/05/23 ed.
30. Eisenberg MA, Andrea J, Meehan W, Mannix R. Time interval between concussions and symptom duration. Pediatrics. 2013;132:8–17.
31. Corwin DJ, Zonfrillo MR, Master CL, Arbogast KB, Grady MF, Robinson RL, et al. Characteristics of prolonged concussion recovery in a pediatric subspecialty referral population. J Pediatr. 2014;165(6):1207–15.
32. Guskiewicz KM, McCrea M, Marshall SW, Cantu RC, Randolph C, Barr W, et al. Cumulative effects associated with recurrent concussion in collegiate football players: the NCAA concussion study. JAMA. 2003;290:2549–55. 2003/11/20 ed.
33. Slobounov S, Slobounov E, Sebastianelli W, Cao C, Newell K. Differential rate of recovery in athletes after first and second concussion episodes. Neurosurgery. 2007;61:338–44; discussion 344.
34. Slobounov S, Cao C, Sebastianelli W, Slobounov E, Newell K. Residual deficits from concussion as revealed by virtual time-to-contact measures of postural stability. Clin Neurophysiol. 2008;119:281–9.
35. Erlanger D, Feldman D, Kutner K, Kaushik T, Kroger H, Festa J, et al. Development and validation of a web-based neuropsychological test protocol for sports-related return-to-play decision-making. Arch Clin Neuropsychol. 2003;18:293–316. 2003/11/01 ed.
36. Iverson GL, Gaetz M, Lovell MR, Collins MW. Cumulative effects of concussion in amateur athletes. Brain Inj. 2004;18:433–43. 2004/06/16 ed.

37. Gronwall D, Wrightson P. Cumulative effect of concussion. Lancet. 1975;2:995–7. 1975/11/22 ed.
38. Moser RS, Schatz P. Enduring effects of concussion in youth athletes. Arch Clin Neuropsychol. 2002;17:91–100. 2003/11/01 ed.
39. Covassin T, Stearne D, Elbin R. Concussion history and postconcussion neurocognitive performance and symptoms in collegiate athletes. J Athl Train. 2008;43:119–24.
40. Iverson GL, Brooks BL, Lovell MR, Collins MW. No cumulative effects for one or two previous concussions. Br J Sports Med. 2006;40:72–5. 2005/12/24 ed.
41. Broglio SP, Ferrara MS, Piland SG, Anderson RB, Collie A. Concussion history is not a predictor of computerised neurocognitive performance. Br J Sports Med. 2006;40:802–5. 2006/08/25 ed.
42. Collie A, McCrory P, Makdissi M. Does history of concussion affect current cognitive status? Br J Sports Med. 2006;40:550–1.
43. Macciocchi SN, Barth JT, Littlefield L, Cantu RC. Multiple concussions and neuropsychological functioning in collegiate football players. J Athl Train. 2001;36:303–6.
44. Bruce JM, Echemendia RJ. History of multiple self-reported concussions is not associated with reduced cognitive abilities. Neurosurgery. 2009;64:100–6; discussion 106. 2009/01/16 ed.
45. Heilbronner RL, Bush SS, Ravdin LD, Barth JT, Iverson GL, Ruff RM, et al. Neuropsychological consequences of boxing and recommendations to improve safety: a National Academy of Neuropsychology education paper. Arch Clin Neuropsychol. 2009;24:11–9. 2009/04/28 ed.
46. Hollis SJ, Stevenson MR, McIntosh AS, Shores EA, Collins MW, Taylor CB. Incidence, risk, and protective factors of mild traumatic brain injury in a cohort of Australian nonprofessional male rugby players. Am J Sports Med. 2009;37:2328–33.
47. Schulz MR, Marshall SW, Mueller FO, Yang J, Weaver NL, Kalsbeek WD, et al. Incidence and risk factors for concussion in high school athletes, North Carolina, 1996-1999. Am J Epidemiol. 2004;160:937–44.
48. Guskiewicz KM, Weaver NL, Padua DA, Garrett Jr WE. Epidemiology of concussion in collegiate and high school football players. Am J Sports Med. 2000;28:643–50.
49. Zemper ED. Two-year prospective study of relative risk of a second cerebral concussion. Am J Phys Med Rehabil. 2003;82(9):653–9.
50. Longhi L, Saatman KE, Fujimoto S, Raghupathi R, Meaney DF, Davis J, et al. Temporal window of vulnerability to repetitive experimental concussive brain injury. Neurosurgery. 2005;56:364–74.
51. Meehan WP, Zhang J, Mannix R, Whalen MJ. Increasing recovery time between injuries improves cognitive outcome after repetitive mild concussive brain injuries in mice. Neurosurgery. 2012;71:885–91.
52. Cantu RC. Second-impact syndrome. Clin Sports Med. 1998;17:37–44. 1998/02/26 ed.
53. Schneider R. Head and neck injuries in football: mechanisms, treatment, and prevention. Baltimore: Williams & Wilkings; 1973.
54. Saunders RL, Harbaugh RE. The second impact in catastrophic contact-sports head trauma. JAMA. 1984;252:538–9. 1984/07/27 ed.
55. McCrory P. Does second impact syndrome exist? Clin J Sport Med. 2001;11:144–9. 2001/08/10 ed.
56. Randolph C, Kirkwood MW. What are the real risks of sport-related concussion, and are they modifiable? J Int Neuropsychol Soc. 2009;15:512–20. 2009/07/04 ed.
57. Kirkwood MWW, Randolph C, Yeates KOO. Sport-related concussion: a call for evidence and perspective amidst the alarms. Clin J Sport Med. 2012;22:383–4.
58. Bruce DA, Alavi A, Bilaniuk L, Dolinskas C, Obrist W, Uzzell B. Diffuse cerebral swelling following head injuries in children: the syndrome of "malignant brain edema". J Neurosurg. 1981;54:170–8.

59. Ellemberg D, Henry LC, Macciocchi SN, Guskiewicz KM, Broglio SP. Advances in sport concussion assessment: from behavioral to brain imaging measures. J Neurotrauma. 2009;26:2365–82. 2009/09/01 ed.
60. McAllister TW, Saykin AJ, Flashman LA, Sparling MB, Johnson SC, Guerin SJ, et al. Brain activation during working memory 1 month after mild traumatic brain injury: a functional MRI study. Neurology. 1999;53(6):1300–8.
61. McAllister TW, Sparling MB, Flashman LA, Guerin SJ, Mamourian AC, Saykin AJ. Differential working memory load effects after mild traumatic brain injury. Neuroimage. 2001;14:1004–12.
62. Chen J, Johnston K, Frey S, Petrides M, Worsley K, Ptito A. Functional abnormalities in symptomatic concussed athletes: an fMRI study. Neuroimage. 2004;22:68–82.
63. Jantzen KJ, Anderson B, Steinberg FL, Kelso JA. A prospective functional MR imaging study of mild traumatic brain injury in college football players. AJNR Am J Neuroradiol. 2004;25:738–45. 2004/05/14 ed.
64. Vagnozzi R, Signoretti S, Tavazzi B. Temporal window of metabolic brain vulnerability to concussion: a pilot 1H-magnetic resonance spectroscopic study in concussed athletes—part III. Neurosurgery. 2008;62:1286–96.
65. Lipton ML, Gulko E, Zimmerman ME, Friedman BW, Kim M, Gellella E, et al. Diffusion-tensor imaging implicates prefrontal axonal injury in executive function impairment following very mild traumatic brain injury. Radiology. 2009;252:816–24.
66. Wilde EA, McCauley SR, Hunter JV, Bigler ED, Chu Z, Wang ZJ, et al. Diffusion tensor imaging of acute mild traumatic brain injury in adolescents. Neurology. 2008;70:948–55.
67. Zhang L, Ravdin LD, Relkin N, Zimmerman RD, Jordan B, Lathan WE, et al. Increased diffusion in the brain of professional boxers: a preclinical sign of traumatic brain injury? Am J Neuroradiol. 2003;24:52–7.
68. Chappell MH, Uluä AM, Zhang L, Heitger MH, Jordan BD, Zimmerman RD, et al. Distribution of microstructural damage in the brains of professional boxers: a diffusion MRI study. J Magn Reson Imaging. 2006;24:537–42.
69. Nuwer MR, Hovda DA, Schrader LM, Vespa PM. Routine and quantitative EEG in mild traumatic brain injury. Clin Neurophysiol. 2005;116:2001–25.
70. De Beaumont L, Lassonde M, Leclerc S, Théoret H. Long-term and cumulative effects of sports concussion on motor cortex inhibition. Neurosurgery. 2007;61:327–9. 2007/09/01 ed.
71. Gaetz M, Goodman D, Weinberg H. Electrophysiological evidence for the cumulative effects of concussion. Brain Inj. 2000;14:1077–88. 2001/01/09 ed.
72. De Beaumont L, Brisson B, Lassonde M, Jolicoeur P. Long-term electrophysiological changes in athletes with a history of multiple concussions. Brain Inj. 2007;21:631–44. 2007/06/20 ed.
73. Broglio SP, Pontifex MB, O'Connor P, Hillman CH. The persistent effects of concussion on neuroelectric indices of attention. J Neurotrauma. 2009;26:1463–70.
74. Corsellis JA, Bruton CJ, Freeman-Browne D. The aftermath of boxing. Psychol Med. 1973;3:270–303.
75. McKee AC, Cantu RC, Nowinski CJ, Hedley-Whyte ET, Gavett BE, Budson AE, et al. Chronic traumatic encephalopathy in athletes: progressive tauopathy after repetitive head injury. J Neuropathol Exp Neurol. 2009;68:709–35.
76. Guskiewicz KM, Marshall SW, Bailes J, McCrea M, Cantu RC, Randolph C, et al. Association between recurrent concussion and late-life cognitive impairment in retired professional football players. Neurosurgery. 2005;57:719–26. 2005/10/22 ed.
77. Martland HSH. Punch drunk. JAMA. 1928;91:1103–7.
78. Roberts GW, Allsop D, Bruton C. The occult aftermath of boxing. J Neurol Neurosurg Psychiatry. 1990;53:373–8.
79. Jordan B, Relkin N, Ravdin L, Jacobs A, Bennett A, Gandy S. Apolipoprotein E epsilon4 associated with chronic traumatic brain injury in boxing. JAMA. 1997;278:136–40.

80. Iverson GL. Chronic traumatic encephalopathy and risk of suicide in former athletes. Br J Sports Med. 2014;48:162–5.
81. Guskiewicz K, Marshall S, Bailes J, McCrea M, Harding Jr H, Matthews A, et al. Recurrent concussion and risk of depression in retired professional football players. Med Sci Sports Exerc. 2007;39:903–9. 2007/06/05 ed.
82. Randolph C. Is chronic traumatic encephalopathy a real disease? Curr Sports Med Rep. 2014;13:33–7.
83. Karantzoulis S, Randolph C. Modern chronic traumatic encephalopathy in retired athletes: what is the evidence? Neuropsychol Rev. 2013;23(4):350–60.
84. Omalu BI, DeKosky ST, Hamilton RL, Minster RL, Kamboh MI, Shakir AM, et al. Chronic traumatic encephalopathy in a National Football League player: part I. Neurosurgery. 2005;57:128–34.
85. Omalu BI, DeKosky ST, Hamilton RL, Minster RL, Kamboh MI, et al. Chronic traumatic encephalopathy in a national football league player: part II. Neurosurgery. 2006;59:1086–92; discussion 1092–3.
86. Gardner A, Iverson GL, McCrory P. Chronic traumatic encephalopathy in sport: a systematic review. Br J Sports Med. 2014;48:84–90.
87. Gavett BE, Stern RA, McKee AC. Chronic traumatic encephalopathy: a potential late effect of sport-related concussive and subconcussive head trauma. Clin Sports Med. 2011;30:179–88, xi.
88. McKee AC, Stein TD, Nowinski CJ, Stern RA, Daneshvar DH, Alvarez VE, et al. The spectrum of disease in chronic traumatic encephalopathy. Brain. 2012;136:43–64.
89. Gavett BE, Cantu RC, Shenton M, Lin AP, Nowinski CJ, McKee AC, et al. Clinical appraisal of chronic traumatic encephalopathy: current perspectives and future directions. Curr Opin Neurol. 2011;24:525–31.
90. Omalu B, Bailes J, Hamilton RL, Kamboh MI, Hammers J, Case M, et al. Emerging histomorphologic phenotypes of chronic traumatic encephalopathy in American athletes. Neurosurgery. 2011;69:173–83; discussion 183.
91. Stern RA, Daneshvar DH, Baugh CM, Seichepine DR, Montenigro PH, Riley DO, et al. Clinical presentation of chronic traumatic encephalopathy. Neurology. 2013;81:1122–9.
92. Love S, Solomon GS. Talking with parents of high school football players about chronic traumatic encephalopathy: a concise summary. Am J Sports Med. 2015;43(5):1260–4.
93. Baron SL, Hein MJ, Lehman E, Gersic CM. Body mass index, playing position, race, and the cardiovascular mortality of retired professional football players. Am J Cardiol. 2012;109:889–96.
94. DeKosky ST, Ikonomovic MD, Gandy S. Traumatic brain injury—football, warfare, and long-term effects. N Engl J Med. 2010;363(14):1293–6.
95. Baugh CM, Stamm JM, Riley DO, Gavett BE, Shenton ME, Lin A, et al. Chronic traumatic encephalopathy: neurodegeneration following repetitive concussive and subconcussive brain trauma. Brain Imaging Behav. 2012;6:244–54.
96. Greenwald R, Gwin J, Chu J, Crisco J. Head impact severity measures for evaluating mild traumatic brain injury risk exposure. Neurosurgery. 2008;62:789–98.
97. Crisco JJ, Wilcox BJ, Machan JT, McAllister TW, Duhaime AC, Duma SM, et al. Magnitude of head impact exposures in individual collegiate football players. J Appl Biomech. 2012;28:174–83.
98. Crisco JJ, Wilcox BJ, Beckwith JG, Chu JJ, Duhaime AC, Rowson S, et al. Head impact exposure in collegiate football players. J Biomech. 2011;44:2673–8.
99. Guskiewicz K, Mihalik J. Measurement of head impacts in collegiate football players: relationship between head impact biomechanics and acute clinical outcome after concussion. Neurosurgery. 2007;61:1244–53.
100. Broglio SP, Sosnoff JJ, Shin S, He X, Alcaraz C, Zimmerman J. Head impacts during high school football: a biomechanical assessment. J Athl Train. 2009;44:342–9. 2009/07/14 ed.

101. Bailes JE, Petraglia AL, Omalu BI, Nauman E, Talavage T. Role of subconcussion in repetitive mild traumatic brain injury. J Neurosurg. 2013;119:1235–45.
102. Mihalik J, Bell D, Marshall S, Guskiewicz K. Measurement of head impacts in collegiate football players: an investigation of positional and event-type differences. Neurosurgery. 2007;61:1229–35.
103. Schnebel B, Gwin JT, Anderson S, Gatlin R. In vivo study of head impacts in football: a comparison of National Collegiate Athletic Association Division I versus high school impacts. Neurosurgery. 2007;60:490–6. 2007/03/01 ed.
104. Johnson VE, Stewart W, Smith DH. Widespread τ and amyloid-β pathology many years after a single traumatic brain injury in humans. Brain Pathol. 2012;22:142–9.
105. Kutner KC, Erlanger DM, Tsai J, Jordan B, Relkin NR. Lower cognitive performance of older football players possessing apolipoprotein E epsilon4. Neurosurgery. 2000;47:651–7; discussion 657–8.
106. Stern RA, Riley DO, Daneshvar DH, Nowinski CJ, Cantu RC, McKee AC. Long-term consequences of repetitive brain trauma: chronic traumatic encephalopathy. PM R. 2011;3:S460–7.
107. Schneider GE. Is it really better to have your brain lesion early? A revision of the "Kennard Principle". Neuropsychologia. 1979;17:557–83.
108. Stamm JM, Bourlas AP, Baugh CM, Fritts NG, Daneshvar DH, Martin BM, et al. Age of first exposure to football and later life cognitive impairment in former NFL players. Neurology. 2015;84(11):1114–20.
109. Covassin T, Schatz P, Swanik CB. Sex differences in neuropsychological function and post-concussion symptoms of concussed collegiate athletes. Neurosurgery. 2007;61:341–5. 2007/09/01 ed.
110. Covassin T, Elbin RJ. The female athlete: the role of gender in the assessment and management of sport-related concussion. Clin Sports Med. 2011;30:125–31, x.

Skull Fractures and Structural Brain Injuries

7

Kevin T. Huang, Muhammad M. Abd-El-Barr, and Ian F. Dunn

Introduction

In comparison to concussion and other forms of nonstructural brain injury, skull fractures and other forms of structural head injury are uncommon in young athletes. They represent, however, a spectrum of pathologies; mild injuries require observation alone, while others are life threatening and may require emergent surgical intervention. As such, an understanding of the nature and management of these lesions is important for any modern medical practitioner dealing with young patients with exposure to head trauma in any setting.

Classification

Skull fractures can be described by their location (frontal, temporal, parietal, occipital, basilar), pattern (linear, comminuted if complex and branching, or diastatic if resulting in the opening of a preexisting suture line), exposure to the outside environment (open vs. closed), and degree of displacement (depressed vs. nondepressed) (Fig. 7.1). In cases of depressed skull fracture specifically, the terms simple and compound are frequently used instead of closed and open, respectively. Structural brain injury represents a heterogeneous set of pathologies that represent any significant mass lesion or disruption of normal cerebral anatomy. These include epidural/extradural hematoma (EDH), subdural hematoma (SDH), traumatic subarachnoid hemorrhage (tSAH), and intracerebral/intraparenchymal hemorrhage.

K.T. Huang, MD (✉) • M.M. Abd-El-Barr, MD, PhD • I.F. Dunn, MD
Brigham and Women's Hospital/Boston Children's Hospital, Harvard Medical School, Boston, MA, USA
e-mail: khuang3@partners.org; amabd-el-barr@partners.org; idunn@partners.org

M. O'Brien, W.P. Meehan III (eds.), *Head and Neck Injuries in Young Athletes*, Contemporary Pediatric and Adolescent Sports Medicine,
DOI 10.1007/978-3-319-23549-3_7

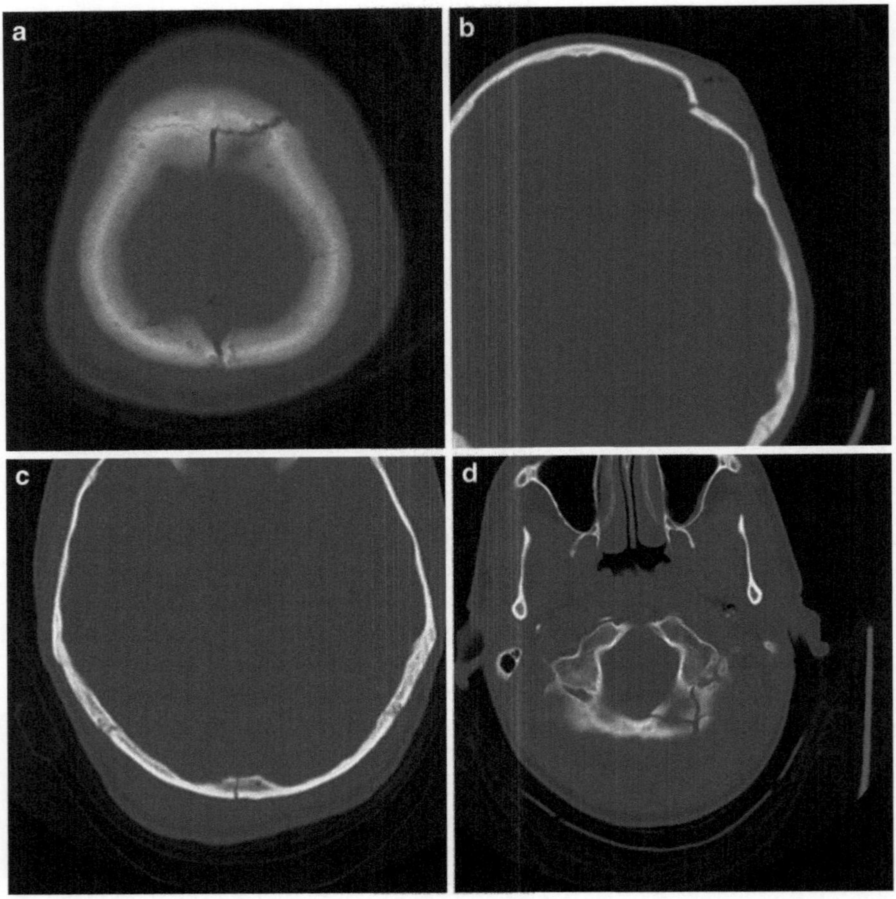

Fig. 7.1 (**a**, *top left*) A traumatic diastatic fracture involving the sagittal suture and left coronal suture in a 53-year-old male after a fall. (**b**, *top right*) A depressed left frontal skull fracture in a 9-year-old following a golf club strike to the head; note the subcutaneous and intracranial air indicating the open nature of the injury. (**c**, *bottom left*) A linear fracture of the occipital bone in a 22-year-old following a motor vehicle-related injury. (**d**, *bottom right*) An image taken from the same scan and same patient as in (**c**), showing that the fracture has tracked inferiorly and has comminuted involvement of the skull base

Epidemiology and Etiology

The epidemiology of traumatic brain injury (TBI) as a whole is limited by a number of factors, including non-standardized definitions, underreporting of cases (in particular from patients who may not seek medical attention), differences in specific population focus across studies, and, until relatively recently, lack of coordinated efforts to monitor epidemiologic data on a broad scale. Despite this, there is a greater appreciation that sports are a major contributor to the incidence of structural injuries, especially in the young. A retrospective review of the National Hospital Ambulatory Medical Care Survey revealed that 14 % of emergency room visits for life-threatening injuries were sports related, with children having a higher percentage compared to adults (32 % vs. 9 %) [65].

Data on skull fractures in particular are clouded by their frequent coincidence with other types of TBI. In studies that examine the incidence of TBI, the separate incidence of overlying skull fractures is not consistently reported. It is important to keep in mind that epidemiology of these lesions remain difficult when interpreting data regarding their incidence in the population.

The incidence of skull fractures across all ages, as measured by presentation to the US emergency departments, has been estimated at 16 cases per 100,000 per year (3.5 % of all those presenting to attention for head injuries) [45]. However, measured incidences show considerable variation, with some researchers reporting an incidence of 66 per 100,000 per year in adults of the United Kingdom and others citing a 6 % incidence of comminuted skull fractures alone among patients presenting with head injury [40, 93]. Children are particularly prone to skull fracture, with some estimating that greater than 20 % of children presenting to attention in the emergency room for head injury have evidence of a skull fracture [36].

As is consistent across almost all types of head injury, skull fractures have a strong predilection for the young male, with an estimated 2:1 to 3:1 male to female ratio [8, 93]. Though few studies explicitly have evaluated skull fractures as a separate entity from other types of TBI, it is presumed that the causes of skull fracture mimic those of head injury overall, in which transportation-related incidents, occupational hazards, falls, and assaults feature prominently [8, 46, 59, 88]. It should be noted that the presence of an overlying skull fracture has been shown to dramatically increase the risk of finding an underlying intracranial pathology in both adults and children, as much as 20-fold in some studies [17, 23, 75, 99].

Most studies do not feature sports-related injuries as a major contributor to measured incidences of skull fractures [5]. The converse is also typically true, and most sports-related head injuries do not feature skull fractures or other structural brain injuries. Nonetheless, skull fractures are not unheard of in sports and are commonly seen in patients with severe injuries that require inpatient admission. As many as 40 % of inpatient admissions for sports-related head injury have evidence of a skull fracture [53, 58]. Common mechanisms for these injuries include high-energy collisions (skiing, football, hockey), impacts from hard, high-velocity projectiles (golf, shooting), or falls from heights (cycling, climbing, horseback-riding) [30, 58]. Interestingly, although head injuries in this sport are extremely rare, some limited evidence suggests that among sports-related head injuries presenting to the emergency department, those that are golf related have an association with skull fractures. This is presumably due to a unique combination of hard, high-velocity objects with small surface areas (golf balls and club heads) and no routine use of protective headgear [58, 76, 96]. Despite some work into identifying skull fractures incidences in individual sports, however, it is important to emphasize that little evidence has yet been gathered on the epidemiology of skull fractures in the overall population of young athletes.

The incidence of most types of traumatic intracranial hemorrhage is lower than that of skull fractures due to the higher necessary kinetic energy to generate these injuries. It is common for patients with traumatic intracranial hemorrhage to have overlying skull fractures, but the converse is not necessarily true. Among patients presenting with TBI, incidence estimates range from 2.7 to 4 % for EDH, approximately 11 % for SDH, and 8.2 % for intraparenchymal hemorrhage [10–12]. The incidence of tSAH is significantly higher than those of other types of intracranial hemorrhage. An estimated 30–60 % of admissions for TBI will feature some type of tSAH present on computed tomography (CT) imaging [26, 52, 62, 69]. As with skull fractures, the mechanisms for intracranial hemorrhage are similar to those for TBI as a whole: transportation-related (most often motor vehicle-related) injuries, falls, occupational hazards, and violence/assault [10–12, 62].

Though sports-related injuries are not known to be a leading cause of these lesions in previously reported literature, the incidence of intracranial hemorrhage in sports-related TBI has not been systematically examined to our knowledge. Sports-related intracranial hematoma formation is not unheard of, however, and they are implicated in the majority of fatalities and catastrophic morbidity across a variety of sports [3, 15, 30, 49, 106]. Brain injuries account for an estimated 69 % of football-related fatalities in the United States, with 75 % of these occurring in high school-level players [15]. SDHs account for the overwhelming majority (86 %) of those brain injury-related fatalities and are also implicated in the majority of boxing-related fatalities [66]. This association is not necessarily true for fatalities across all sports, however, and intracranial hemorrhage accounts for approximately half of amateur baseball-related fatalities and only a tiny portion of serious basketball-related injury [4, 24].

Biomechanics and Pathophysiology

Numerous studies have demonstrated the resilience of the human skull to a variety of biomechanical loads. Unembalmed cadaveric studies have demonstrated that the human skull can withstand blunt force loads of up to 14.1 kN (3170 lb, mean: 6.4 kN = 1439 lb) and energies of up to 68.5 J (50.5 foot-pounds, mean: 28.0 *J* = 20.7 foot-pounds) before fracture [103]. These values are roughly consistent across different cadaveric studies [25]. These measurements, however, are not necessarily representative of all anatomic regions of the human skull. The pterion and squamous temporal bone are known to be particularly weak, with lower peak forces needed to induce fracture [102]. Special consideration also needs to be given to the pediatric skull, which not only has thinner bone but also unfused cranial sutures in infants. In cadaveric studies of infants, falls from heights of 82 cm (~32 in.) have been shown to consistently produce skull fractures [98]. Skull thickness grows steadily in children, with 85–90 % of peak skull thickness present by the second decade of life and peak skull thickness typically achieved by the third decade of life [1, 34].

Of note, there exist differences in the generation of different types of skull fractures [64]. Linear fractures are typically the result of pure energy absorption by the skull after contact with a hard object, with little dispersion of the kinetic energy toward translation, rotation, or angulation. Depressed skull fractures often result from contact with smaller objects, which focus the energy to a smaller region of the skull. This focus can be significant enough to disrupt the bone underlying the site of impact in a circumferential manner, resulting in separation from the surrounding bone and depression of the fracture. Cases of basilar skull fracture can result from either transmission of mechanical forces from remote sites of impact, which can disrupt some of the relatively weaker structures of the skull base, or from direct pressure upon the bones of the face or skull base.

The pathophysiology of intracranial hemorrhage inevitably involves the disruption of the integrity of an intracranial vessel due to either direct laceration by a bone fragment or propagation of kinetic energy leading to shearing forces upon the vessel itself. The type and location of the vessel dictate the nature of subsequent hemorrhage.

In instances of EDH, the disrupted vessel lies between the skull and underlying dura and classically involves laceration of the middle meningeal artery due to an overlying skull fracture of the pterion (though venous bleeding from the middle meningeal vein, diploic veins, or venous sinuses have also been known to occur) [11, 68].

In cases of SDH, the disrupted vessels are located just beneath the dura but still on top of the arachnoid membrane. The classically involved vessels in cases of SDH are the bridging subdural veins and, in cases of young athletes without preexisting structural brain disease, are not easily damaged. Laceration of these vessels require either an overlying skull fracture or foreign object that has been propelled inward to lacerate the dura itself or a very high-energy impact such as from a high-speed motor vehicle collision. As such, acute traumatic SDH is associated with very significant injuries and prognosis is poor, with mortality estimates ranging from 40 to 60 % [12, 37, 55, 100]. In both SDH and EDH, the immediate concern is the risk of mass effect of the hematoma upon underlying brain tissue, which, if severe enough, will cause herniation and subsequent damage of critical neural structures.

A recent review attempted to set thresholds for acceleration values needed to produce SDH in football players. Reviewing cadaveric studies, animal studies, and finite-element simulations, a threshold of approximately 5000 rad/s [2] was set for rotational acceleration (RA) and 3000*g* for translational acceleration (TA) to cause venous rupture and subsequent SDH [28].

tSAH, on the other hand, is a much more common occurrence, but its precise etiology is unclear. In particular, though the natural history and etiology of aneurysmal and spontaneous SAH have been well documented, comparatively less has been written about the pathophysiology of SAH following trauma. It has been proposed that tSAH results from hemorrhage of pial vessels or possibly diffusion of blood from cerebral contusions into the subarachnoid space [91]. When present, the blood itself is rarely of sufficient quantity to cause significant mass effect on its own, but the chemical irritation of the blood is well known to produce significant headaches. Perhaps more significantly, there is a concern that tSAH predisposes the patient to delayed vasospasm and subsequent cerebral ischemia as is seen in cases of

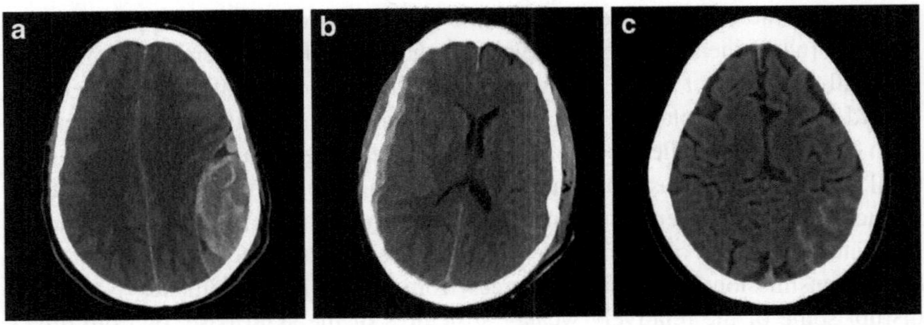

Fig. 7.2 (**a**, *left*) A large, left parietal epidural hematoma a 40-year-old male following falling down a flight of stairs. Note the characteristic ellipsoid appearance of the lesion and the associated midline shift. (**b**, *middle*) A right frontotemporal subdural hematoma in a 56-year-old male involved in a motorcycle accident. Note that the hematoma spreads across multiple suture lines. (**c**, *right*) Traumatic subarachnoid hemorrhage in the left occipital lobe in a 32-year-old male following a fall down a flight of stairs. Note the presence of hyper-attenuating substance tracking along the cortical sulci on the left compared to the open ones on the right

aneurysmal SAH [35, 89] (Fig. 7.2). These concerns are somewhat controversial, however, and many have proposed that tSAH is a process that is biologically distinct from aneurysmal SAH, with lower associated risks of vasospasm [31]. An additional controversy is whether tSAH predisposes patients to posttraumatic hydrocephalus, presumably through damage to cerebrospinal fluid (CSF) absorption pathways by hemorrhagic materials [90]. Other studies, however, have failed to find any correlation between the presence of tSAH and the development of posttraumatic hydrocephalus [74].

Initial Evaluation and Diagnosis

When assessing a patient with a suspected skull fracture or intracranial hematoma, there are several points that need to be considered in the initial assessment and workup. As with many forms of potentially serious trauma, timing to proper evaluation of the patient is key. As has been demonstrated in the literature on EDH in particular, the time between trauma and operation is consistently listed as one of the major predictors of outcome and mortality (while gender, age, mechanism of injury, EDH location, and shape are not) [7, 54, 78].

History taking should be thorough but focused and obtained from reliable witnesses if the patient is unable to accurately describe the incident themselves. Key factors to elucidate include:

- Exact timing of the trauma (reports of general times of day, for instance, "earlier this evening," can be misleading and are often insufficient)
- Sequence of events surrounding the trauma, with consideration of the possibility that a change in mental status (from some unrelated pathology) leads to the trauma instead of the converse

- Mechanism of injury (including good approximation of speeds and energies involved in the trauma)
- Precise anatomic location of any cranial trauma (with special attention to possibility for the head to be launched from the primary impact and make a secondary impact)
- Other bodily injuries, particularly significant ones that can "distract" the patient from relevant pain along the craniospinal axis, or other injuries that may impact the findings on neurologic examination
- Post-trauma course, with special attention to mental status, amnesia, occurrence of any seizure or seizure-like episodes, and any potential therapies or workup that may already have been initiated
- Focused review of systems, including nausea, vomiting, seizure, changes in mental status, any new-onset neurologic deficits, and reports of clear, salty fluid in the ears, nose, or throat which may be indicative of a CSF leak
- Brief social history, with the understanding that the patient's consumption of alcohol, tobacco, and illicit drugs can significantly impact their presentation and hospital course
- Past medical history, including an assessment of baseline health and with particular focus on previous neurosurgical procedures or preexisting neurologic disease such as hydrocephalus, epilepsy, or recent history of head injury

In addition to the history, the physical examination can often provide key insights that may influence management. In addition to a proper trauma survey and neurologic examination (details of which are beyond the scope of this chapter), there are several important factors that are important not to miss as part of the initial examination. These include:

- Vital sign abnormalities, in particular bradycardia, hypertension, and respiratory irregularities that may signal impending or ongoing increases in intracranial pressure.
- Brief assessment of the patient's mental status and level of consciousness. Determination of a patient's Glasgow Coma Scale (GCS) score is important, and repeated studies have validated the utility of GCS in predicting outcomes and influencing management [11, 18, 38, 62].
- Careful inspection of the entirety of the scalp, with clearing of any dirt or blood products if they obstruct proper inspection. Inspection of only the injury sites described in the patient history is often *insufficient*, and patient hair can very easily hide lacerations, hematomas, and bony defects unless explicitly examined.
- Palpation for any cranial defects, step-offs, or inappropriate mobility. In certain cases of complex or depressed skull fracture, mobility of liberalized bone fragments can be easily appreciated.
- Inspection for any signs of basilar skull fracture, including periorbital or postauricular ecchymosis or hematoma, and any new-onset deficits of any of the cranial nerves.
- Examination of the tympanic membranes and nares for any signs of blood or CSF.

Neurologic examination should be quick but thorough, with focus given to detection of new-onset deficits. Any abnormalities must be interpreted in the context of the patient's other injuries, current mental status, and baseline status of health.

In cases where structural brain or skull injury is suspected, computed tomography (CT) scan is the imaging modality of choice for further workup due to its speed and high sensitivity for both bony and hemorrhagic lesions. Plain skull radiograph is insufficient as a radiologic investigation of structural brain injury. Moreover, though some have proposed their utility as a screening tool for intracranial hemorrhage (based on the strong association between skull fractures and underlying structural imaging previously noted in this chapter), their usage in this manner remains controversial [17, 36, 42]. Magnetic resonance imaging (MRI), though possessing a superior ability to detect intracranial blood products, is typically too slow or unavailable for routine use in assessing head trauma.

In the setting of moderate to severe brain injury, focal neurologic deficit, or obvious skull fracture, prompt evaluation with a CT scan is necessary to assess for structural lesions. The decision to obtain imaging in cases of mild head injury, however, can be sometimes be more nuanced. Various guidelines exist for determining the need for CT scan in the setting of mild brain injury [39, 44, 72, 84, 86]. The Canadian CT Head Rule, one of the more widely applied schemas that has compared favorably against competing sets of guidelines, specifies that cases of mild head injury require a head CT only if they have [87]:

- GCS score < 15 at 2 h following injury
- Suspected open or depressed skull fracture
- Any signs of basilar skull fracture
- Two or more episodes of vomiting
- Age greater than or equal to 65 years
- Amnesia that covers greater than 30 min before the impact
- Dangerous mechanism (pedestrian struck by motor vehicle, occupant ejected from a motor vehicle, fall from height greater than 3 ft or 5 stairs)

Though other guidelines differ in their specific cutoffs for imaging, all agree that radiologic evaluation should be conducted in a prompt fashion if there is any suspicion for underlying structural skull or brain injury [39, 44]. It is also important to keep in mind that neuroimaging is also necessary in head trauma patients if the patient's mental status is impaired and a proper neurologic examination is unattainable (and thus a new neurologic deficit cannot be reliable excluded).

Based on findings of the CT scan, further imaging may be indicated. In particular, if CT scan demonstrates skull fracture extension over any of the dural venous sinuses or through vessel-containing foramina, CT angiography can be performed to assess for vessel integrity and patency [16, 105].

In addition to imaging, in cases of severe head injury, intracranial pressure monitoring may also be indicated. Continuous intracranial pressure monitoring, when combined with measurements of mean arterial pressure, can help assess cerebral perfusion pressure, an important, modifiable, predictor of outcomes in severe head injury [2, 19, 50]. Moreover, intracranial pressure monitoring can also be useful in the early detection of delayed-onset hemorrhage and expanding intracranial masses, which may require surgical intervention.

Intracranial pressure monitoring can be performed through installation of an invasive or noninvasive monitor by a trained neurosurgeon and is indicated in all salvageable head injury patients with GCS scores 3–8 (after resuscitation) and an abnormal CT scan [6]. Monitoring is also indicated in salvageable patients who meet two or more of the following criteria:

- Age > 40 years
- Unilateral or bilateral motor posturing (decerebrate or decorticate posturing)
- Systolic blood pressures < 90 mmHg

In all instances of severe head trauma, prompt consultation with a neurotrauma specialist can help guide further possible workup and also facilitate transition of these patients from the emergent setting to a properly equipped and staffed intensive care unit.

Treatment

The treatment for skull fractures and associated structural brain injuries varies based on the severity of the pathology. When necessary, treatment for these lesions relies heavily on surgical intervention, as the pathology is anatomic in nature. There should be no hesitation to seek prompt neurosurgical consultation if the primary practitioner feels that operative intervention may be required or if they feel they require additional expertise or assistance.

Skull Fractures

Closed, nondepressed linear skull fractures without evidence of underlying structural parenchymal lesions do not require surgical intervention and can be managed expectantly (Table 7.1). Care should be geared toward reassurance and management of any potential coinciding nonstructural injuries.

Open, nondepressed skull fractures without evidence of underlying hematomas can also typically be managed nonoperatively. The existence of an open communication to the outside world does raise the concern for increased infection risk, and in such cases thorough irrigation and approximation of the wound are prudent. Care should be taken, however, to ensure that there exists no disruption of the underlying dura and that the brain parenchyma has not been directly exposed to environmental pathogens.

Table 7.1 Overview of skull fractures

	Nondepressed	Depressed
Closed	*Features*: Can be linear or comminuted, can have extension into the facial bones or skull base	*Features*: Fracture fragments with inward displacement into the cranial vault, no evidence of communication with outside environment
	Mechanism: High-energy collision	*Mechanism*: Impact from a hard object with a smaller surface area and significant force
	Management: Evaluate and rule out any associated underlying injures (cerebrospinal fluid leak, vascular disruption, intracranial hemorrhage, etc.). If no other injuries, expectant management	*Management*: Operative elevation and washout if fracture displaced greater than the distance of the adjoining skull. Follow for risk of infection and seizures
Open	*Features*: Can be linear or comminuted, must have communication with outside air through disruption of the skin and galea	*Features*: Fracture fragments with inward displacement, evidence of open communication with outside environment
	Mechanism: High-energy impact and associated deep skull laceration	*Mechanism*: Impact from a hard object with a smaller surface area and significant force and associated deep skull laceration
	Management: Irrigation and closure	*Management*: If displacement greater than width of adjoining skull, operative elevation, debridement, and closure. Follow closely for risk of infection and seizures

Very little data exist on the management of simple (closed) depressed skull fractures due to their relative rarity compared to compound (open) depressed fractures [5, 17]. Current practice advocates surgical elevation if the degree of depression surpasses the full thickness of the surrounding skull. The thought is that significant displacement of the fracture will result in increased pressure and irritation of the underlying cortical surface (possibly raising in the incidence of posttraumatic epilepsy) and will also result in poor cosmetic appearance upon healing of the fracture [9]. However, as mentioned above, very little data exists to support this practice, and authors have proposed that surgery should be pursued only in cases of unacceptable cosmetic appearance or dural disruption [48, 85].

Similarly, there still exists some controversy regarding the optimal management of compound depressed skull fractures. Current guidelines recommend operative intervention (featuring elevation of the fracture and aggressive debridement) in cases where the fractured bone fragment has been displaced greater than the thickness of the surrounding calvarium [9]. This is based on a relatively high rate of reported infections (~11 %) and posttraumatic epilepsy (15 %) in these patients [47, 48]. As with the case for simple depressed fractures, however, there exists little high-quality evidence to guide this practice, and authors have reported successful nonoperative management in certain select groups of patients, in particular those without evidence of dural violation [40, 92].

Though most skull fractures heal without issue, in the pediatric population, some fractures can exhibit gradual extension over time. These lesions, referred to simply as growing skull fractures, are heavily associated with very young children (those less than 3 years of age) and are seen in patients with both an overlying skull fracture and, importantly, an underlying dural defect [33, 95]. The pathogenesis of the fracture involves progressive erosion of both bone and brain tissue and is thought to be caused by a combination of uncontained CSF pulsations escaping through the dural opening, growing leptomeningeal cysts, and normal brain growth [71, 104]. The occurrence of growing skull fractures is rare, with an estimated incidence of <0.05 % to 1.6 % of all skull fractures [27]. When detected, repair of the dural defect and cranioplasty are important in limiting the disease process [27, 33, 71, 95, 104].

As is true with all forms of surgical intervention, individual patient context should inform a clinician's treatment plan. Surgical fixation may prove beneficial even in patients with minimally depressed skull fractures who are either unable to accept the cosmetic defect or are insistent upon aggressive return to contact sports.

Epidural/Extradural Hematoma

Traumatic EDH has traditionally been considered a neurosurgical emergency which may require emergent intervention. Operative treatment typically involves evacuation of the hematoma and then identification of any potential sources of bleeding in order to achieve adequate hemostasis of the source, which is typically a bleeding meningeal artery.

Operative intervention is categorically recommended in all lesions that are greater than 30 cm^3 in estimated total volume. Nonoperative management is reserved for only those lesions that are (1) less than 30 cm^3 in volume, (2) produce less than 5 mm of midline shift, (3) present with a GCS score greater than 8, and (4) are not associated with focal neurologic deficits [11, 13, 22]. Serial monitoring with neuroimaging and close observation in a dedicated neurosurgical center is advised.

Mortality following EDH has been estimated at ~10 % for adults and 5 % for children [21, 41, 60, 73]. It is important to seek prompt attention when these lesions are detected or suspected, particularly when there is reason to believe that compression of critical neural structures is involved. In patients with EDH and evidence of herniation, delays in treatment have consistently shown to increase mortality rates [20, 37, 82].

Acute Subdural Hematoma

Management of acute traumatic SDH differs from that of EDH in that bleeding is more often venous rather than arterial and the risk of rapid expansion is lower. As such, nonsurgical management plays a much larger role in care of patients with SDH. Indications for surgery include significant mass effect as demonstrated on neuroimaging (greater than 1 cm thickness or a midline shift greater than 0.5 cm), strong clinical evidence to suggest an expanding, compressive lesion (patients with asymmetric and/or fixed and dilated pupils, measured ICP>20 mmHg, or patients with GCS score<9 and who have a measured 2 point drop in GCS score between the time of injury and hospitalization) [12]. These indications, however, must also be weighed in the setting of goals of care for the patient and whether the extent of a patient's injuries renders surgery futile. In weighing these considerations, it should be kept in mind that younger patients are known to experience better outcomes following surgery for SDH, with patients 18–30 years old experiencing a third of the morality seen in patients >50 years of age [56].

Traumatic Subarachnoid Hemorrhage

There still exists much uncertainty regarding the significance of tSAH in brain injury. Though it has been established that the presence of tSAH is an independent predictor of worse outcomes following TBI, it is unclear if there is any causal component to this correlation [43, 51, 83, 89, 101]. Moreover, as has been discussed above, tSAH is known to have a much lower incidence of secondary vasospasm as compared to aneurysmal SAH. Thus, standard treatment protocols for aneurysmal SAH do not necessarily apply to cases of tSAH.

The presence of subarachnoid blood alone does not require operative treatment and can be managed nonsurgically. Care should be taken, however, to consider the possibility that SAH can arise from underlying pathologies that may require intervention, such as cerebral aneurysms or arteriovenous malformations. Pharmacologic intervention in cases of tSAH remains controversial. Though certain reports have demonstrated benefits to the use of nimodipine, a calcium channel blocker, in cases of tSAH, a systematic review of the available literature has failed to find any therapeutic benefit [94].

Use of Protective Headgear

Though proper treatment can lead to good outcomes in some patients with serious structural injury, prevention of the initial injury is obviously preferable. One of the key factors in both reducing the severity of injury and also the prevention of injury altogether is the use of helmets and protective headgear. Protective headgear use has been shown to decrease the incidence of skull fractures across a variety of sports, including skiing, snowboarding, American football, cyclists, baseball, hockey, and equestrian sports [4, 15, 57, 70, 80, 97].

There has been an increased interest in designing protective helmets to decrease the rate of skull fractures, intracranial hemorrhages, and concussions, especially in contact sports. This has been especially true in football, where almost 70 % of fatalities have been due to brain injuries. Due to a peak of brain-related injuries in the 1960s, the National Operating Committee on Standards for Athletic Equipment (NOCSAE) was founded in 1969, and the first safety standards for football helmets were implemented in 1973 [15]. It is important to note that C.W. Gadd's severity index, which forms the basis of the NOCSAE helmet assurance specifications, places a very important weight to translational acceleration (TA). However, recent evidence suggests that rotational acceleration (RA) may be more important in causing SDHs in football players. Thus, it is not surprising that a recent biomechanical study of the helmets used by two high school players who suffered SDHs did not fall short of the outdated NOCSAE guidelines [28]. Although current helmet design has clearly demonstrated the ability to reduce skull fractures, their ability to prevent concussion has not been well proven as of yet. The biomechanics of collision sports are complex, and more advanced methods will be needed to design helmets and other protective gear to optimize injury risk reduction.

Regulated and widespread adoption of protective headgear in these sports has already led to significant reductions in reported rates of skull fractures and serious sports-related brain injuries. Helmets do not prevent all instances of serious injury, and devastating intracranial injuries have been known to occur in young athletes who engage in regular contact sports with standard, non-defective headgear [29]. Nevertheless, helmets have been shown to reduce the *risk* of these serious injuries, and, whenever possible, athletes should be encouraged to consistently and properly use helmets when engaging in both practice and competitive play.

Return to Play

The majority of current return-to-play guidelines are designed for patients with concussions or mild TBI and are not specific for those with skull fractures or structural brain injury [14, 63, 79]. Thus, there are relatively little data to guide how a structural skull or brain lesion should affect an athlete's return-to-play guidelines. This issue is further complicated by the fact that the presence of skull fracture alone does not necessarily place an injury in any particular category in most of the head injury classification schemes as many, though not all, are based on symptoms or GCS score alone [3, 32, 61, 77, 79, 99].

Nevertheless, as has been discussed in this chapter, skull fractures and structural brain injury are typically serious injuries associated with significant morbidity and potentially mortality. Most will be associated with moderate to severe head injury, and, by definition, all of them represent some disruption in the normal anatomy of the brain and skull. After such an injury, extreme caution should be exercised in the timing of any sort of return to play or even if return to play will be possible at all (at any point in time). It is up to the individual clinician to best evaluate the extent of a patient's initial injury and the state of their current recovery following such an injury. Notably, having had a craniotomy is not an absolute contraindication to return to play, and successful return-to-play following craniotomy has been documented at amateur and professional levels for contact sports such as football, boxing, and ice hockey [67, 81]. Graduated return to play in a stepwise fashion is a prudent measure, and it is inadvisable for a patient to return to contact athletics if still symptomatic or if the structural abnormality has not been fully resolved [81].

Conclusions

Skull fractures and structural brain injuries represent an important source of morbidity and mortality in cases of TBI, though sports and athletics account for only a small portion of the annual incidence of these lesions. However, it is clear that young athletes are at risk of suffering these injuries. More work must be aimed at preventing such injuries with rules that protect the player and improved protective equipment. When such injuries unfortunately occur, a thorough but efficient history and physical exam are key to helping elucidate the underlying diagnosis. The management of these injures is frequently operative, and prompt neurosurgical consultation should be sought in cases of compound skull fracture or suspected intracranial hemorrhage.

References

1. Adeloye A, Kattan KR, Silverman FN. Thickness of the normal skull in the American Blacks and Whites. Am J Phys Anthropol. 1975;43:23–30.
2. Andrews PJ, Sleeman DH, Statham PF, McQuatt A, Corruble V, Jones PA, et al. Predicting recovery in patients suffering from traumatic brain injury by using admission variables and physiological data: a comparison between decision tree analysis and logistic regression. J Neurosurg. 2002;97:326–36.
3. Bailes JE, Cantu RC. Head injury in athletes. Neurosurgery. 2001;48:26–45; discussion 45–6.
4. Boden BP, Tacchetti R, Mueller FO. Catastrophic injuries in high school and college baseball players. Am J Sports Med. 2004;32:1189–96.
5. Braakman R. Depressed skull fracture: data, treatment, and follow-up in 225 consecutive cases. J Neurol Neurosurg Psychiatry. 1972;35:395–402.
6. Brain Trauma F, American Association of Neurological S, Congress of Neurological S, Joint Section on N, Critical Care AC, Bratton SL, et al. Guidelines for the management of severe traumatic brain injury. VI. Indications for intracranial pressure monitoring. J Neurotrauma. 2007;24 Suppl 1:S37–44.
7. Bricolo AP, Pasut LM. Extradural hematoma: toward zero mortality. A prospective study. Neurosurgery. 1984;14:8–12.
8. Bruns Jr J, Hauser WA. The epidemiology of traumatic brain injury: a review. Epilepsia. 2003;44 Suppl 10:2–10.

9. Bullock MR, Chesnut R, Ghajar J, Gordon D, Hartl R, Newell DW, et al. Surgical management of depressed cranial fractures. Neurosurgery. 2006;58:S56–60; discussion Si–iv.
10. Bullock MR, Chesnut R, Ghajar J, Gordon D, Hartl R, Newell DW, et al. Surgical management of traumatic parenchymal lesions. Neurosurgery. 2006;58:S25–46; discussion Si–iv.
11. Bullock MR, Chesnut R, Ghajar J, Gordon D, Hartl R, Newell DW, et al. Surgical management of acute epidural hematomas. Neurosurgery. 2006;58:S7–15; discussion Si–iv.
12. Bullock MR, Chesnut R, Ghajar J, Gordon D, Hartl R, Newell DW, et al. Surgical management of acute subdural hematomas. Neurosurgery. 2006;58:S16–24; discussion Si–iv.
13. Bullock R, Smith RM, van Dellen JR. Nonoperative management of extradural hematoma. Neurosurgery. 1985;16:602–6.
14. Cantu RC, Aubry M, Dvorak J, Graf-Baumann T, Johnston K, Kelly J, et al. Overview of concussion consensus statements since 2000. Neurosurg Focus. 2006;21:E3.
15. Cantu RC, Mueller FO. Brain injury-related fatalities in American football, 1945-1999. Neurosurgery. 2003;52:846–52; discussion 852–3.
16. Carter DA, Mehelas TJ, Savolaine ER, Dougherty LS. Basal skull fracture with traumatic polycranial neuropathy and occluded left carotid artery: significance of fractures along the course of the carotid artery. J Trauma. 1998;44:230–5.
17. Chan KH, Mann KS, Yue CP, Fan YW, Cheung M. The significance of skull fracture in acute traumatic intracranial hematomas in adolescents: a prospective study. J Neurosurg. 1990;72:189–94.
18. Chang EF, Meeker M, Holland MC. Acute traumatic intraparenchymal hemorrhage: risk factors for progression in the early post-injury period. Neurosurgery. 2006;58:647–56; discussion 647–56.
19. Clifton GL, Miller ER, Choi SC, Levin HS. Fluid thresholds and outcome from severe brain injury. Crit Care Med. 2002;30:739–45.
20. Cohen JE, Montero A, Israel ZH. Prognosis and clinical relevance of anisocoria-craniotomy latency for epidural hematoma in comatose patients. J Trauma. 1996;41:120–2.
21. Cook RJ, Dorsch NW, Fearnside MR, Chaseling R. Outcome prediction in extradural haematomas. Acta Neurochir (Wien). 1988;95:90–4.
22. Cucciniello B, Martellotta N, Nigro D, Citro E. Conservative management of extradural haematomas. Acta Neurochir (Wien). 1993;120:47–52.
23. Dacey Jr RG, Alves WM, Rimel RW, Winn HR, Jane JA. Neurosurgical complications after apparently minor head injury. Assessment of risk in a series of 610 patients. J Neurosurg. 1986;65:203–10.
24. Datti R, Gentile SL, Pisani R. Acute intracranial epidural haematoma in a basketball player: a case report. Br J Sports Med. 1995;29:95–6.
25. Delye H, Verschueren P, Depreitere B, Verpoest I, Berckmans D, Vander Sloten J, et al. Biomechanics of frontal skull fracture. J Neurotrauma. 2007;24:1576–86.
26. Eisenberg HM, Gary Jr HE, Aldrich EF, Saydjari C, Turner B, Foulkes MA, et al. Initial CT findings in 753 patients with severe head injury. A report from the NIH Traumatic Coma Data Bank. J Neurosurg. 1990;73:688–98.
27. Ersahin Y, Gulmen V, Palali I, Mutluer S. Growing skull fractures (craniocerebral erosion). Neurosurg Rev. 2000;23:139–44.
28. Forbes JA, Zuckerman S, Abla AA, Mocco J, Bode K, Eads T. Biomechanics of subdural hemorrhage in American football: review of the literature in response to rise in incidence. Childs Nerv Syst. 2014;30:197–203.
29. Forbes JA, Zuckerman SL, He L, McCalley E, Lee YM, Solomon GS, et al. Subdural hemorrhage in two high-school football players: post-injury helmet testing. Pediatr Neurosurg. 2013;49:43–9.
30. Friermood TG, Messner DG, Brugman JL, Brennan R. Save the trees: a comparative review of skier-tree collisions. J Orthop Trauma. 1994;8:116–8.
31. Fukuda T, Hasue M, Ito H. Does traumatic subarachnoid hemorrhage caused by diffuse brain injury cause delayed ischemic brain damage? Comparison with subarachnoid hemorrhage caused by ruptured intracranial aneurysms. Neurosurgery. 1998;43:1040–9.

32. Gennarelli TA, Spielman GM, Langfitt TW, Gildenberg PL, Harrington T, Jane JA, et al. Influence of the type of intracranial lesion on outcome from severe head injury. J Neurosurg. 1982;56:26–32.
33. Gupta SK, Reddy NM, Khosla VK, Mathuriya SN, Shama BS, Pathak A, et al. Growing skull fractures: a clinical study of 41 patients. Acta Neurochir (Wien). 1997;139:928–32.
34. Hansman CF. Growth of interorbital distance and skull thickness as observed in roentgenographic measurements. Radiology. 1966;86:87–96.
35. Harders A, Kakarieka A, Braakman R. Traumatic subarachnoid hemorrhage and its treatment with nimodipine. German tSAH Study Group. J Neurosurg. 1996;85:82–9.
36. Harwood-Nash DC, Hendrick EB, Hudson AR. The significance of skull fractures in children. A study of 1,187 patients. Radiology. 1971;101:151–6.
37. Haselsberger K, Pucher R, Auer LM. Prognosis after acute subdural or epidural haemorrhage. Acta Neurochir (Wien). 1988;90:111–6.
38. Hatashita S, Koga N, Hosaka Y, Takagi S. Acute subdural hematoma: severity of injury, surgical intervention, and mortality. Neurol Med Chir (Tokyo). 1993;33:13–8.
39. Haydel MJ, Preston CA, Mills TJ, Luber S, Blaudeau E, DeBlieux PM. Indications for computed tomography in patients with minor head injury. N Engl J Med. 2000;343:100–5.
40. Heary RF, Hunt CD, Krieger AJ, Schulder M, Vaid C. Nonsurgical treatment of compound depressed skull fractures. J Trauma. 1993;35:441–7.
41. Heinzelmann M, Platz A, Imhof HG. Outcome after acute extradural haematoma, influence of additional injuries and neurological complications in the ICU. Injury. 1996;27:345–9.
42. Hofman PA, Nelemans P, Kemerink GJ, Wilmink JT. Value of radiological diagnosis of skull fracture in the management of mild head injury: meta-analysis. J Neurol Neurosurg Psychiatry. 2000;68:416–22.
43. Hukkelhoven CW, Steyerberg EW, Habbema JD, Farace E, Marmarou A, Murray GD, et al. Predicting outcome after traumatic brain injury: development and validation of a prognostic score based on admission characteristics. J Neurotrauma. 2005;22:1025–39.
44. Ingebrigtsen T, Romner B, Kock-Jensen C. Scandinavian guidelines for initial management of minimal, mild, and moderate head injuries. The Scandinavian Neurotrauma Committee. J Trauma. 2000;48:760–6.
45. Jager TE, Weiss HB, Coben JH, Pepe PE. Traumatic brain injuries evaluated in U.S. emergency departments, 1992-1994. Acad Emerg Med. 2000;7:134–40.
46. Jennett B. Epidemiology of head injury. J Neurol Neurosurg Psychiatry. 1996;60:362–9.
47. Jennett B, Miller JD. Infection after depressed fracture of skull. Implications for management of nonmissile injuries. J Neurosurg. 1972;36:333–9.
48. Jennett B, Miller JD, Braakman R. Epilepsy after monmissile depressed skull fracture. J Neurosurg. 1974;41:208–16.
49. Jordan BD, Zimmerman RD. Computed tomography and magnetic resonance imaging comparisons in boxers. JAMA. 1990;263:1670–4.
50. Juul N, Morris GF, Marshall SB, Marshall LF. Intracranial hypertension and cerebral perfusion pressure: influence on neurological deterioration and outcome in severe head injury. The Executive Committee of the International Selfotel Trial. J Neurosurg. 2000;92:1–6.
51. Kakarieka A, Braakman R, Schakel EH. Clinical significance of the finding of subarachnoid blood on CT scan after head injury. Acta Neurochir (Wien). 1994;129:1–5.
52. Kakarieka A, Schakel EH, Fritze J. Clinical experiences with nimodipine in cerebral ischemia. J Neural Transm Suppl. 1994;43:13–21.
53. Kelly KD, Lissel HL, Rowe BH, Vincenten JA, Voaklander DC. Sport and recreation-related head injuries treated in the emergency department. Clin J Sport Med. 2001;11:77–81.
54. Knuckey NW, Gelbard S, Epstein MH. The management of "asymptomatic" epidural hematomas. A prospective study. J Neurosurg. 1989;70:392–6.
55. Koc RK, Akdemir H, Oktem IS, Meral M, Menku A. Acute subdural hematoma: outcome and outcome prediction. Neurosurg Rev. 1997;20:239–44.
56. Kotwica Z, Brzezinski J. Acute subdural haematoma in adults: an analysis of outcome in comatose patients. Acta Neurochir (Wien). 1993;121:95–9.

57. Kraus JF, Anderson BD, Mueller CE. The effectiveness of a special ice hockey helmet to reduce head injuries in college intramural hockey. Med Sci Sports. 1970;2:162–4.
58. Lindsay KW, McLatchie G, Jennett B. Serious head injury in sport. Br Med J. 1980;281:789–91.
59. Macpherson BC, MacPherson P, Jennett B. CT evidence of intracranial contusion and haematoma in relation to the presence, site and type of skull fracture. Clin Radiol. 1990;42:321–6.
60. Maggi G, Aliberti F, Petrone G, Ruggiero C. Extradural hematomas in children. J Neurosurg Sci. 1998;42:95–9.
61. Marshall LF, Marshall SB, Klauber MR, Van Berkum CM, Eisenberg H, Jane JA, et al. The diagnosis of head injury requires a classification based on computed axial tomography. J Neurotrauma. 1992;9 Suppl 1:S287–92.
62. Mattioli C, Beretta L, Gerevini S, Veglia F, Citerio G, Cormio M, et al. Traumatic subarachnoid hemorrhage on the computerized tomography scan obtained at admission: a multicenter assessment of the accuracy of diagnosis and the potential impact on patient outcome. J Neurosurg. 2003;98:37–42.
63. McCrory P, Meeuwisse WH, Aubry M, Cantu B, Dvorak J, Echemendia RJ, et al. Consensus statement on concussion in sport: the 4th international conference on concussion in sport held in Zurich, November 2012. J Am Coll Surg. 2013;216:e55–71.
64. Meaney DFO, Stephen E, Gennarelli TA. Biomechanical basis of traumatic brain injury. In: Winn HR, editor. Youmans neurologic surgery, vol. 4. 6th ed. Philadelphia: Elsevier Saunders; 2011. p. 3277–87.
65. Meehan 3rd WP, Mannix R. A substantial proportion of life-threatening injuries are sport-related. Pediatr Emerg Care. 2013;29:624–7.
66. Miele VJ, Bailes JE, Cantu RC, Rabb CH. Subdural hematomas in boxing: the spectrum of consequences. Neurosurg Focus. 2006;21:E10.
67. Miele VJ, Bailes JE, Martin NA. Participation in contact or collision sports in athletes with epilepsy, genetic risk factors, structural brain lesions, or history of craniotomy. Neurosurg Focus. 2006;21:E9.
68. Mohanty A, Kolluri VR, Subbakrishna DK, Satish S, Mouli BA, Das BS. Prognosis of extradural haematomas in children. Pediatr Neurosurg. 1995;23:57–63.
69. Morris GF, Bullock R, Marshall SB, Marmarou A, Maas A, Marshall LF. Failure of the competitive N-methyl-D-aspartate antagonist Selfotel (CGS 19755) in the treatment of severe head injury: results of two phase III clinical trials. The Selfotel Investigators. J Neurosurg. 1999;91:737–43.
70. Moss PS, Wan A, Whitlock MR. A changing pattern of injuries to horse riders. Emerg Med J. 2002;19:412–4.
71. Muhonen MG, Piper JG, Menezes AH. Pathogenesis and treatment of growing skull fractures. Surg Neurol. 1995;43:367–72; discussion 372–3.
72. Papa L, Stiell IG, Clement CM, Pawlowicz A, Wolfram A, Braga C, et al. Performance of the Canadian CT head rule and the New Orleans criteria for predicting any traumatic intracranial injury on computed tomography in a United States level I trauma center. Acad Emerg Med. 2012;19:2–10.
73. Pillay R, Peter JC. Extradural haematomas in children. S Afr Med J. 1995;85:672–4.
74. Poca MA, Sahuquillo J, Mataro M, Benejam B, Arikan F, Baguena M. Ventricular enlargement after moderate or severe head injury: a frequent and neglected problem. J Neurotrauma. 2005;22:1303–10.
75. Quayle KS, Jaffe DM, Kuppermann N, Kaufman BA, Lee BC, Park TS, et al. Diagnostic testing for acute head injury in children: when are head computed tomography and skull radiographs indicated? Pediatrics. 1997;99:E11.
76. Rahimi SY, Singh H, Yeh DJ, Shaver EG, Flannery AM, Lee MR. Golf-associated head injury in the pediatric population: a common sports injury. J Neurosurg. 2005;102:163–6.
77. Rimel RW, Giordani B, Barth JT, Jane JA. Moderate head injury: completing the clinical spectrum of brain trauma. Neurosurgery. 1982;11:344–51.

78. Rivas JJ, Lobato RD, Sarabia R, Cordobes F, Cabrera A, Gomez P. Extradural hematoma: analysis of factors influencing the courses of 161 patients. Neurosurgery. 1988;23:44–51.
79. Ropper AH, Gorson KC. Clinical practice. Concussion. N Engl J Med. 2007;356:166–72.
80. Rughani AI, Lin CT, Ares WJ, Cushing DA, Horgan MA, Tranmer BI, et al. Helmet use and reduction in skull fractures in skiers and snowboarders admitted to the hospital. J Neurosurg Pediatr. 2011;7:268–71.
81. Saigal R, Batjer HH, Ellenbogen RG, Berger MS. Return to play for neurosurgical patients. World Neurosurg. 2014;82:485–91.
82. Sakas DE, Bullock MR, Teasdale GM. One-year outcome following craniotomy for traumatic hematoma in patients with fixed dilated pupils. J Neurosurg. 1995;82:961–5.
83. Servadei F, Murray GD, Teasdale GM, Dearden M, Iannotti F, Lapierre F, et al. Traumatic subarachnoid hemorrhage: demographic and clinical study of 750 patients from the European brain injury consortium survey of head injuries. Neurosurgery. 2002;50:261–7; discussion 267–9.
84. Smits M, Dippel DW, de Haan GG, Dekker HM, Vos PE, Kool DR, et al. External validation of the Canadian CT head rule and the New Orleans criteria for CT scanning in patients with minor head injury. JAMA. 2005;294:1519–25.
85. Steinbok P, Flodmark O, Martens D, Germann ET. Management of simple depressed skull fractures in children. J Neurosurg. 1987;66:506–10.
86. Stiell IG, Clement CM, Rowe BH, Schull MJ, Brison R, Cass D, et al. Comparison of the Canadian CT head rule and the New Orleans criteria in patients with minor head injury. JAMA. 2005;294:1511–8.
87. Stiell IG, Wells GA, Vandemheen K, Clement C, Lesiuk H, Laupacis A, et al. The Canadian CT head rule for patients with minor head injury. Lancet. 2001;357:1391–6.
88. Tagliaferri F, Compagnone C, Korsic M, Servadei F, Kraus J. A systematic review of brain injury epidemiology in Europe. Acta Neurochir (Wien). 2006;148:255–68; discussion 268.
89. Taneda M, Kataoka K, Akai F, Asai T, Sakata I. Traumatic subarachnoid hemorrhage as a predictable indicator of delayed ischemic symptoms. J Neurosurg. 1996;84:762–8.
90. Tian HL, Xu T, Hu J, Cui YH, Chen H, Zhou LF. Risk factors related to hydrocephalus after traumatic subarachnoid hemorrhage. Surg Neurol. 2008;69:241–6; discussion 246.
91. Ullman JSM, Brent C, Eisenberg HM. Traumatic subarachnoid hemorrhage. In: Bederson JB, editor. Subarachnoid hemorrhage: pathophysiology and management. Park Ridge: American Association of Neurological Surgeons; 1997.
92. van den Heever CM, van der Merwe DJ. Management of depressed skull fractures. Selective conservative management of nonmissile injuries. J Neurosurg. 1989;71:186–90.
93. van Staa TP, Dennison EM, Leufkens HG, Cooper C. Epidemiology of fractures in England and Wales. Bone. 2001;29:517–22.
94. Vergouwen MD, Vermeulen M, Roos YB. Effect of nimodipine on outcome in patients with traumatic subarachnoid haemorrhage: a systematic review. Lancet Neurol. 2006;5:1029–32.
95. Vignes JR, Jeelani NU, Jeelani A, Dautheribes M, Liguoro D. Growing skull fracture after minor closed-head injury. J Pediatr. 2007;151:316–8.
96. Wang A, Cohen AR, Robinson S. The "swing-ding": a golf-related head injury in children. J Neurosurg Pediatr. 2011;7:111–5.
97. Wasserman RC, Buccini RV. Helmet protection from head injuries among recreational bicyclists. Am J Sports Med. 1990;18:96–7.
98. Weber W. Experimental studies of skull fractures in infants. Z Rechtsmed. 1984;92:87–94.
99. Williams DH, Levin HS, Eisenberg HM. Mild head injury classification. Neurosurgery. 1990;27:422–8.
100. Wong CW. Criteria for conservative treatment of supratentorial acute subdural haematomas. Acta Neurochir (Wien). 1995;135:38–43.
101. Wong GK, Yeung JH, Graham CA, Zhu XL, Rainer TH, Poon WS. Neurological outcome in patients with traumatic brain injury and its relationship with computed tomography patterns of traumatic subarachnoid hemorrhage. J Neurosurg. 2011;114:1510–5.

102. Yoganandan N, Pintar FA. Biomechanics of temporo-parietal skull fracture. Clin Biomech (Bristol, Avon). 2004;19:225–39.
103. Yoganandan N, Pintar FA, Sances Jr A, Walsh PR, Ewing CL, Thomas DJ, et al. Biomechanics of skull fracture. J Neurotrauma. 1995;12:659–68.
104. Zegers B, Jira P, Willemsen M, Grotenhuis J. The growing skull fracture, a rare complication of paediatric head injury. Eur J Pediatr. 2003;162:556–7.
105. Zhao X, Rizzo A, Malek B, Fakhry S, Watson J. Basilar skull fracture: a risk factor for transverse/sigmoid venous sinus obstruction. J Neurotrauma. 2008;25:104–11.
106. Zuckerman SL, Kuhn A, Dewan MC, Morone PJ, Forbes JA, Solomon GS, et al. Structural brain injury in sports-related concussion. Neurosurg Focus. 2012;33(E6):1–12.

Chiari Malformations and Other Anomalies

8

Muhammad M. Abd-El-Barr and Mark R. Proctor

Introduction

Athletes are certainly susceptible to sports-specific injuries, but like any other patient, they may also harbor underlying congenital and acquired spinal cord and brain anomalies that may complicate their care and return to play. Chiari malformations, spinal cord cysts and syringes, tethered spinal cord, and spinal cord tumors are some of the pathologies that may be preexisting or detected in an evaluation after a sports-related injury. In this age of increased medical imaging, many of these anomalies are found incidentally in patients who are often asymptomatic. In this chapter, we review the essential background about these anomalies, evaluation techniques, possible treatments, and requirements for the return of these athletes to their sport of choice.

Chiari Malformations

Background

Chiari malformations are abnormalities of the hindbrain originally described by the Austrian pathologist Hans Chiari in the early 1890s. These malformations range from herniation of the cerebellar tonsils through the foramen magnum (Chiari I) to

M.M. Abd-El-Barr, MD, PhD (✉)
Brigham and Women's Hospital/Boston Children's Hospital, Harvard Medical School, Boston, MA, USA
e-mail: amabd-el-barr@partners.org

M.R. Proctor, MD
Vice-Chair of Neurosurgery, Boston Children's Hospital/Harvard Medical School, Boston, MA, USA
e-mail: Mark.Proctor@childrens.harvard.edu

M. O'Brien, W.P. Meehan III (eds.), *Head and Neck Injuries in Young Athletes*, Contemporary Pediatric and Adolescent Sports Medicine,
DOI 10.1007/978-3-319-23549-3_8

complete agenesis of the cerebellum (Chiari IV). It is important to note that these are not a continuum or a grading scale but four separate and unrelated entities described and named somewhat uncreatively by the same person. The most common Chiari malformations are Type 1 and Type 2. Type 1 Chiari malformations consist of downward displacement of the cerebellar tonsils into the upper cervical spinal canal and are the ones that will be commonly encountered in clinical practice. The Chiari Type II (CMII) malformations are exclusively seen in the context of myelomeningocele ("open spinal bifida") and hydrocephalus and are therefore not going to be incidentally discovered in an athlete.

Chiari I malformations are one of more common incidental findings seen in neurosurgical practice, with an incidence of approximately 1–4 % of individuals undergoing magnetic resonance imaging (MRI) [12]. By analyzing over 20,000 MRIs of the brain and cervical spine, Meadows et al. found that 175 (0.8 %) patients had evidence of Chiari I malformation, which they defined as tonsillar herniation greater than or equal to 5 mm below the foramen magnum [1]. Similarly, by analyzing over 14,000 brain and cervical MRIs, Strahle et al. found an incidence of 3.6 % using the same criteria at a tertiary referral center [2].

The mean age of diagnosis and onset of symptoms is 25 ± 15 years, which coincides with the age of participation in sports for most athletes [3, 4]. Some patients may have what is called "tonsillar ectopia," another normal variant in which the cerebellar tonsils are descended <5 mm beyond the foramen magnum, and is essentially never of clinical significance in the athlete. The Chiari malformation is so common that some authors have recently suggested it should be called the Chiari anomaly [5].

Evaluation

Chiari I malformations are thought to be due to a mismatch in size between the brain and skull. Due to a possible congenital mesodermal insufficiency during skull development, a small posterior fossa develops, and due to the compactness of the posterior fossa, the cerebellar tonsils herniate [6, 7]. Patients may be asymptomatic, or present with symptoms due to their tonsillar herniation, an associated syrinx which can be present, or both. The descended cerebellar tonsils can cause compression of the cerebellum, brain stem, and upper cervical spinal cord [2, 8]. This crowding is thought to cause the most common symptom, namely, headaches. These headaches, which are described as "tussive," are exacerbated by transient increases in intracranial pressure such as when the patient coughs, laughs, or has some other transient spike in intracranial pressure related to physical exertion. These headaches are usually located in the occiput at the craniocervical junction, and the patient may describe them as either occipital headaches or neck pain. Other clinical findings from the compression which are less common include cranial nerve findings from brain stem compression, such as snoring, difficulty swallowing, double vision, or sleep apnea [9].

The compression at the level of the foramen magnum, in addition to causing direct pressure effects, can also disrupt normal egress of cerebrospinal fluid (CSF) of the fourth ventricle of the brain into the foramen magnum. When this happens, the Chiari malformation can lead to the development of syringomyelia, or a dilated cystic space within the spinal cord (see "Syringomyelia" section) [2].

When a Chiari I malformation is seen on a spine MRI, one must be careful to exclude mass lesions, hydrocephalus, or other conditions of the brain that may cause downward herniation of the cerebellar tonsils. The normal position of the cerebellar tonsils should not exceed 5 mm below the foramen magnum, based on studies of normal MRIs [10], which is usually taken as a line connecting the basion to the opisthion on a midsagittal image [11] (Fig. 8.1). Care should be taken to look for evidence of platybasia, basilar invagination, and atlanto-occipital assimilation as they may herald cervical instability [12]. There is also evidence that it not just the absolute magnitude of tonsillar descent that is concerning: tonsils that are peg-like or pointed are more concerning than those that are rounded and smooth [11, 13]. A syrinx secondary to Chiari I malformation, which is usually located in the cervical spine as opposed to lower in the spine, can also be seen in patients with Chiari I malformations (50–70 %) (Fig. 8.2). Therefore, in patients with a significant Chiari I malformation, it is prudent for them to undergo imaging of the spinal axis as well [11, 13].

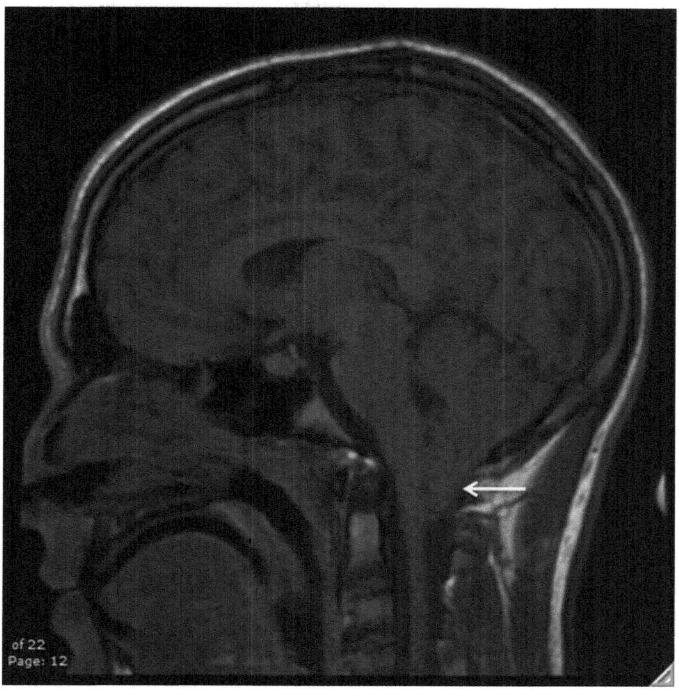

Fig. 8.1 Midsagittal T1-weighted MRI reveals a Chiari malformation with characteristic tonsillar herniation (*white arrow*)

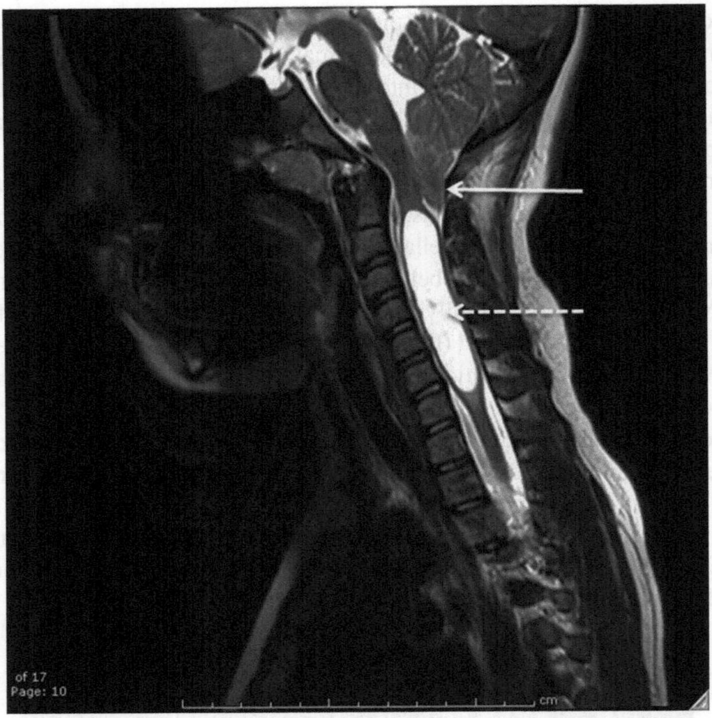

Fig. 8.2 Midsagittal T2-weighted MRI revealing a Chiari malformation (*solid white arrow*) with associated cervical syrinx (*dotted white arrow*)

Flow studies are occasionally employed in patients with CMI. The tight foramen magnum is thought to cause disturbance in CSF flow dynamics, and there is evidence that this can be seen on flow-sensitive phase contrast MRI sequences [14]. There is evidence that this CSF flow disturbance may be causally related to the formation of the syringomyelia [15]. Some authors have used this modality to determine the need for surgery and to measure the success of their surgical treatment [16]. Overall, it is not a critical study and generally does not add more information than the clinical symptomatology.

Treatment

It is important to delineate the etiology of a patient's complaints, as many symptoms can be multifactorial, and the presence of a Chiari malformation does not always imply that it is the cause of the symptoms. In fact, most CMI are asymptomatic. For instance, many patients suffering a concussion undergo imaging of the brain, and an incidental Chiari malformation may be discovered because of its high prevalence in the population. Genuinely symptomatic patients can benefit from surgery, but most neurosurgeons agree that an asymptomatic Chiari malformation does not require surgery [5, 8, 17].

What are the reasons to consider operating on an athlete with asymptomatic Chiari malformation? One concern is that the Chiari malformation can become symptomatic over time, and therefore, the surgery should be performed prophylactically [18, 19]. This is not an adequate reason to perform surgery, as the condition can always be treated if symptoms develop. The more concerning issue is that a patient with a significant Chiari malformation could present with a catastrophic central nervous system (CNS) injury after trauma owing to preexisting spinal cord or brain stem compression from the malformation. There are anecdotal case reports of this phenomenon occurring [20, 21], but no prospective study has ever shown an asymptomatic Chiari presenting with catastrophic neurological injury. Therefore, the true incidence of this event is probably quite low, and several studies that have looked prospectively at patients with Chiari malformation have suggest that the natural history is benign [5, 8, 22]. The surgery to decompress a Chiari does carry some risks, and the very low risk of spinal cord injury in the asymptomatic patient needs to be weighed against the risks and potential complications of surgery. Although the literature has yet to define the exact degree of concern that a sport medicine clinician should have in this situation, most neurosurgeons do not advocate prophylactic surgery for asymptomatic Chiari malformations in competitive athletes. A recent retrospective review of over 100 patients diagnosed with Chiari malformations seen at our institution revealed that none of these patients sustained an injury resulting in death, paralysis, or coma in over 1500 athletic seasons. Similarly, in over 150 collision sports seasons, none of these athletes sustained an injury resulting in death, paralysis, or coma [4].

Return to Play

In general, in a patient with a Chiari malformation that is asymptomatic and has no associated syrinx, it is felt that there is no significant contraindication to return to play. It is our practice to allow these athletes to participate but to also inform the athletes and their families of the potential concerns that the Chiari malformation may become symptomatic or, as anecdotally reported, be implicated in the causation of severe neurologic injury. These decisions are complex enough that a multidisciplinary team consisting of a neurosurgeon and a sports medicine physician should be considered, although the vast majority of athletes will not experience adverse effects from participating in sports with this condition. We do not limit patients who have required surgical decompression but are now neurologically intact from future participation in any sport.

Syringomyelia

Syringomyelia is a condition in which the spinal cord is distended by the accumulation of fluid inside of the cord. The central canal, which runs the length of the spinal cord, is thought to be an extension of fluid-filled ventricular system of the brain. It had previously been thought to be collapsed after birth, but in the current era of increased high-quality MRIs being done on patients, it is being seen more regularly [23]. On the opposite end of the spectrum is the large syringomyelia cavity, which may be associated with conditions such as Chiari malformation, tethered spinal cord, spinal cord tumor, prior spinal cord injury, or prior infection around the spinal cord [2]. In general, it is easy to distinguish the normal dilated central canal from a pathological syrinx, as the former is centrally located and does not distend the spinal cord. Between these two extremes are occasional patients with slightly larger central canal expansion of unclear significance and prognosis that probably benefit from neurosurgical evaluation [14].

Evaluation

Imaging characteristics of the benign dilated central canal should include the absence of any other CNS pathology, a normal caliber of the spinal cord, and if contrast is administered, no enhancement. When this finding is discovered, it is often advisable that the entire spinal axis be imaged, to rule out a Chiari malformation or spinal cord tethering (Fig. 8.3).

A careful history will rule out preexisting conditions, such as Chiari-type symptoms as defined previously, prior meningitis, or prior spinal cord injury. If a syrinx is large enough to compress the crossing fibers in the spinal cord that are transmitting pain and temperature sensation subserved by the lateral spinothalamic pathway, patients may have a cape-like "suspended" sensory loss to pain and temperature or a pain syndrome marked by unusual burning or dysesthetic pain. Back pain, which is a common finding in athletes, is relatively unusual in patients with syringomyelia unless there is concomitant scoliosis. Physical exam findings can include reflex

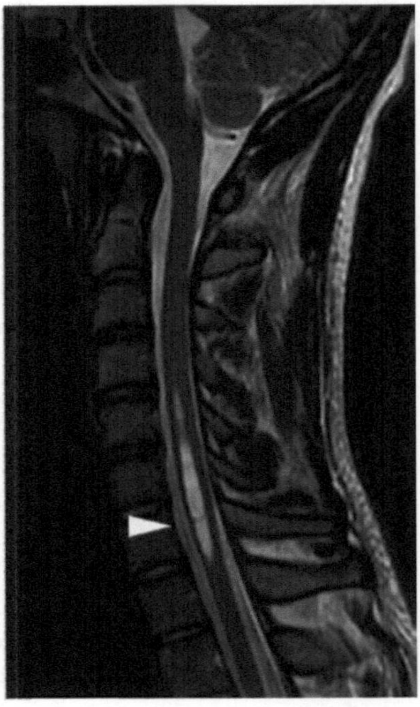

Fig. 8.3 Idiopathic syrinx (*white arrow*) with no associated Chiari malformation or tethered cord (not shown)

changes, including loss of an abdominal reflex, or hyperreflexia in the legs as compared to the reflexes in the arms. There are some case reports of a large syrinx causing more serious problems such as hemiplegia [24].

Treatment

It is not uncommon for a neurosurgeon to see athletes referred for syringomyelia, especially after imaging for back pain. The vast majority of these syrinxes are benign dilatations of the central canal [2, 23] and require no further imaging or treatment. As stated previously, it is important, especially for large syringes, that the extremes of the spinal axis be imaged to rule out a Chiari malformation or a tethered spinal cord. In the absence of concerning findings on the physical exam, or concerning details in the history, no treatment or additional investigation is required for these findings. When a true syringomyelia is present, the treatment must be designed to treat the underlying conditions. For instance, if the syrinx is the result of CSF circulation alterations caused by a significant Chiari malformation, surgical decompression of the Chiari malformation is encouraged. This surgical decompression often leads to regression of the resultant syringomyelia [17, 25]. Direct surgery on a syrinx is often unnecessary and unsuccessful [26, 27].

In general, any syrinx-associated conditions, including tumor, tethered cord, postinfectious or secondary to traumatic spinal cord injury, or Chiari malformation, require referral to a neurosurgeon.

Return to Play

Athletes should not be restricted from play because of a benign dilatation of the central canal. The athlete should be reassured that this is a normal anatomic variant, and as long as there are no associated findings on imaging, no further workup is required [23, 28].

It is important that if there is an underlying condition causing a syringomyelia, this underlying condition be treated. The syrinx usually will regress after dealing with the underlying condition, and the recommendations about return to play will in general coincide with the recommendations associated with this underlying condition.

Spinal Cysts

Spinal cysts are different from syringomyelia in that they are areas of fluid external to the spinal cord, rather than within the spinal cord. They may occur in different areas of the spinal cord, and due to their heterogeneity in presentation and rarity, generalizations about management are difficult. Arachnoid cysts, which are contained beneath the dura, are often found ventrally in the cervical spine and dorsally in the thoracic and lumbar spine [29]. When associated with an expansion of the dural sac along the nerve root, these cysts are called perineural cysts, and if in the lumbosacral spine, these are called Tarlov cysts [30]. Meningoceles are extradural cysts that occur in the caudal end of the dural sac, and patients often present with deep tailbone pain, but also occasionally with bowel and bladder dysfunction.

Evaluation, Treatment, and Return to Play

A comprehensive review of all the different spinal cysts and their management is beyond the scope of this chapter. However, due to their rarity and nuances, a neurosurgical consultation is recommended for patients found to have such lesions. Most patients will not require surgical intervention and will be allowed to return to play. Again, a case-by-case evaluation and multidisciplinary approach is needed when dealing with these lesions.

Tethered Cord

Tethered spinal cord refers to any condition in which the spinal cord is pathologically attached to the bones or soft tissues of the back. Most of these conditions are discovered in infancy or early childhood due to the presence of lumbar or sacral cutaneous stigmata such as a dimple, hairy patch, fatty mass, discoloration of the skin, or other unusual findings such as a skin appendage. Later presentations in childhood or in teenage years are thought to be due to symptoms from tension on the lower spinal cord, including back pain, bowel and bladder control difficulties, limb asymmetry or scoliosis, or neurologic dysfunction [31, 32]. These later presentations might be seen in the athlete and present to the sports medicine physician. In addition, tethering can rarely be seen in the cervical region, often the result of prior pathology such as surgery or neck injury, and therefore not likely to present without prior knowledge. However, congenital tethering of the cervical region can occur (Fig. 8.4).

In the absence of external signs, establishing the diagnosis of tethered spinal cord is difficult in younger children, as it is difficult to detect bowel or bladder dysfunction or for the child to express pain in a definable way. Symptoms usually present during growth spurts, with the first wave of detectable symptoms at 4–6 years on average. Pain in the back or lower extremities, limb asymmetry, and scoliosis are potential reasons that athletes with this condition may present to a sports medicine physician. Of note, it would be extremely rare for upper extremity pain or neurological findings to be the result of tethering in the lumbar area. In general, objective findings on the neurologic examination that are not easily explained, or pain that persists despite routine treatments aimed at core and lower extremity strengthening, should prompt imaging to look for a tethered spinal cord. Importantly, the cutaneous lesions described above are usually more subtle and difficult to detect in older children or teenagers.

Imaging may show thickening and fatty infiltration of the filum terminale, which may or may not occur with a lower-than-normal termination of the spinal cord at the L1–2 level [33]. Some tethering lesions are extremely complex and may include

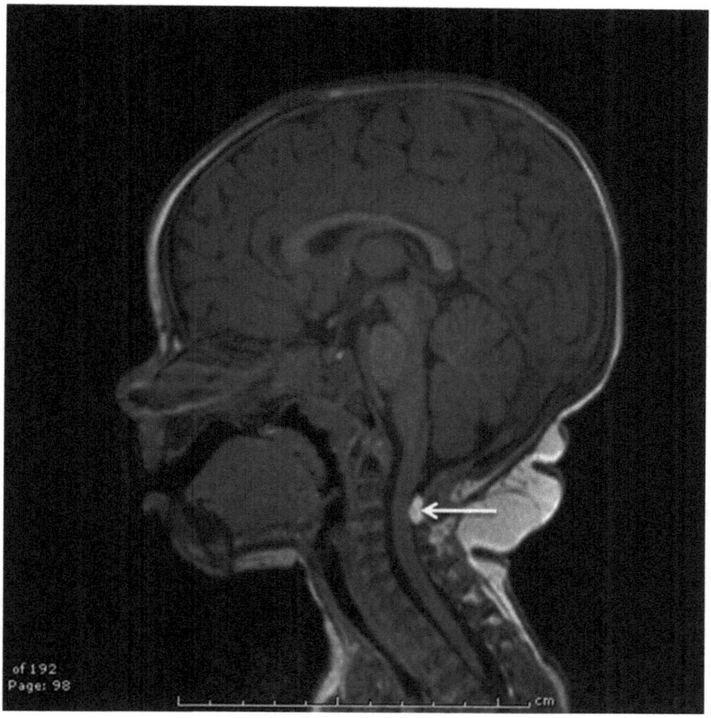

Fig. 8.4 19-month-old female presented with taffy mass on the neck and found to have evidence of cervical tethering due to dorsal cervical lipoma (*white arrow*)

large masses of fat, congenital tumors, and other congenital abnormalities. Because tethering is most likely to affect the base of the spinal cord, the lower sacral nerves are most vulnerable. Urodynamic studies are often considered as an objective test to look for neuropathic bladder changes, especially if urinary incontinence or unexplained symptoms of urinary urgency or frequency exist. We have found these studies to be helpful in making the diagnosis in younger children as well as a measure of how well treatment assessed this problem [34].

Treatment

We generally do not recommend treatment for an asymptomatic skeletally mature patient with spinal tethering. Careful analysis by a neurosurgeon is necessary as surgery may be indicated if the patient has abnormalities on the neurologic exam or on other objective tests such as urodynamic evaluations of the nerve supply to the urogenital system. Surgical treatment may be relatively straightforward such as de-tethering at the point of tethering. Interestingly, in complex patients who have undergone prior de-tetherings, major spinal column surgeries such as vertebral column resection to shorten the spine are now being performed, with long-term outcomes still unclear [35].

Return to Play

Patients that are found to have spinal tethering on imaging should be referred to a neurosurgeon. Asymptomatic patients should not be discouraged from participation in sports. There have been rare cases of patients presenting with rapid neurologic deterioration because of participation in activities that put stretch on the spinal cord or spinal cord nerves. When a tethered spinal cord is detected in asymptomatic athletes, we have recommended periodic clinical follow-up until full axial growth of the patient has occurred. The patients and families should also be counseled regarding the potential for the development of symptoms over time, and the risks and benefits of prophylactic surgery reviewed. After surgery, the course is generally benign and the athlete would have no limitations [33].

Prior Spinal Cord Injury

Spinal injury can generally be classified into one of three categories: (1) spinal column injury alone without any injury to the spinal cord, which is covered in another section of this book; (2) a spinal cord trauma causing permanent neurologic and/or radiographic abnormalities; and (3) transient neurological injury followed by complete recovery, with no evidence clinically or radiographically of spinal cord injury [36]. This latter injury, often called spinal cord concussion, cervical cord neuropraxia, or transient quadriparesis, seems to be a functional injury similar to a concussion and is a relatively frequent occurrence in young athletes [36–38].

Evaluation

MRI is the study of choice to evaluate the spinal cord after injury. This is because MRI is the only test that can look accurately at the soft tissues and can both reveal injury to the spinal cord and detect other lesions such as a herniated disc, while radiographs and computed tomography (CT) scans may be normal. MRI may also undercover functional stenosis, which is a relative spinal cord compression in the setting of normal plain radiographic or CT findings. In these cases, the spinal canal is compressed by soft tissue abnormalities such as disk herniation or ligamentous hypertrophy, or intrinsic spinal pathology such as syrinx or tumor [39], which are not seen by other imaging modalities.

Athletes who have suffered a transient neuropraxia but have normal MRI imaging do not appear to be at any increased risk for catastrophic spinal cord injury [37, 40]. However, if there is an underlying anatomic lesion such as herniated cervical disk or spinal canal stenosis, the athlete's risk of spinal cord injury with subsequent trauma is increased.

Treatment and Return to Play

Any permanent neurologic injury or radiographic findings of structural changes in the spinal cord would likely preclude an athlete in participating in high-impact sports. Once an injury to the cord has occurred, even if there has been functional recovery, the reserve capacity of the spinal cord is unknown. The risk of second injury is increased, and unfortunately, it is impossible to predict which patients would be able to tolerate another injury without significant functional effects.

If the spinal cord and neurologic exam are normal but spinal canal stenosis exists, the abnormality may be amenable to surgical correction. Once the anatomic abnormality has been corrected, the athlete may be able to return to play if the surgery did not involve fusing multiple letters of the spine (generally, loss of one motion segment would be tolerated, but loss of two or more would not be). In certain cases, the athlete can return to some activities, but not other higher risk activities that involve the likelihood of severe flexion or extension movements of the neck and/or back [36]. We believe that most athletes with a transient neurologic deficit with normal imaging and clinical examination can return to play without increased risk of subsequent injury [40].

Spinal Cord Tumors

It is rare for patients with intrinsic tumors of the spinal cord or intradural tumors that compress the spinal cord to present to a sports medicine physician, but it does occur [41]. More commonly, patients with tumors of the bone or soft tissues may present with symptoms of spinal cord compression, topics discussed elsewhere. Patients with intraspinal tumors often present with local or radiating pain and, as expected, frequently have neurologic abnormalities when examined.

Symptoms that should prompt imaging include pain that is worse at night (due to tumor swelling when recumbent as well as nocturnal release of oncological growth factors) [42], radiating pain that is worse with activity, as well as any unexplained abnormalities in the neurologic examination.

Treatment and Return to Play

When a spinal cord tumor is diagnosed, the patient should be referred promptly to a neurosurgeon. Often times, surgery is needed for cytoreduction, decompression of the spinal canal, and biomechanical stability.

Return to play after surgery depends on the extent and success of surgery for the tumor, the length of bony exposure required, the subsequent stability of the spine, and the neurologic status of the patient. As expected, return to play must be individualized by the treating surgeon (Fig. 8.5).

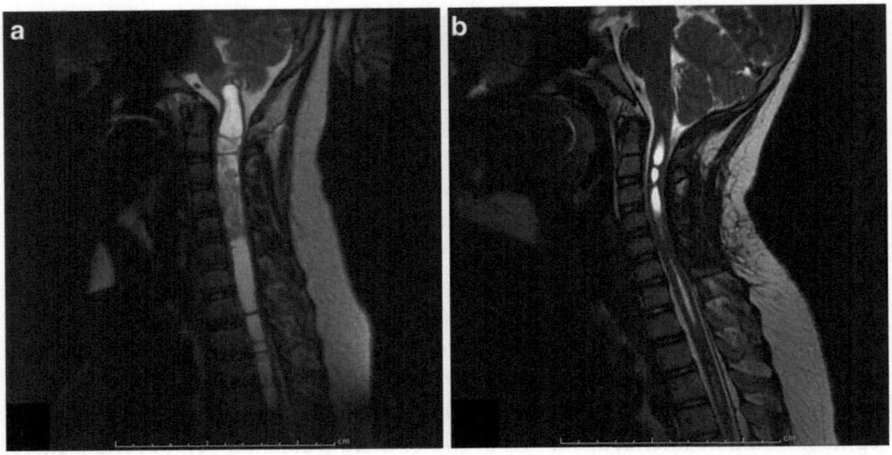

Fig. 8.5 (**a**) Midsagittal MRI of a 14-year-old male who presented with several weeks of neck pain and found to have large intramedullary cervical tumor with associated syrinxes above and below tumor. (**b**) Postoperatively, patient did very well with only some upper limb numbness. Note the near total resolution of the tumor associated syrinxes

Summary

Spinal abnormalities can have an impact on an athlete's ability to participate in sports. One of the challenges in the current era is distinguishing the clinically relevant lesions from those that are incidental, which is substantially more prevalent with the increased use of medical imaging.

A multidisciplinary approach, using the expertise of sports medicine physicians, neurosurgeons, and ancillary staff such as physical therapists, is tantamount for the proper care of the athlete found to have a spinal abnormality.

At this point, the recommendations regarding sports and cervical spine pathology are largely based on consensus and experience. As we gather more data and clinical experience regarding sports participation in patients found to have spinal abnormalities, we hope that these recommendations can be refined further.

References

1. Meadows J, Kraut M, Guarnieri M, Haroun RI, Carson BS. Asymptomatic Chiari Type I malformations identified on magnetic resonance imaging. J Neurosurg. 2000;92(6):920–6.
2. Strahle J, Muraszko KM, Kapurch J, Bapuraj JR, Garton HJ, Maher CO. Chiari malformation Type I and syrinx in children undergoing magnetic resonance imaging. J Neurosurg Pediatr. 2011;8(2):205–13.
3. Miele VJ, Bailes JE, Martin NA. Participation in contact or collision sports in athletes with epilepsy, genetic risk factors, structural brain lesions, or history of craniotomy. Neurosurg Focus. 2006;21(4):E9.
4. Meehan 3rd WP, Jordaan M, Prabhu SP, Carew L, Mannix RC, Proctor MR. Risk of athletes with chiari malformations suffering catastrophic injuries during sports participation is low. Clin J Sport Med. 2015;25(2):133–7.

5. Novegno F, Caldarelli M, Massa A, et al. The natural history of the Chiari Type I anomaly. J Neurosurg Pediatr. 2008;2(3):179–87.
6. Marin-Padilla M. Cephalic axial skeletal-neural dysraphic disorders: embryology and pathology. Can J Neurol Sci. 1991;18(2):153–69.
7. Marin-Padilla M, Marin-Padilla TM. Morphogenesis of experimentally induced Arnold—Chiari malformation. J Neurol Sci. 1981;50(1):29–55.
8. Strahle J, Muraszko KM, Kapurch J, Bapuraj JR, Garton HJ, Maher CO. Natural history of Chiari malformation Type I following decision for conservative treatment. J Neurosurg Pediatr. 2011;8(2):214–21.
9. Khatwa U, Ramgopal S, Mylavarapu A, et al. MRI findings and sleep apnea in children with Chiari I malformation. Pediatr Neurol. 2013;48(4):299–307.
10. Aboulezz AO, Sartor K, Geyer CA, Gado MH. Position of cerebellar tonsils in the normal population and in patients with Chiari malformation: a quantitative approach with MR imaging. J Comput Assist Tomogr. 1985;9(6):1033–6.
11. Chiapparini L, Saletti V, Solero CL, Bruzzone MG, Valentini LG. Neuroradiological diagnosis of Chiari malformations. Neurol Sci. 2011;32 Suppl 3:S283–6.
12. Elster AD, Chen MY. Chiari I malformations: clinical and radiologic reappraisal. Radiology. 1992;183(2):347–53.
13. Tubbs RS, Pugh JA, Oakes WJ. Chiari malformations. In: Winn HR, editor. Youmans neurological surgery. 6th ed. New York: Elsevier; 2011. p. 1918–27.
14. Hofmann E, Warmuth-Metz M, Bendszus M, Solymosi L. Phase-contrast MR imaging of the cervical CSF and spinal cord: volumetric motion analysis in patients with Chiari I malformation. Am J Neuroradiol. 2000;21(1):151–8.
15. Oldfield EH, Muraszko K, Shawker TH, Patronas NJ. Pathophysiology of syringomyelia associated with Chiari I malformation of the cerebellar tonsils. Implications for diagnosis and treatment. J Neurosurg. 1994;80(1):3–15.
16. Armonda RA, Citrin CM, Foley KT, Ellenbogen RG. Quantitative cine-mode magnetic resonance imaging of Chiari I malformations: an analysis of cerebrospinal fluid dynamics. Neurosurgery. 1994;35(2):214–23; discussion 223–4.
17. Rocque BG, George TM, Kestle J, Iskandar BJ. Treatment practices for Chiari malformation type I with syringomyelia: results of a survey of the American Society of Pediatric Neurosurgeons. J Neurosurg Pediatr. 2011;8(5):430–7.
18. Wan MJ, Nomura H, Tator CH. Conversion to symptomatic Chiari I malformation after minor head or neck trauma. Neurosurgery. 2008;63(4):748–53; discussion 753.
19. Yarbrough CK, Powers AK, Park TS, Leonard JR, Limbrick DD, Smyth MD. Patients with Chiari malformation Type I presenting with acute neurological deficits: case series. J Neurosurg Pediatr. 2011;7(3):244–7.
20. Callaway GH, O'Brien SJ, Tehrany AM. Chiari I malformation and spinal cord injury: cause for concern in contact athletes? Med Sci Sports Exerc. 1996;28(10):1218–20.
21. Makela JP. Arnold-Chiari malformation type I in military conscripts: symptoms and effects on service fitness. Mil Med. 2006;171(2):174–6.
22. Benglis Jr D, Covington D, Bhatia R, et al. Outcomes in pediatric patients with Chiari malformation Type I followed up without surgery. J Neurosurg Pediatr. 2011;7(4):375–9.
23. Magge SN, Smyth MD, Governale LS, et al. Idiopathic syrinx in the pediatric population: a combined center experience. J Neurosurg Pediatr. 2011;7(1):30–6.
24. Frogameni AD, Widoff BE, Jackson DW. Syringomyelia causing acute hemiparesis in a college football player. Orthopedics. 1994;17(6):552–3.
25. Schijman E, Steinbok P. International survey on the management of Chiari I malformation and syringomyelia. Childs Nerv Syst. 2004;20(5):341–8.
26. Batzdorf U, Klekamp J, Johnson JP. A critical appraisal of syrinx cavity shunting procedures. J Neurosurg. 1998;89(3):382–8.
27. Roy AK, Slimack NP, Ganju A. Idiopathic syringomyelia: retrospective case series, comprehensive review, and update on management. Neurosurg Focus. 2011;31(6):E15.
28. Singhal A, Bowen-Roberts T, Steinbok P, Cochrane D, Byrne AT, Kerr JM. Natural history of untreated syringomyelia in pediatric patients. Neurosurg Focus. 2011;31(6):E13.

29. Evangelou P, Meixensberger J, Bernhard M, et al. Operative management of idiopathic spinal intradural arachnoid cysts in children: a systematic review. Childs Nerv Syst. 2013;29(4):657–64.
30. Lucantoni C, Than KD, Wang AC, et al. Tarlov cysts: a controversial lesion of the sacral spine. Neurosurg Focus. 2011;31(6):E14.
31. Hertzler 2nd DA, DePowell JJ, Stevenson CB, Mangano FT. Tethered cord syndrome: a review of the literature from embryology to adult presentation. Neurosurg Focus. 2010;29(1):E1.
32. Filippidis AS, Kalani MY, Theodore N, Rekate HL. Spinal cord traction, vascular compromise, hypoxia, and metabolic derangements in the pathophysiology of tethered cord syndrome. Neurosurg Focus. 2010;29(1):E9.
33. Kim AH, Kasliwal MK, McNeish B, Silvera VM, Proctor MR, Smith ER. Features of the lumbar spine on magnetic resonance images following sectioning of filum terminale. J Neurosurg Pediatr. 2011;8(4):384–9.
34. Maher CO, Bauer SB, Goumnerova L, Proctor MR, Madsen JR, Scott RM. Urological outcome following multiple repeat spinal cord untethering operations. Clinical article. J Neurosurg Pediatr. 2009;4(3):275–9.
35. Hsieh PC, Stapleton CJ, Moldavskiy P, et al. Posterior vertebral column subtraction osteotomy for the treatment of tethered cord syndrome: review of the literature and clinical outcomes of all cases reported to date. Neurosurg Focus. 2010;29(1):E6.
36. Bailes JE, Petschauer M, Guskiewicz KM, Marano G. Management of cervical spine injuries in athletes. J Athl Train. 2007;42(1):126–34.
37. Bailes JE. Experience with cervical stenosis and temporary paralysis in athletes. J Neurosurg Spine. 2005;2(1):11–6.
38. Vaccaro AR, Klein GR, Ciccoti M, et al. Return to play criteria for the athlete with cervical spine injuries resulting in stinger and transient quadriplegia/paresis. Spine J. 2002;2(5):351–6.
39. Proctor MR, Cantu RC. Head and neck injuries in young athletes. Clin Sports Med. 2000;19(4):693–715.
40. Dailey A, Harrop JS, France JC. High-energy contact sports and cervical spine neuropraxia injuries: what are the criteria for return to participation? Spine. 2010;35(21 Suppl):S193–201.
41. O'Brien M, Curtis C, D'Hemecourt P, Proctor M. Case report: a case of persistent back pain and constipation in a 5-year-old boy. Phys Sportsmed. 2009;37(1):133–7.
42. Hermann DM, Barth A, Porchet F, Hess CW, Mumenthaler M, Bassetti CL. Nocturnal positional lumboischialgia: presenting symptom of lumbar spinal tumours. J Neurol. 2008;255(11):1836–7.

Muscular and Ligamentous Cervical Spine Injuries

9

Kate Dorney and Rebekah Mannix

Anatomy of the Cervical Spine

The bony cervical spine and spinal cord are stabilized and further supported by groups of ligaments and muscles. The cervical spine ligaments include the anterior longitudinal and posterior longitudinal ligaments, the nuchal ligament complex, the capsular ligaments, and the ligamentum flavum. The anterior and posterior longitudinal ligaments stabilize the vertebral bodies. The nuchal ligament complex (supraspinous, interspinous, and infraspinous ligaments), capsular ligaments, and the ligamentum flavum stabilize the posterior column. Disruption of these ligaments can result in cervical spine instability.

The musculature of the cervical spine is further broken down into anterior and posterior neck muscles. The anterior neck muscles include the platysma, sternocleidomastoid, anterior vertebral muscles, and lateral vertebral muscles. The posterior neck muscles include the trapezius, splenius capitis, semispinalis capitis, and levator scapulae.

The anterior neck muscles serve an important role in head and neck movement, particularly in flexion and lateral bending and rotation. The platysma, which is the most superficial muscle in the anterior neck, is a broad thin muscle that overlies the other muscles and neck structures. The sternocleidomastoid arises from the sternum and the medial third of the clavicle and passes obliquely across the side of the neck to insert into the mastoid process. It flexes, laterally bends, and rotates the neck. The anterior vertebral muscles, which include the longus colli, longus capitis, rectus capitis anterior, and rectus capitis lateralis, attach to the vertebrae and occipital region of the skull and assist in neck flexion, rotation, and lateral bending. The

K. Dorney, MD (✉) • R. Mannix, MD, MPH
Division of Emergency Medicine, Boston Children's Hospital,
300 Longwood Ave, Boston, MA 02115, USA
e-mail: kate.dorney@childrens.harvard.edu; rebekah.mannix@childrens.harvard.edu

M. O'Brien, W.P. Meehan III (eds.), *Head and Neck Injuries in Young Athletes*,
Contemporary Pediatric and Adolescent Sports Medicine,
DOI 10.1007/978-3-319-23549-3_9

lateral vertebral muscles (also known as the scalene muscles) attach from the cervical vertebrae to the first or second ribs and act as weak movers of the neck as well as accessory muscles of respiration.

As a group, the posterior neck muscles maintain posture and act as neck stabilizers and extensors. In general, the posterior muscle group is stronger than the anterior cervical muscle group. The trapezius is a flat, triangular muscle that covers the posterior portion of the neck, shoulders, and thorax. It originates in the occiput, nuchal ligament, spinous processes of C7-T12, and supraspinal ligaments and inserts into the lateral clavicle, acromion, and scapular spine. It maintains cervical posture and is an important mover and stabilizer of the scapula. The splenius capitis and semispinalis capitis arise from the lower cervical and upper thoracic vertebrae and insert at the skull base. The levator scapulae originates in the first four cervical vertebral bodies and inserts into the superomedial corner of the scapula.

Epidemiology

While the precise incidence of cervical strains and sprains is unknown, 14.9 % of sport-related injuries occur to the head and neck, the vast majority as strains and sprains [1].

Evaluation

Although the overall incidence of significant cervical spine injuries in sports is low, the potential devastating consequences if such an injury is missed mandate strict vigilance by all primary responders at an athletic event. As such, the first priority when evaluating an athlete with a potential neck injury is to assess for an unstable bony or ligamentous injury. As it can be difficult at the time of injury on the athletic field to determine the extent of cervical injury or to differentiate between a fully recoverable injury, such as cervical cord neuropraxia, and a permanent case of quadriplegia, the athlete with the concerning findings must be immobilized at the head and neck and transported to a medical facility for further evaluation [2]. For further information on the acute response to head and neck injuries, please see accompanying chapter, “Sideline Response and Transport.”

Once it has been established that no unstable injuries exist, the evaluation of cervical muscle strains and stable ligamentous sprains can proceed. Key factors to examine include vital signs, inspection of neck/shoulders and back, palpation of spine, active and passive range of motion, strength testing, and a thorough neurological examination.

Inspection of the neck should be performed from all views (anterior, posterior, and lateral). The examiner should evaluate for any external signs of trauma, such as abrasions, lacerations, contusions, or erythema that may indicate the location of underlying injury. In addition, the inspection should assess for any rotational deformity or, if the condition is chronic, muscle atrophy. Palpation for bony tenderness or palpable deformities can indicate bony or ligamentous injury. Palpable muscle spasm can provide information about which muscles and underlying structures may be involved. If there is no concern for unstable spinal injury, active range of motion should be assessed before passive, in order to reduce the potential for further injury on passive testing. First, assess active range of motion for cervical flexion, extension, lateral bending, and lateral rotation. This is most simply accomplished by asking the athlete to touch chin to chest and then look upwards. The patient is then asked to touch the ear to the ipsilateral shoulder while keeping the shoulder relaxed. Normal range of lateral bending is approximately 45° [3]. Lateral rotation can be assessed by asking the athlete to twist the chin toward the right and left. The normal range of lateral rotation is 60–80° [3]. Next, test the neck muscles for strength in flexion, extension, lateral bending, and rotation. A detailed neurologic exam is important as it may elicit neurologic deficits, which can be subtle and might suggest a soft tissue injury such as ligamentous sprain or intervertebral disc herniation.

For athletes with concerning injuries that are transported to the hospital for further evaluation, the history and physical are key elements to help dictate need for further testing or imaging. Details from the history can provide insight into possible diagnoses. Important elements to cover include the chief complaint, nature of the pain, and full characterization of neck pain including location, radiation, onset, nature, temporal pattern, aggravating or relieving factors, and any associated symptoms. Information about the mechanism of injury can provide clues to typical associated patterns of injury. Flexion injuries tend to compress anterior elements while disrupting posterior elements; associated injuries include anterior wedge vertebral body fractures, chip fractures, anterior dislocations, rupture of the posterior ligaments or ligamentum flavum. Extension injuries tend to compress the posterior elements and disrupt the anterior elements with associated injuries including bony injury to spinous processes, facets, and neural arch or rupture of the anterior longitudinal ligament and anterior disc. Compression injuries are more likely to occur when the neck is in slight flexion rather than neutral position [4].

While obtaining the past medical history, it is especially important to ascertain information on previous injuries or on any predisposing medical conditions. More common examples of predisposing conditions include Trisomy 21, Klippel-Feil syndrome, achondroplasia, Morquio syndrome, Marfan syndrome, Larsen syndrome, or any history of cervical spine surgery or arthritis as this may increase the frequency of significant injury to the cervical spine. A comprehensive review of systems is important to include in the history and can provide further clues to the nature and severity of possible cervical spine injury as well as other possible injuries.

Determining return to play is a difficult challenge and tends to be determined on an individual basis after the extent of the injury is assessed [5]. Proposed minimum criteria include no neck tenderness or spasm; no neck or arm pain; no numbness, weakness, or paresthesias at rest or on axial compression; and full range of motion without pain [6].

Imaging Considerations

In case of tenderness or other symptoms potentially suggestive of cervical spine injury such as neurologic deficit on exam or persistent paresthesias, typical evaluation includes three view cervical spine radiography series including cross-table lateral (in collar) followed by AP and open-mouth odontoid views. Studies have shown that the cross-table lateral view on its own is not enough to rule out significant injury as 20 % of unstable cervical spine injuries are missed when this is used in isolation [2]. That being said, while the standard of care in the adult population is to obtain a CT of the cervical spine if there is concern for injury, in a large, retrospective cohort of children with blunt trauma-related bony or ligamentous cervical spine injury, cervical spine X-ray had a sensitivity of 90 % in detecting the abnormality [7]. For the vast majority of pediatric athletes presenting with neck trauma, the standard three view cervical spine X-ray may be adequate.

However, if there are abnormalities on the neurological examination concerning for spinal cord injury, a lateral cervical spine radiograph is obtained while the patient remains immobilized in the cervical collar. Generally, additional XR views are not obtained if there is an abnormality found on the lateral view XR and the patient instead has a CT scan or MRI to further define the extent of the injuries, specifically to determine the presence of spinal cord compression by bone, disc, or hematoma [2]. CT is often the optimum imaging modality if there is high suspicion for significant acute injury after the initial evaluation. In general, MRI is best to delineate ligamentous integrity in patients with neurologic symptoms or prolonged duration of symptoms.

Flexion/extension X-rays can be used in alert, cooperative patients, particularly in the subacute and chronic setting, to assess for ligamentous injury. Flexion and extension should be actively performed by the cooperative patient in a methodical, slow fashion and only to the point of pain or neurologic symptoms so as to avoid inadvertent injury. Findings on flexion/extension films concerning for ligamentous injury include motion of the vertebral body relative to its position on the plain lateral view (>3.5 mm horizontal displacement between adjacent disks), anterior intervertebral disc-space narrowing, anterior angulation and displacement of the vertebral body, and/or fanning of the spinous processes [8].

Unique Considerations to the Pediatric Athlete

There are several anatomic and radiographic characteristics of the pediatric cervical spine that can make evaluating for the possibility of cervical spine injuries more difficult in the pediatric athlete. The nature of the development of the spinal cord also tends to predispose younger children toward different types and locations of injury than their adolescent or adult counterparts.

In terms of spinal column development, the vertebral bodies of children are composed of bone and cartilaginous growth centers that are smaller and more elastic than those of adults. The vertebral bodies typically achieve adult-like proportions by approximately 10 years of age [9]. Children also have more horizontally oriented cervical facets, increased capsular and spinal ligament laxity, and less developed paracervical musculature, all which result in relative hypermobility of the cervical spine [9]. Because of all of these features, the fulcrum of the cervical spine tends to descend as the spine matures—school-aged kids younger than 8 years of age tend to have a fulcrum between cervical vertebrae 1 through 3, while older children between the ages of 8 and 12 have a fulcrum between cervical vertebrae 3 and 5. Children older than 12 years of age have a fulcrum between cervical vertebrae 5 and 6 which is similar to that found in adults [5].

In the pediatric athlete, a phenomenon called pseudosubluxation exists whereby there is some asymmetry of the posterior cervical line between C1 and C3 but no ligamentous injury or instability. It is a normal developmental variant that resolves with time and with maturation of the spinal column. True subluxation can be differentiated from pseudosubluxation by evaluating the posterior cervical line (also known as the Swischuk line) between the anterior aspects of the C1 and C3 spinous processes. True subluxation should be suspected if the posterior cervical line misses the anterior aspect of the C2 spinous processes by 2 mm or more [10].

Ligamentous Injuries

After an acute trauma, the pediatric athlete is at risk for ligamentous injury to the cervical spine. Ligamentous injuries can be difficult to detect as they are not always obvious on initial radiographic views of the cervical spine; thus, a high clinical suspicion must be maintained. Ligamentous injuries to the cervical spine include cervical vertebral subluxation, acute atlantoaxial instability, atlantoaxial rotary subluxation, and spinal cord injury without radiographic abnormality.

Cervical Vertebral Subluxation

Cervical vertebral subluxation typically results from an injury during which axial compression is combined with cervical flexion. This mechanism results in injury to the posterior supporting ligaments that causes anterior translation of the superior vertebral body. A common example of axial compression combined with cervical flexion occurs when a football player spears another player with their helmet.

Patients with cervical vertebral subluxation often complain of neck pain and stiffness. This injury is not usually associated with neurologic deficits. As mentioned above, this injury can occur despite unremarkable standard cervical spine radiographs; however, the patient will typically complain of persistent neck pain. MRI of the cervical spine best delineates the integrity of the ligamentous structures and thus is the typical way this diagnosis is made, although MRI is not as sensitive for cervical ligamentous injuries as it is for ligamentous injuries elsewhere. Therefore, consideration of flexion/extension X-rays should occur if injury remains suspected despite normal cervical spine radiographs and there is limited MR availability.

Patients with cervical vertebral subluxation are generally treated with stabilization in collar followed by posterior cervical fusion as soon as feasible to prevent chronic instability and risk of future injury.

Acute Atlantoaxial Instability

Acute atlantoaxial instability typically results from trauma that forces the neck into extreme flexion causing disruption (or rupture) of the transverse ligament of the odontoid process. Disruption or rupture of the transverse ligament allows the odontoid process to move posteriorly and compress the spinal cord.

There is a broad range of symptoms that patients can present with depending on degree of mobility of the odontoid process and how much the spinal cord is compressed. Symptoms can range from neck pain to weakness to full paralysis. Diagnosis is made on lateral radiographs of the cervical spine when the space between the posterior aspect of the anterior arch of the atlas and the anterior aspect of the odontoid process is greater than 5 mm in children or greater than 3 mm in adults [11].

Acute atlantoaxial instability is an unstable injury that requires definitive treatment (typically posterior fusion) followed by immobilization.

Atlantoaxial Rotary Subluxation

Atlantoaxial rotary subluxation (also known as Grisel syndrome) is a common form of torticollis seen in children that typically occurs following minor trauma, head and neck surgery, or an upper respiratory tract infection [8].

Patients with atlantoaxial rotary subluxation typically present with painful torticollis with head turned to one side and the neck laterally flexed in the opposite direction. Occipital neuralgia and occasionally symptoms of vertebrobasilar artery insufficiency can also be present [12]. There is a four-tier classification system associated with progressive widening of the atlanto-dens interval [10]:

- I: Intact transverse ligament
- II: Disruption of transverse ligament
- III: Disruption of transverse ligament and alar ligament
- IV: Posterior rotatory displacement of the atlas on C2

Diagnosis of atlantoaxial rotary subluxation can be inferred on XR but is confirmed via cervical spine CT. After a traumatic injury, if atlantoaxial rotary subluxation is suspected, flexion and extension films should not be performed, although they are often quite helpful in the diagnosis in the absence of trauma. On a standard lateral view X-ray, an atlanto-dens interval (ADI) up to 4.5 mm in flexion may be normal in children, while an ADI of >3 mm can suggest injury in older athletes [13]. If flexion/extension films cannot be performed and standard view cervical spine radiography is not diagnostic, CT is helpful. On CT, C1 is not oriented in line with the head. Treatment in the pediatric population is via traction if there are no associated neurologic symptoms. Given the risk of recurrence of deformity, close follow-up is required, often with flexion/extension radiographs after the traction is removed. Fusion is indicated in patients with neurologic involvement, if the deformity is refractory to above treatment or if it recurs despite immobilization [12].

Spinal Cord Injury Without Radiographic Abnormality

Spinal cord injury without radiographic abnormality (SCIWORA) is a spinal cord injury without abnormality depicted on conventional radiography or CT scan. SCIWORA is thought to be related to a transient ligamentous deformation of the cervical spinal column due to the relative hypermobility of the pediatric cervical spine [5, 10]. It is seen most frequently in the pediatric population and is estimated to account for up to two thirds of severe cervical injuries in patient under 8 years of age [12]. Diagnosis is made via MRI in patients with normal radiography but persistent (albeit transient) neurologic deficit. Treatment is spine immobilization for 1–3 weeks [12]. The prognosis in terms of neurologic outcome for patients with SCIWORA is determined primarily by their admission neurologic status, i.e., patients with complete deficits tend to have difficult recovery; however, patients with mild deficits tend to recover well [14].

Special Consideration in Patients with Trisomy 21

A large proportion of patients with Trisomy 21 now participate in the Special Olympics. A unique consideration in this patient population is that up to 40 % of children with Trisomy 21 may have underlying hypermobility of the cervical spine. This hypermobility predisposes them to ligamentous injury despite relatively minor trauma. The most common injury is subluxation at the atlantoaxial joint (C1-2) followed by atlanto-occipital subluxation. Because of this, cervical spine stability assessment is recommended in all patients with Trisomy 21 who participate in athletic activities. This assessment is especially important in those activities involving trauma to the head and neck such as soccer. Rigid guidelines to outline which children require treatment and who should be excluded from participation do not yet exist [2].

Muscular Injuries

After an acute trauma, the pediatric athlete is at risk for muscular injury to the cervical spine in addition to ligamentous injury. Muscular injury to the cervical spine is often a diagnosis of exclusion after imaging modalities have confirmed no evidence of bony or ligamentous injury. Muscular injuries to the cervical spine include cervical strain or sprain and whiplash.

Cervical Strain/Sprain

The most common form of cervical injury is injury to the soft tissues of the cervical spine and paracervical muscles. Isolated strains and sprains do not involve injury to the nerves or bones and are most often caused by motor vehicle accidents, falls, or injuries sustained in contact-collision sports and recreational activities. Forced flexion of the head and neck is the most common etiology of cervical ligamentous sprains [9]. Athletes involved in wrestling, football, and rugby are most susceptible [9].

Upon presentation, athletes often complain of cervical pain without radiation or neurologic symptoms. Typically, there is limitation in cervical range of motion and muscle spasm or tenderness with normal neurologic exam.

Because of the potential for dangerous injury to the cervical spine after trauma, all potential neck injuries must be carefully evaluated. These patients should be immobilized pending complete examination and imaging studies if indicated. Patients with isolated cervical strain or sprain have normal radiographic imaging of cervical spine on standard X-ray views.

Treatment is individualized based upon severity, but options include NSAIDs or acetaminophen, immobilization in cervical collar (rigid collar generally if persistent midline cervical spine tenderness or soft collar if only paraspinal tenderness), and heat. Initially, physical activity is restricted. Eventually, once pain and range of motion are improved, referral to a physical therapist is recommended. Physical therapy programs for cervical rehabilitation focus on restoring cervical range of motion and paracervical muscle strength [9]. Typically, athletes are counseled to avoid returning to play until they are asymptomatic with normal cervical range of motion and strength.

Whiplash

Whiplash occurs after an acceleration-deceleration injury to the cervical spine that can be seen in motor vehicle accidents or athletic endeavors (especially football, hockey, or rugby). The mechanism is thought to be strong compressive and translational forces on the joints and soft tissues, which results in an abnormal S-shaped movement pattern of the lower cervical spine.

Athletes typically present with head, neck, and/or upper thoracic pain and decreased range of motion that typically occurs at the time of injury but often continues to worsen over the subsequent 48 h. On exam, whiplash is often associated with cervical muscle spasm but not with neurologic signs and symptoms.

Because of the potential for dangerous injury to the cervical spine, patients with tenderness on exam require imaging of the cervical spine to evaluate for significant injury. Patients are typically imaged via the standard cervical spine X-ray series, which is typically negative aside from only preexisting degenerative changes or decreased cervical spine lordosis secondary to spasm. Generally, these patients do not need MRI or CT unless they present with a neurologic deficit or there is suspected damage to the spinal cord.

Treatment of whiplash includes a multifaceted approach including analgesia (NSAIDs, acetaminophen), heat, and physical therapy.

References

1. Yard EE, Collins CL, Comstock RD. A comparison of high school sports injury surveillance data reporting by certified athletic trainers and coaches. J Athl Train. 2009;44(6):645–52.
2. Proctor MR, Cantu RC. Head and neck injuries in young athletes. Clin Sports Med. 2000;19(4):693–715.
3. Mo T. The neck and upper limb. Stamford: Appleton and Lange; 1997.
4. Banerjee R, Palumbo MA, Fadale PD. Catastrophic cervical spine injuries in the collision sport athlete, Part 1: epidemiology, functional anatomy, and diagnosis. Am J Sports Med. 2004;32(4):1077–87.
5. Jagannathan J, Dumont AS, Prevedello DM, Shaffrey CI, Jane Jr JA. Cervical spine injuries in pediatric athletes: mechanisms and management. Neurosurg Focus. 2006;21(4):E6.
6. Cantu RC. Head and spine injuries in youth sports. Clin Sports Med. 1995;14(3):517–32.
7. Nigrovic LE, Rogers AJ, Adelgais KM, Olsen CS, Leonard JR, Jaffe DM, et al. Utility of plain radiographs in detecting traumatic injuries of the cervical spine in children. Pediatr Emerg Care. 2012;28(5):426–32.
8. DeLee JC, Drez D, editors. DeLee and Drez's orthopaedic sports medicine: principles and practice. 3rd ed. St. Louis: WB Saunders; 2009.
9. Herman MJ. Cervical spine injuries in the pediatric and adolescent athlete. Instr Course Lect. 2006;55:641–6.
10. Mortazavi M, Gore PA, Chang S, Tubbs RS, Theodore N. Pediatric cervical spine injuries: a comprehensive review. Childs Nerv Syst. 2011;27(5):705–17.
11. Ralston ME, Chung K, Barnes PD, Emans JB, Schutzman SA. Role of flexion-extension radiographs in blunt pediatric cervical spine injury. Acad Emerg Med. 2001;8(3):237–45.
12. Wheeless C. Atlantoaxial subluxation. Durham: Duke University; 2011.
13. Pizzutillo PD. Spinal considerations in the young athlete. Instr Course Lect. 1993;42:463–72.
14. Pang D, Pollack IF. Spinal cord injury without radiographic abnormality in children—the SCIWORA syndrome. J Trauma. 1989;29(5):654–64.

Burners, Stingers, and Cervical Cord Neurapraxia/Transient Quadriparesis

10

Preetha A. Kurian, Deborah I. Light, and Hamish A. Kerr

Introduction

Transient neurological injuries of the cervical spine present as sensory and motor deficits that are temporally limited, typically resolving within minutes but occasionally lasting up to weeks. Complete recovery from these injuries occurs by definition, but it is not always immediately apparent whether a young athlete has sustained a transient or a more severe neurological injury. The medical provider must therefore be well versed in the assessment and management of cervical neurological injuries and in distinguishing transient from more severe or catastrophic injury. It is likewise important to recognize and distinguish between the various transient injury types in athletes. They differ in management, in return to play decisions, and in the need for further assessment of the potential future risk of more serious injury.

Injuries to the cervical spine occur relatively commonly in collision sports and have been estimated to occur in approximately 10 % of American football players [1]. While some patterns of spinal injury are more common in one collision sport than in another, the mechanisms of injury are likely common in all sports. The majority of the available data in young athletes come from the study of such sports as American football, rugby, and hockey, and transient cervical neurological injuries have been well described in young participants of these sports [2–6]. Permanent or catastrophic neurological injury has also been well described in this population [5, 7–9], and this concern has led to ongoing interest in and debate over the role, if any, that transient injuries may play in the risk of subsequent catastrophic neurological injury [1] in the young athlete. The aim of this chapter is to provide an

P.A. Kurian • D.I. Light, MD • H.A. Kerr, MD (✉)
Department of Internal Medicine and Pediatrics, Albany Medical College, Albany Medical Center, 724 Watervliet-Shaker Road, Latham, NY 12110, USA
e-mail: kurianp@mail.amc.edu; lightd@mail.amc.edu; KerrH@mail.amc.edu

M. O'Brien, W.P. Meehan III (eds.), *Head and Neck Injuries in Young Athletes*, Contemporary Pediatric and Adolescent Sports Medicine,
DOI 10.1007/978-3-319-23549-3_10

overview of transient cervical neurological injuries including anatomy, mechanisms of injury, evaluation and management, current opinions on return to play, and possible implications for risk of future catastrophic injury.

Clinical Anatomy

Managing and treating neurological injuries to the cervical spine requires a basic understanding of the regional anatomy and mechanisms of injury. The spinal cord exits the skull through the foramen magnum and is protected by the bony spinal canal formed by the seven cervical vertebrae. Nerve roots exit the spinal canal through neural foramina, and can become injured at this point of exit. The brachial plexus is formed from the nerve roots of C5–T1 and is only partially protected by the bone and soft tissue structures of the neck and shoulder. The anatomy of the cervical spine is structured to handle a variety of forces while still permitting a wide range of motion. Compressive or axial forces are mainly resisted by the vertebral bodies and intervertebral disks. Shear forces are countered by paraspinal and ligamentous structures, and tensile forces are resisted by the annulus fibrosus and longitudinal ligaments [10, 11]. When the forces applied exceed the capacity of these structures to resist them, injury to the underlying neurological structures can occur. Young athletes are likely to have more intrinsic mobility of the cervical spine [12–14], and it has been suggested that this may allow extreme forces to stretch or compress the spinal cord beyond its tolerance without necessarily causing simultaneous damage to the bony structures. Spinal cord injury without radiographic abnormality (SCIWORA) was described initially by Pang in 1982 as spinal cord injury without evidence of spinal fracture or instability on plain radiographs or CT imaging [15]. SCIWORA severity may range from mild and transient to severe and prolonged, and MRI findings may predict the severity of injury [16]. Extremes of flexion or extension may cause these varying degrees of neurological injury to the spinal cord, even when the mobile pediatric cervical spine itself tolerates the movement without obvious injury.

Most cervical spine neurological injuries in sports involve flexion or extension of the cervical spine under an axial load, or traction on the cervical nerve roots or brachial plexus. Flexion injuries, such as those sustained from spearing in football or scrum collapses in rugby, can cause transient spinal cord injury, but in adults they may be more likely to result in structural failure of the cervical spine and catastrophic injury. In children they may be more likely to cause transient neurapraxia, given the greater mobility of the connective tissue in the pediatric cervical spine [13, 17]. Extension injuries are a more common cause of transient spinal cord injury in adults. Traction or compression of the cervical nerve roots or brachial plexus, as can occur during tackles or falls, can result in peripheral nerve injury. A transient disruption of function can occur following a traumatic nerve injury and is termed neurapraxia. More severe injury may disrupt both the axon and the myelin sheath and lead to Wallerian degeneration of the axon, termed axonotmesis. Complete disruption of the nerve including the axon, myelin sheath, and epineurium is termed neurotmesis [6, 18].

Transient Injury to Peripheral Nerve: Burners and Stingers

Burners or stingers are characterized by transient, unilateral reversible pain or paresthesia radiating down the affected upper extremity and are thought to represent a neurapraxia of the peripheral nerve [19]. Weakness of muscles such as the deltoid, biceps, or supraspinatus may also be present. Typically, this is in the distribution of the C5–C6 nerve root; however, there is usually no cervical tenderness, and full range of motion of the neck is preserved [20]. Classically, these symptoms last only a few minutes and spontaneously resolve. However, in some instances, athletes suffer from what is known as the chronic burner syndrome, defined as neurapraxia associated with persistent weakness and a high recurrence rate [21, 22].

As many as 65 % of football players will sustain a stinger at some point during their collegiate career [11, 23, 24]. In a retrospective study, looking at 152 professional rugby players, 72 % suffered from one or more stinger injuries, and 95 % continued to play with no time lost from training or games [25]. Even greater numbers do not report their injuries out of fear of being pulled from the game or because of the view that such injuries are trivial in comparison to other spinal injuries [23, 24, 26].

Injury Mechanism(s)

Stingers are peripheral nerve injuries as opposed to spinal cord injuries (which are central nerve injuries), most commonly affecting the cervical C5–C6 nerve distributions. The pathophysiology of stingers has remained somewhat controversial, and it is likely that they represent several different types of injury. The site of injury may involve either the cervical nerve root or upper brachial plexus. The former is the more commonly reported site in adults and professional athletes and has been reported to be associated with underlying cervical stenosis or disk disease [21, 27, 28]. It has also been suggested that this may be secondary to the anatomic differences between the two locations. The brachial plexus has epineurium and perineurium tissue, in addition to a plexiform structure, allowing it to absorb tensile and compressive forces better than the more exposed cervical roots [28, 29].

Three different mechanisms of injury resulting in a burner/stinger have been postulated (see Fig. 10.1):

1. *Traction.* The first mechanism is a traction or brachial plexus stretch injury, which occurs with depression of the ipsilateral shoulder with concomitant flexion of the neck creating a stretch on the brachial plexus and nerve roots [24, 30, 31].
2. *Direct blow.* The second proposed mechanism is direct trauma to the supraclavicular region or Erb's point, causing a direct compressive effect on the nerve [20, 24, 32].
3. *Compression.* The third described mechanism is an extension-compression mechanism created by hyperextension of the neck and lateral bend to the affected side, effectively creating a narrowing of the intervertebral foramen and compression of

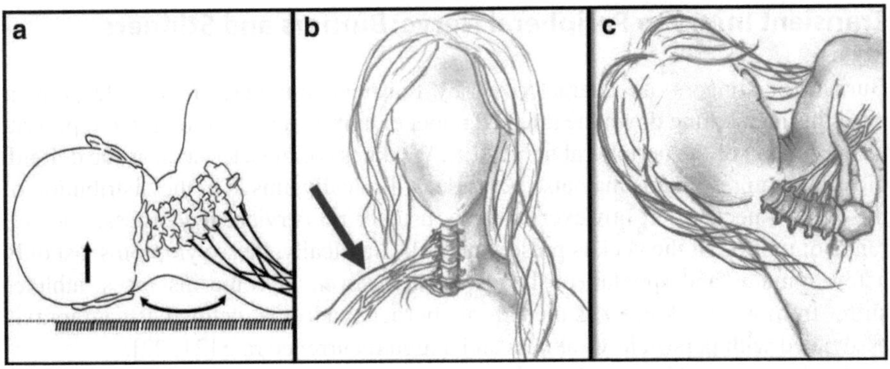

Fig. 10.1 Illustrations of three mechanisms of burner/stinger: (**a**) traction (*arrows* show direction of movement), (**b**) direct blow to Erb's point (*arrow*), (**c**) compression (Images courtesy William H. Light Ph.D. (panel **a**) and Achala Talati D.O. (panels **b** and **c**))

the nerve root [33]. Levitz et al. implicate this mechanism as the main cause of chronic burner syndrome in 83 % of athletes, with 94 % of these athletes having associated cervical disk disease or degenerative changes [21, 27, 34].

A more recent retrospective study of Canadian football by Charbonneau et al. looked at 244 collegiate football players, noting the annual incidence of stingers to be 26 %, or 64 players in the 2010 season [26]. The most common mechanism of injury in this study was a direct blow to the shoulder. Prior to this study, the most commonly reported mechanism was the extension-compression mechanism [23, 27]. The authors postulated that this may be secondary to improved education and coaching of tackling techniques, which reduced cervical spine injuries by taking the impact to the shoulder rather than the head, but may have also placed the athlete at greater risk for brachial plexus injuries [26].

Evaluation

Initial Evaluation (On Field)

An athletic trainer responding to an athlete showing signs of distress or inability to move their arm will often conduct an initial assessment on the field. An athlete can be asked to describe what happened and what they currently feel. It is imperative to hear whether symptoms are unilateral or bilateral. Transient unilateral symptoms are less concerning, as is the absence of neck pain [35, 36]. A rudimentary strength assessment of wrist extension, biceps, deltoid, and supraspinatus can be conducted quickly with the athlete asked to resist wrist and elbow extension and resist shoulder abduction. Any deficits should prompt removal of the athlete from field of play [36–38].

Initial Evaluation (Field Side or Training Room)

In an athlete presenting with sensory symptoms in an upper extremity, it must first be determined whether the symptoms are isolated and unilateral. Any bilateral symptoms or lower extremity involvement should instead prompt suspicion for a spinal cord injury. Strength and range of motion of the neck and upper extremity should be assessed, and reflexes of the triceps, biceps, and brachioradialis should be elicited. The Spurling maneuver, in which the head is rotated to the affected side and an axial load is applied, may be positive for reproduction of radiating pain or paresthesias in athletes who have sustained an injury to the cervical nerve root, but will likely be negative in the setting of a more distal brachial plexus injury. Radiating pain reproduced by tapping on Erb's point (Fig. 10.1, panel b) may suggest direct trauma as a mechanism of peripheral nerve injury.

Players with prompt resolution of unilateral sensory symptoms and without any weakness may be allowed to continue playing [38]. Any weakness, asymmetry of reflexes, or positive Spurling sign should prompt removal from play and further evaluation for structural cervical spine abnormalities.

Further Evaluation (Emergency Department or Office Follow-Up)

Radiographic evaluation including cervical X-ray and magnetic resonance imaging (MRI) is recommended after a first stinger if symptoms persist beyond 1 h, if there is associated neck pain, or if the neurological exam suggests a particular nerve-root distribution [20, 39]. X-ray is helpful in identifying instability on flexion or extension as well as evidence of foraminal stenosis. MRI should be performed in any athlete presenting with persistent weakness and can identify disk herniation or, as in the case of chronic burner syndrome, foraminal narrowing and disk disease [21].

Electrodiagnostic testing such as electromyography (EMG) may be helpful in evaluating the athlete with prolonged symptoms, particularly motor weakness, and is ideally performed at least 4 weeks after injury [28, 40]. Electrodiagnostics may also be helpful in distinguishing between cervical nerve root and brachial plexus injury, as well as between neurapraxic and axonal injury [41] (see Table 10.1). This can aid in predicting time to recovery and prognosis, as neurapraxia portends a more favorable recovery [40]. A completely normal EMG is not a prerequisite for return to play, particularly if the athlete demonstrates full clinical recovery of strength and range of motion [28].

Table 10.1 Classification of burners based on Seddon's criteria [18]

	Grade 1: Neurapraxia	Grade 2: Axonotmesis	Grade 3: Neurotmesis
Severity	Mild	Moderate	Severe
EMG findings	Focal demyelination but no axonal loss	Axonal injury resulting in positive waves and fibrillation potentials	Acute denervation
		Axon is disrupted, but epineurium is intact	Disrupts axons, endoneurium, perineurium, and epineurium
Recovery	Minutes–6 weeks	Recovery may take months	Ranges from complete recovery to none

Return to Play

Unfortunately, there is no uniform guideline for return to play after a burner or stinger; however, several practical factors should be considered. In general, an athlete must have full resolution of symptoms, pain-free range of motion, and normal strength [40]. If an athlete fulfills these criteria and this is their first stinger, they may return to play in the same game [29]. However, if symptoms last greater than 24 h, or there is a history of multiple stingers, then further evaluation should be considered before allowing return to play. Although it is not known how many stingers a player can safely sustain before risking permanent deficits, some experts suggest that athletes acquiring multiple stingers (e.g., more than 3) within a season should be considered for removal for the season, if not permanently [40]. Absolute contraindications to return to play include persistent weakness, persistent pain, EMG abnormalities (aside from reinnervation), reduced cervical range of motion, or evidence of myelopathy [20, 40]. Routine cervical imaging for burners or stingers in asymptomatic players is typically not recommended [29, 31, 40].

Transient Injury to the Cervical Spinal Cord

When transient neurological injury occurs to the cervical spinal cord itself, it is termed cervical cord neurapraxia. This clinical entity was described by Torg et al. in 1986 [42] and by definition involves transient functional disruption of the spinal cord from a traumatic mechanism, with subsequent complete recovery of baseline neurological function. Depending on associated motor symptoms, this has also been termed transient quadriplegia or transient quadriparesis. This injury is most commonly described in American football players, but has also been described in Rugby players [2, 43]. Affected athletes may experience numbness, tingling, or burning below the level of the injury, which either is bilateral or involves more than just the upper extremity on the affected side. Motor weakness or paralysis may also be present. Symptoms typically last several minutes but can persist up to 48 h and perhaps longer in pediatric patients [13]. A grading system based on symptom duration was developed by Torg, with Grade I injury persisting less than 15 min, Grade II 15 min to 24 h, and Grade III lasting greater than 24 h. Adults generally do not complain of associated neck pain aside from neuropathic burning pain, whereas younger children may more commonly present with neck pain [13, 14].The risk of cervical cord neurapraxia appears to increase with increasing levels of play. In a study of high school and college American football players, the incidence of cervical cord neurapraxia increased from high school to collegiate levels of play, with an annual incidence of 0.17 per 100,000 and 2.05 per 100,000, respectively [44]. Torg has previously reported an overall incidence of 7 per 10,000 elite American football players [42].

Mechanism

Penning first proposed a mechanism of injury for cervical neurapraxia in 1962, suggesting hyperextension of the cervical spine, which causes folding of the dura mater and ligamentum flavum with protrusion into the spinal canal, as well as approximation of the posterior inferior edge of a vertebral body with the anterior superior aspect of the lamina of the inferior vertebra [45–47]. This effectively causes a decrease in the diameter of the cervical spinal canal, with transient compression of the spinal cord. Hyperflexion mechanisms, theoretically with similar transient narrowing of the AP diameter of the spinal canal, have also been reported, particularly in pediatric athletes [13]. In fact, cervical cord neurapraxia is likely a mild form of SCIWORA, which is well described in children and is thought to be a result of a hypermobile cervical spine and cervical ligaments which allow movement that is sufficient to injure the cord without structural damage to the bones or surrounding connective tissues [16]. In patients with preexisting cervical spinal stenosis (congenital or acquired), the pincer mechanism may be amplified, and this has been shown to be a risk factor for recurrence [48].

Evaluation and Management

The approach to an athlete with any neurological symptoms suggestive of acute spinal cord injury should involve immediate spinal immobilization until traumatic cervical spine instability can be definitively ruled out. Plain radiographs in flexion and extension may reveal evidence of ligamentous injury or instability. Computed tomography (CT) can reveal evidence of bony injury. Any athlete with evidence of cervical cord injury should be considered for MRI, which in addition to revealing cord injury or compressive pathology (such as hematoma) can also help to establish whether there is underlying spinal stenosis which may be a predisposing factor for reinjury. Return to play decisions following an episode of cervical cord neurapraxia are an area of ongoing debate and, as discussed below, may be informed by assessment for preexisting or acquired cervical spine abnormalities.

Prevention of Cervical Neurological Injury

Modifiable Factors

Modifiable factors for prevention of both reversible and irreversible neurological injury in sport include proper equipment, proper tackling techniques, and rules modification/enforcement.

Rule changes in both American football and ice hockey have been shown to decrease the overall rate of spine injuries. The practice of spear tackling in American football, or using the helmet as the initial contact point in tackling and thereby axially loading the cervical spine in a flexed position, was banned by the National

Collegiate Athletic Association (NCAA) and the National Federation of State High School Athletic Associations in the mid-1970s. During that time, a decrease in severe cervical spine injury rates was noted at both the high school and college level [49]. In ice hockey, the practice of checking from behind has been shown to result in flexion injuries to the cervical spine, and penalties for this practice were instituted in the mid-1980s in Canada [3, 5]. A decrease in spinal injuries was also noted after implementation of these rules change [5]. Quarrie et al. showed that an educational intervention via CDROM video for coaches ("Rugby Smart") in New Zealand ultimately helped reduce the incidence of serious spinal cord injury [50].

Coaches should review proper tackling techniques, specifically avoiding the dropping of the shoulder and allowing the head and neck to be driven into extension [24]. The athlete should be able to make eye contact with their opponent in order to ensure a more vertical tackling position [24]. Postural dysfunction (stooped shoulder, head forward posture) may cause brachial plexus irritation to persist after a stinger. Chest-out posturing and thoracic outlet obstruction exercises allow the intervertebral foramina to open to its maximum [51].

Equipment modification, such as the use of thicker shoulder pads, neck rolls, or Cowboy Collars in American football, has been used to try to decrease cervical injury [52]. Such measures decrease extension and lateral flexion, as well as provide more padding for Erb's point and thus minimize direct impact to the area, but the evidence is limited as to the efficacy of such measures for preventing stingers or cervical cord neurapraxia [52]. While no protective equipment has been definitely shown to prevent severe spinal injury in collision sports, all players should have properly fitting equipment that should be worn according to the standards in place for each sport [32].

Developmental Cervical Stenosis

Cervical stenosis has been shown by some authors to be a risk factor for permanent neurological injury in contact sports [53]. The diagnosis of cervical stenosis was previously made by measuring the canal diameter on a cervical plain film. However, this method has been shown to be subject to error due to magnification artifact, which may be present to different degrees on different films. Pavlov and Torg [54] therefore proposed evaluating the width of the canal by comparing it with the vertebral body width on the same film. This Torg ratio (or Pavlov ratio) is calculated by dividing the distance between the midpoint of the posterior aspect of the vertebral body to the nearest point on the spinolaminar line by the sagittal diameter of the vertebral body (see Fig. 10.2). In a retrospective cohort study, Torg found that a ratio of 0.8 or less was 93 % sensitive for predicting an episode of cervical cord neurapraxia [55]. However, it was found to have a poor positive predictive value of 0.2 %. Herzog subsequently showed this ratio to be a poor predictor of true functional spinal stenosis as well, with a positive predictive value of only 12 % [56]. It is now widely accepted that MRI or myelography demonstrating the degree of "functional stenosis," or the amount of spinal fluid that is visible around the cord, is a far more accurate, though more expensive, assessment of true spinal stenosis.

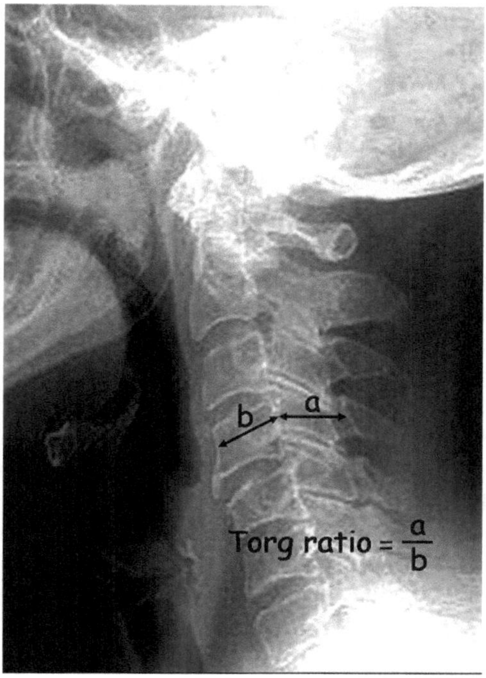

Fig. 10.2 Torg ratio. The distance between the midpoint of the posterior aspect of the vertebral body to the nearest point on the spinolaminar line (**a**) is divided by the sagittal diameter of the vertebral body (**b**)

Cervical Stenosis and Stingers

There is evidence of an association between cervical spinal stenosis and risk of sustaining a stinger injury, particularly via the nerve-root compressive mechanism. Meyer et al. demonstrated that players with cervical stenosis as assessed by the Torg ratio had a threefold higher risk of sustaining a stinger than those without stenosis [27]. In contrast, Castro et al. in their study of 165 collegiate athletes noted no difference in initial stinger frequency in players with cervical stenosis compared to players without stenosis. They did note that players with a history of repeated stingers often did have lower Torg ratios [47, 57]. Page et al. examined the utility of preparticipation screening radiographs of the cervical spine in 125 athletes and found the Torg ratio to have a positive predictive value of only 22 % for subsequent stinger experience [31]. The Torg ratio is therefore not an accurate predictor of an athlete's risk for developing a stinger and should not be used as a screening tool [19, 31, 55].

Cervical Stenosis and Cervical Cord Injury

There is debate as to whether players who have had an episode of cervical cord neurapraxia should be allowed to return to play. As mentioned above, an association between spinal stenosis and transient cervical cord neurapraxia has been demonstrated [42, 58]. Torg reported a 56 % recurrence rate in football players who returned to play after an episode of cervical cord neurapraxia [59] but also found no evidence that these players were at increased risk of sustaining a permanent neurological injury [60, 61]. It is not recommended that athletes undergo screening radiographs for cervical stenosis [62]; however, diagnostic radiographs should be obtained as part of an evaluation for an athlete who has experienced an episode of cervical cord neurapraxia. If a low Torg ratio is noted, this should then be followed up by MRI of the cervical spine to determine whether functional spinal stenosis is present [63–67].

It is less clear whether the Torg ratio can be applied similarly to the younger adolescent athlete, who may in fact be more likely to sustain a transient spinal cord injury in the absence of stenosis due to greater cervical spine mobility. Boockvar et al. [13] described 13 children ages 7–15 who experienced cervical cord neurapraxia, none of whom were found to have an abnormal Torg ratio. The Torg ratio has not been adequately studied as a screening tool in the pediatric population, and the cutoff values described by Torg for professional football players may not be appropriate for the developing adolescent spine [68].

Expert opinion varies as to the approach to return to play for athletes found to have true functional spinal stenosis after a transient spinal cord injury. Some suggest that in a player who has fully recovered and has no evidence of cervical spine instability, the presence of stenosis represents only a relative contraindication to play and should be discussed with the player [6]. Others have suggested that it represents an absolute contraindication [65]. Regardless, this decision must be made in collaboration with the athlete, who must be fully informed of the potential risks.

Acquired Cervical Stenosis: Spear Tackler's Spine

This entity was first described by Torg in 1993 based on an analysis of 15 athletes from the National Football Head and Neck Injury Registry; 4 of whom sustained permanent neurological injury, and 11 of whom had transient neurological symptoms [46]. All of these players were found to have a history of employing spear tackling techniques, loss of the normal cervical lordosis on X-ray, evidence of posttraumatic changes on X-ray, and developmental narrowing of the cervical spine based on a Torg ratio of less than 0.8. Based on these findings, it was recommended that Spear Tackler's Spine be considered an absolute contraindication to participation in collision sports, or any sport which places the athlete at risk of axial loading of the cervical spine [46].

Summary

Contact and collision sports entail risks of neurological injury. Thankfully, many of these injuries are transient in nature, though debate still exists as to whether transient injuries or the factors that predispose to them also incur a risk of future more permanent injury. It is important for physicians to be comfortable distinguishing among these different neurological injuries, as their management and follow-up is based on injury type, severity, and symptoms. The presence of underlying developmental or acquired cervical spine abnormalities should be considered when making decisions about return to play.

Acknowledgments Thanks to William H. Light Ph.D. and Achala Talati D.O. for contribution to figure illustrations.

References

1. Gill SS, Boden BP. The epidemiology of catastrophic spine injuries in high school and college football. Sports Med Arthrosc. 2008;16(1):2–6.
2. Quarrie KL, Cantu RC, Chalmers DJ. Rugby union injuries to the cervical spine and spinal cord. Sports Med. 2002;32(10):633–53.
3. Benson BW, Meeuwisse WH. Ice hockey injuries. Med Sport Sci. 2005;49:86–119.
4. Rihn JA, Anderson DT, Lamb K, Deluca PF, Bata A, Marchetto PA, et al. Cervical spine injuries in American football. Sports Med. 2009;39(9):697–708.
5. Tator CH, Provvidenza C, Cassidy J. Spinal injuries in Canadian ice hockey: an update to 2005. Clin J Sport Med. 2009;19:451–6.
6. Torg JS. Cervical spine injuries and the return to football. Sports Health. 2009;1(5):376–83.
7. Torg JS, Truex Jr R, Quedenfeld TC, Burstein A, Spealman A, Nichols 3rd C. The National Football Head and Neck Injury Registry. Report and conclusions 1978. JAMA. 1979;241(14): 1477–9.
8. Torg JS, Vegso JJ, Sennett B, Das M. The National Football Head and Neck Injury Registry. 14-year report on cervical quadriplegia, 1971 through 1984. JAMA. 1985;254(24):3439–43.
9. McIntosh AS. Rugby injuries. Med Sport Sci. 2005;49:120–39.
10. Banerjee R, Palumbo MA, Fadale PD. Catastrophic cervical spine injuries in the collision sport athlete, Part 1: epidemiology, functional anatomy, and diagnosis. Am J Sports Med. 2004;32(4):1077–87.
11. Wilson JB, Zarzour R, Moorman CT. Spinal injuries in contact sports. Curr Sports Med Rep. 2006;5(1):50–5.
12. Bailey DK. The normal cervical spine in infants and children. Radiology. 1952;59(5):712–9.
13. Boockvar JA, Durham SR, Sun PP. Cervical spinal stenosis and sports-related cervical cord neurapraxia in children. Spine. 2001;26(24):2709–12.
14. Clark AJ, Auguste KI, Sun PP. Cervical spinal stenosis and sports-related cervical cord neurapraxia. Neurosurg Focus. 2011;31(5), E7.
15. Pang D, Wilberger Jr JE. Spinal cord injury without radiographic abnormalities in children. J Neurosurg. 1982;57(1):114–29.
16. Pang D. Spinal cord injury without radiographic abnormality in children, 2 decades later. Neurosurgery. 2004;55(6):1325–42; discussion 1342–3.
17. Jones TM, Anderson PA, Noonan KJ. Pediatric cervical spine trauma. J Am Acad Orthop Surg. 2011;19(10):600–11.
18. Weinberg J, Rokito S, Silber JS. Etiology, treatment, and prevention of athletic "stingers". Clin Sports Med. 2003;22(3):493–500, viii.
19. Olson DE, McBroom SA, Nelson BD, Broton MS, Pulling TJ. Unilateral cervical nerve injuries: brachial plexopathies. Curr Sports Med Rep. 2007;6(1):43–9.
20. Concannon LG, Harrast MA, Herring SA. Radiating upper limb pain in the contact sport athlete: an update on transient quadriparesis and stingers. Curr Sports Med Rep. 2012;11(1):28–34.
21. Levitz CL, Reilly PJ, Torg JS. The pathomechanics of chronic, recurrent cervical nerve root neurapraxia. The chronic burner syndrome. Am J Sports Med. 1997;25(1):73–6.
22. Krivickas LS, Wilbourn AJ. The pathomechanics of chronic, recurrent cervical nerve root neurapraxia: the chronic burner syndrome. Am J Sports Med. 1998;26(4):603–4.
23. Sallis R. Burners: an underreported Injury. Phys Sportsmed. 1992;20(11):47–55.
24. Feinberg JH. Burners and stingers. Phys Med Rehabil Clin N Am. 2000;11(4):771–84.
25. Cunnane M, Pratten M, Loughna S. A retrospective study looking at the incidence of 'stinger' injuries in professional rugby union players. Br J Sports Med. 2011;45(15):A19.

26. Charbonneau RM, McVeigh SA, Thompson K. Brachial neuropraxia in Canadian Atlantic University sport football players: what is the incidence of "stingers"? Clin J Sport Med. 2012;22(6):472–7.
27. Meyer SA, Schulte KR, Callaghan JJ, Albright JP, Powell JW, Crowley ET, et al. Cervical spinal stenosis and stingers in collegiate football players. Am J Sports Med. 1994;22(2):158–66.
28. Weinstein S. Assessment and rehabilitation of the athlete with a stinger. Clin Sports Med. 1998;17(1):127–35.
29. Safran MR. Nerve injury about the shoulder in athletes, Part 2: long thoracic nerve, spinal accessory nerve, burners/stingers, thoracic outlet syndrome. Am J Sports Med. 2004;32(4):1063–76.
30. Kuhlman GS, McKeag DB. The "burner": a common nerve injury in contact sports. Am Fam Physician. 1999;60(7):2035–40, 2042.
31. Page S, Guy JA. Neurapraxia, "stingers," and spinal stenosis in athletes. South Med J. 2004;97(8):766–9.
32. Markey KL, Di Benedetto M, Curl WW. Upper trunk brachial plexopathy. The stinger syndrome. Am J Sports Med. 1993;21(5):650–5.
33. Kelly JD, Aliquo D, Sitler MR, Odgers C, Moyer RA. Association of burners with cervical canal and foraminal stenosis. Am J Sports Med. 2000;28(2):214–7.
34. Shannon B, Klimkiewicz JJ. Cervical burners in the athlete. Clin Sports Med. 2002;21(1): 29–35, vi.
35. Proctor MR, Cantu RC. Head and neck injuries in young athletes. Clin Sports Med. 2000;19(4):693–715.
36. Whiteside JW. Management of head and neck injuries by the sideline physician. Am Fam Physician. 2006;74(8):1357–62.
37. Nissen SJ, Laskowski ER, Rizzo Jr TD. Burner syndrome: recognition and rehabilitation. Phys Sportsmed. 1996;24(6):57–64.
38. Vaccaro AR, Klein GR, Ciccoti M, Pfaff WL, Moulton MJ, Hilibrand AJ, et al. Return to play criteria for the athlete with cervical spine injuries resulting in stinger and transient quadriplegia/paresis. Spine J. 2002;2(5):351–6.
39. Morganti C. Recommendations for return to sports following cervical spine injuries. Sports Med. 2003;33(8):563–73.
40. Standaert CJ, Herring SA. Expert opinion and controversies in musculoskeletal and sports medicine: stingers. Arch Phys Med Rehabil. 2009;90(3):402–6.
41. Di Benedetto M, Markey K. Electrodiagnostic localization of traumatic upper trunk brachial plexopathy. Arch Phys Med Rehabil. 1984;65(1):15–7.
42. Torg JS, Pavlov H, Genuario SE, Sennett B, Wisneski RJ, Robie BH, et al. Neurapraxia of the cervical spinal cord with transient quadriplegia. J Bone Joint Surg Am. 1986;68(9):1354–70.
43. Cantu RC. Cervical spine injuries in the athlete. Semin Neurol. 2000;20(2):173–8.
44. Boden BP, Tacchetti RL, Cantu RC, Knowles SB, Mueller FO. Catastrophic cervical spine injuries in high school and college football players. Am J Sports Med. 2006;34(8):1223–32.
45. Penning L. Some aspects of plain radiography of the cervical spine in chronic myelopathy. Neurology. 1962;12(5):513–9.
46. Torg J, Sennett B, Pavlov H, Leventhal M, Glasgow S. Spear tackler's spine. An entity precluding participation in tackle football and collision activities that expose the cervical spine to axial energy inputs. Am J Sports Med. 1993;21(5):640–9.
47. Castro Jr FP. Stingers, cervical cord neurapraxia, and stenosis. Clin Sports Med. 2003;22(3):483–92.
48. Torg JS, Ramsey-Emrhein JA. Management guidelines for participation in collision activities with congenital, developmental, or postinjury lesions involving the cervical spine. Clin J Sport Med. 1997;7(4):273–91.
49. Torg JS, Guille JT, Jaffe S. Injuries to the cervical spine in American football players. J Bone Joint Surg Am. 2002;84-A(1):112–22.
50. Quarrie KL, Gianotti SM, Hopkins WG, Hume PA. Effect of nationwide injury prevention programme on serious spinal injuries in New Zealand rugby union: ecological study. BMJ. 2007;334(7604):1150.

51. Stracciolini A. Cervical burners in the athlete. Pediatr Case Rev. 2003;3(4):181–8.
52. Gorden JA, Straub SJ, Swanik CB, Swanik KA. Effects of football collars on cervical hyperextension and lateral flexion. J Athl Train. 2003;38(3):209–15.
53. Matsuura P, Waters RL, Adkins RH, Rothman S, Gurbani N, Sie I. Comparison of computerized tomography parameters of the cervical spine in normal control subjects and spinal cord-injured patients. J Bone Joint Surg Am. 1989;71(2):183–8.
54. Pavlov H, Torg JS. Roentgen examination of cervical spine injuries in the athlete. Clin Sports Med. 1987;6(4):751–66.
55. Torg JS, Naranja RJ, Pavlov H, Galinat BJ, Warren R, Stine RA. The relationship of developmental narrowing of the cervical spinal canal to reversible and irreversible injury of the cervical spinal cord in football players. J Bone Joint Surg Am. 1996;78(9):1308–14.
56. Herzog RJ, Wiens JJ, Dillingham MF, Sontag MJ. Normal cervical spine morphometry and cervical spinal stenosis in asymptomatic professional football players. Plain film radiography, multiplanar computed tomography, and magnetic resonance imaging. Spine (Phila Pa 1976). 1991;16(6 Suppl):S178–86.
57. Castro Jr FP, Ricciardi J, Brunet ME, Busch MT, Whitecloud 3rd TS. Stingers, the Torg ratio, and the cervical spine. Am J Sports Med. 1997;25(5):603–8.
58. Torg JS, Corcoran TA, Thibault LE, Pavlov H, Sennett BJ, Naranja Jr RJ, et al. Cervical cord neurapraxia: classification, pathomechanics, morbidity, and management guidelines. J Neurosurg. 1997;87(6):843–50.
59. Torg JS. Management guidelines for athletic injuries to the cervical spine. Clin Sports Med. 1987;6(1):53–60.
60. Torg JS. Cervical spinal stenosis with cord neurapraxia and transient quadriplegia. Clin Sports Med. 1990;9(2):279–96.
61. Torg JS, Ramsey-Emrhein JA. Cervical spine and brachial plexus injuries: return-to-play recommendations. Phys Sportsmed. 1997;25(7):61–88.
62. Torg JS. Cervical spinal stenosis with cord neurapraxia: evaluations and decisions regarding participation in athletics. Curr Sports Med Rep. 2002;1(1):43–6.
63. Cantu RV, Cantu RC. Guidelines for return to contact sports after transient quadriplegia. J Neurosurg. 1994;80(3):592–4.
64. Cantu RC. Stingers, transient quadriplegia, and cervical spinal stenosis: return to play criteria. Med Sci Sports Exerc. 1997;29(7 Suppl):S233–5.
65. Cantu RC. The cervical spinal stenosis controversy. Clin Sports Med. 1998;17(1):121–6.
66. Cantu RV, Cantu RC. Current thinking: return to play and transient quadriplegia. Curr Sports Med Rep. 2005;4(1):27–32.
67. Cantu RC, Bailes JE, Wilberger Jr JE. Guidelines for return to contact or collision sport after a cervical spine injury. Clin Sports Med. 1998;17(1):137–46.
68. Light DI, Kerr HA. Spine injuries in collision/heavy contact sports. In: Micheli L, Stein C, O'Brien M, d'Hemecourt P, editors. Spinal injuries and conditions in young athletes. New York: Springer; 2013. p. 75–87.

Cervical Spine Injuries in Sports

11

Robert V. Cantu and Robert C. Cantu

Epidemiology

More than 30 million children participate in youth sports each year in the United States, and of the estimated 5.5 million children who participate in football, an estimated 28 % are injured each year [1]. A recent study found that nearly 40 % of all life-threatening injuries in children age 6–18 years result from sporting activities [2]. The authors also found one in four cervical spine fractures in pediatric patients are sports related. Cervical spine injuries in younger children differ from those in adults due in part to anatomy. In children, the head is larger relative to the torso, resulting in a higher center of gravity and a larger moment arm acting on the cervical spine. Additionally, children have multiple open vertebral physes and generally more lax ligamentous structures. The combination of these factors results in a higher proportion of injuries involving the upper cervical spine than seen in adults. Mechanism of injury also plays a role in the location of cervical spine injuries. A recent study examining patterns of cervical spine injuries in children found very high forces, such as those seen in motor vehicle collisions (MVC), tended to result in a higher proportion of axial spine (C1–C2) injuries, whereas lower energy mechanisms as seen in most sporting or recreational activities tended to result in more subaxial (C3–C7) injuries [3]. This study found that in children aged 2–7 years, MVC was the most common cause, accounting for 37 % of all cervical spine injuries. In children 8–15 years, however, sports accounted for the same percentage of injuries as MVC's at 23 %. Of those sports injuries 53 % were subaxial.

R.V. Cantu, MD, MS (✉)
Dartmouth Hitchcock Medical Center, One Medical Center Drive, Lebanon, NH 03755, USA
e-mail: robert.v.cantu@hitchcock.org

R.C. Cantu, MD, FACS, FACSM
Emerson Hospital, Concord, MA 01742, USA

Children's Hospital, Boston, MA 02115, USA
e-mail: rcantu@emersonhosp.org

M. O'Brien, W.P. Meehan III (eds.), *Head and Neck Injuries in Young Athletes*,
Contemporary Pediatric and Adolescent Sports Medicine,
DOI 10.1007/978-3-319-23549-3_11

Initial Assessment

On the field management of an athlete who is down and suspected of having a cervical spine injury begins with the ABC's of acute trauma care, prioritizing the patient's airway, breathing, and circulation. If the patient is prone and there is concern for the airway, the athlete should be carefully logrolled into the supine position with one person in charge of maintaining cervical alignment. In sports such as football or hockey where helmets and shoulder pads are worn, they should remain in place during the initial evaluation. This is provided the face mask can be quickly removed, allowing access to the airway. A study by Swenson et al. on ten healthy individuals showed that if the helmet is removed and the shoulder pads remain in place, an increase in cervical lordosis results [4]. Although young children have an increased head-to-torso size, removing just the helmet still results in an increased lordosis [5]. For children ≤6 years of age, however, a backboard with a cutout for the helmet is recommended to maintain neutral alignment. Swartz et al. looked at face mask versus helmet removal and found removing the face mask took less time and resulted in less motion in all three planes [6]. If the helmet has to be removed then the shoulder pads should also be taken off, following the generally accepted "all or none" policy. A recent study has shown that some of the newer football helmets, with increased protection around the mandible, can make basic airway maneuvers such as chin lift more difficult [7] (see Fig. 11.1). Participants attempting to perform bag-mask ventilation on 146 college athlete volunteers reported the helmet as a cause of difficulty in 10.4 % of athletes wearing a modern hockey helmet, and in 79 % of athletes wearing a football helmet [7]. If such a helmet prevents proper management of the airway, then both the helmet and shoulder pads should be removed while maintaining cervical alignment.

The athlete who returns to the sidelines complaining of neck pain requires careful assessment. Generally, any athlete with restricted or painful cervical motion, bony tenderness, or any motor sensory deficit that involves more than a single upper

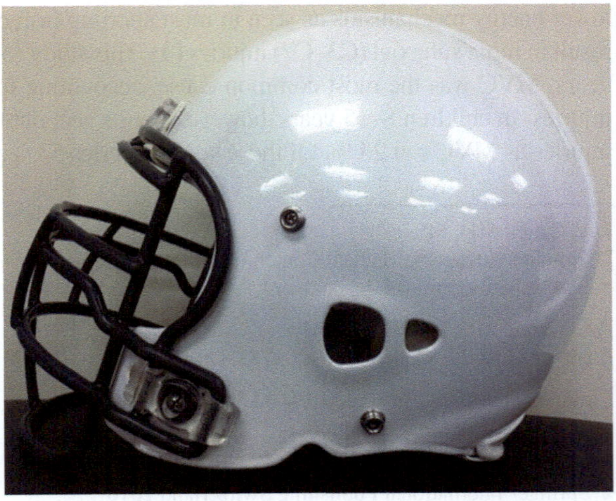

Fig. 11.1 Example of a football helmet with increased protection around base of jaw, making airway maneuvers such as chin lift more difficult

extremity and does not quickly resolve should be removed from competition, placed on spinal precautions, and referred for further evaluation. The athlete who complains of symptoms consistent with a stinger, unilateral upper extremity burning pain and/or weakness typically in a C5–C6 distribution, should be removed from competition until all symptoms have resolved and there is normal and painless cervical range of motion and strength.

Imaging

Imaging of the young athlete with suspected cervical spine injury typically begins with plain radiographs including AP, lateral, and open-mouth odontoid views. Interpreting cervical spine radiographs in children can be challenging due to the developing anatomy where pseudo-subluxation of C2 on C3 and occasionally C3 on C4 can occur (see Fig. 11.2). In one retrospective review of 138 pediatric trauma patients, a 22 % incidence of pseudo-subluxation of C2 on C3 was found [8]. One way to differentiate pseudo-subluxation from true injury is to assess the spinolaminar (Swischuk's) line on the lateral c-spine X-ray. In cases of pseudo-subluxation, the spinolaminar line should pass within 1 mm of the anterior cortex of the posterior arch of C2 (see Fig. 11.3). When this line passes >1.5 mm from the anterior cortex of the posterior arch of C2, acute injury is likely (see Fig. 11.4). The atlantodens interval, the distance from the anterior aspect of the dens to the posterior aspect of the anterior ring of the atlas, can show more variation in children than adults. The atlantodens interval in adults is usually ≤3 mm; however, in children <8 years of age, an atlantodens

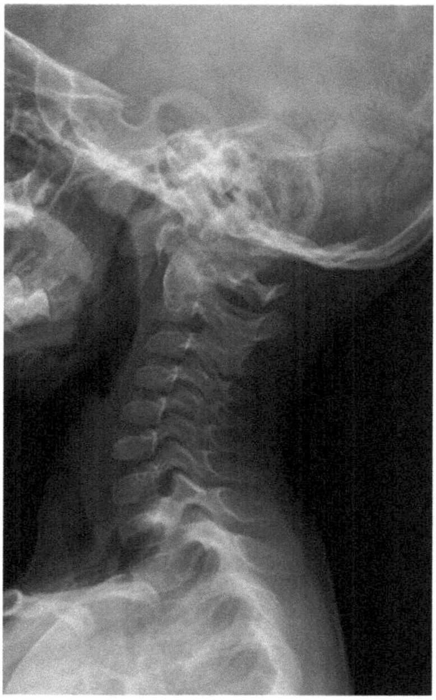

Fig. 11.2 Lateral cervical spine radiograph demonstrating mild pseudo-subluxation of C2 on C3

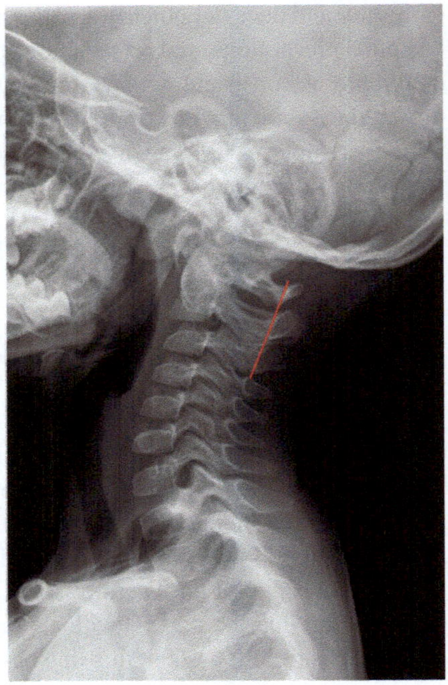

Fig. 11.3 Same X-ray as seen in Fig. 11.2. with Swischuk's (spinolaminar) line showing normal alignment

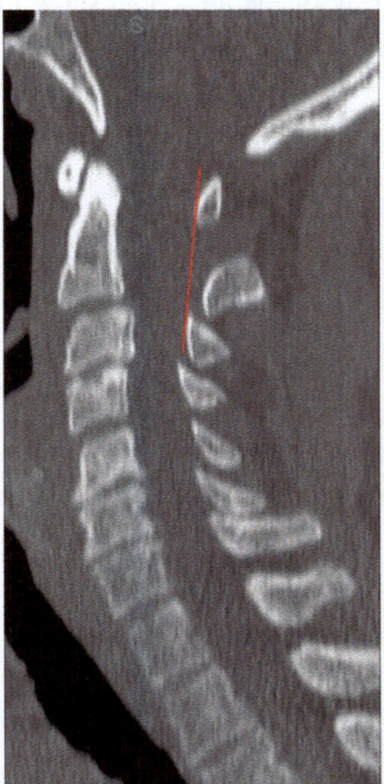

Fig. 11.4 Sagittal image of CT scan showing abnormal spinolaminar line representing injury at C2–C3

interval of 3–5 mm is seen in about 20 % of patients [9]. Understanding normal physes is another challenge unique to children. Unfused C1 ring apophyses, apical odontoid epiphysis, and secondary centers of ossification of the spinous processes can all be mistaken for fractures. Generally normal physes are smooth structures with sclerotic subchondral lines, whereas fractures are more irregular and lack sclerotic lines. In children under age 8 years, anterior wedging of the vertebral bodies up to 3 mm is within normal limits. Wedging can be most pronounced at C3 due to hypermobility of the pediatric cervical spine with increased motion especially at C2–C3.

Although multiple reports have recommended cervical spine CT scan as the preferred screening tool for adult trauma patients, demonstrating quicker time to diagnosis and a shorter stay in the trauma resuscitation area compared to plain films, there remains some question with pediatric patients [10–15]. There is concern, especially in pediatric patients, regarding the radiation dose from CT scanning. A missed cervical spine injury, however, can have lifelong devastating consequences, and therefore CT scan may be used when clinical suspicion for injury is high. A recent review of 1307 pediatric trauma patients compared CT scan to plain X-rays in diagnosing cervical spine fractures [10]. The study found CT scan had a sensitivity of 100 % and a specificity of 98 %, while X-rays had a sensitivity of 62 %. The authors concluded that "CT scans should be the primary modality to image a cervical spine injury." The study also looked at flexion/extension views, and the authors stated that "flexion/extension views did not add to the decision making for C-spine clearance after CT evaluation and are probably not needed" [10]. CT scan is likely most effective in older children and adolescents, where injury patterns are similar to adults. Younger children, however, are more prone to purely ligamentous or soft tissue injury, which may not be appreciated on CT scan. In these patients magnetic resonance imaging (MRI) may be the modality of choice to identify injury. One study of MRI in 64 pediatric cervical spine patients found MRI demonstrated injury in 24 % of patients where X-rays were normal and allowed for spine clearance in three children where CT scan was equivocal [16].

The question of radiation exposure from CT scan in pediatric patients merits consideration. One study prospectively examined radiation exposure in pediatric patients undergoing CT versus conventional radiographs [17]. The authors found a 1.25 higher effective radiation dose with CT scan. Another study comparing CT scan to X-rays found a higher radiation dose with CT for patients with a Glasgow Coma Scale >8, but for those with a GCS <8 the doses were equivalent due to the higher need for repeated radiographs [15]. Although CT scans produce more radiation than plain radiographs, there are ways to shield patients, and by following these protocols, CT exposure can be reduced by 30–50 % in pediatric patients compared to adults with no loss in the quality of images [18, 19]. For most pediatric patients with low suspicion for cervical spine injury, however, three view plain radiographs have been shown to suffice and should constitute the initial radiographic evaluation [20].

Fractures

Cervical spine fractures are relatively rare in athletic events, especially in younger children. Most pediatric cervical fractures result from motor vehicle accidents or falls. In children 8 or less, it is very uncommon to see a subaxial fracture from athletics. The atlantoaxial complex is most at risk in younger children, with the majority of serious injuries involving a ligamentous disruption rather than fracture. Axial compression with extension can potentially cause a fracture of the ring of C1, but the forces required to do so are rarely seen in youth sports. Similarly, odontoid fractures can occur, usually from a rapid deceleration with flexion mechanism, but the forces in youth sports rarely are high enough to cause such injury. When fractures of the odontoid occur, they tend to happen through the synchondrosis of C2 at the base of the odontoid. These fractures tend to displace anteriorly, and reduction can usually be accomplished through immobilization of the cervical spine in extension. In adolescents the cervical anatomy approaches that of adults, and subaxial fractures are occasionally seen with the most common being a compression fracture. More severe burst patterns can also occur. When these compression/burst injuries happen, they tend to occur between C5 and C7, a result of the increased forces on this portion of the spine as the anatomy matures.

The incidence and pattern of cervical spine fracture vary by sport. In the United States, football accounts for the highest number of catastrophic cervical spine injuries due in part to the annual participation in the sport of approximately 1.8 million athletes [21]. The incidence of cervical injury per 100,000 players is actually higher in gymnastics and hockey. The rate of cervical spine injury in football has changed over time. From 1971 to 1975, the National Football Head and Neck Injury Registry recorded 259 cases of cervical fractures (4.14/100,000) and 99 cases of quadriplegia (1.58/100,000) [22]. In 1976 rule changes banning headfirst contact were implemented by the National Collegiate Athletic Association and high school football governing bodies. From 1976 to 1987, the rate of cervical injuries decreased almost 70 % at the high school level from 7.72/100,000 to 2.31/100,000. The rate of quadriplegia decreased 82 %. Over the 25 years, from 1977 to 2001, 223 football players sustained a catastrophic cervical spine injury with either no or incomplete recovery with 183 of those occurring in high school athletes, 29 in college, seven professional, and four recreational players [23].

Understanding the mechanism resulting in cervical spine fracture is important in an effort to reduce the incidence. In football it has been recognized for some time that the headfirst tackle with the neck flexed is a vulnerable position that can lead to axial loading of a straightened spine. When the spine is extended or in neutral position, compressive forces can often be dissipated through the paravertebral musculature and ligaments. When the same force is applied to a straightened spine, the energy is primarily transferred to the vertebrae, and buckling or fracture dislocation of the spine can occur. Most of these fractures occur in the lower cervical spine. As football helmets and face masks evolved in the 1960s, the head was able to be used as a weapon in tackling, and this change likely contributed to the increased rate of cervical spine fractures in the early 1970s. In ice hockey, the rate of catastrophic cervical spine injury was relatively low prior to 1980. From 1982 to 1993, ice hockey saw an increasing rate of cervical injury, again likely related to increased head and face protection making the neck more vulnerable [21]. In ice hockey a common mechanism of cervical spine fracture is headfirst contact into the boards, often when a player has been checked from behind. Rule changes were enacted prohibiting checking from behind a player who no longer has the puck. Data from the Canadian registry suggest that following those changes, major spinal injury and quadriplegia resulting from these illegal techniques decreased [24].

Neuropraxias

Neuropraxias are more common than fractures in youth sports. A "stinger" or "burner injury" is the most common neurologic injury and involves a temporary burning sensation and/or weakness in a single upper extremity. Collision sports such as football and rugby pose the highest risk for stingers. In younger athletes a stinger most commonly results from a forced stretching of the head and neck away from the involved limb resulting in traction to the brachial plexus with the C5 and C6 roots most commonly affected. In older adolescents and adults, the stinger more commonly results from a forced compression of the head and neck toward the involved limb. The shoulder may simultaneously be forced upward, causing a momentary narrowing of the cervical foramen and resulting in a pinching or compression of the nerve root and transient radiculopathy. Kelly et al. have shown that some children have congenital narrowing of the cervical foramen, placing them at increased risk of sustaining a burner [25]. Athletes who have sustained a stinger typically report immediate burning and weakness in the involved extremity and report a "dead arm" sensation. Both sensory and motor function typically return to normal within seconds to minutes with full recovery by 10 min the rule. With repetitive injury permanent damage can occur, and rarely with a severe cervical pinch mechanism, a nerve root(s) can be severed.

Cervical cord neuropraxias are important to differentiate from stingers. Stingers are limited to a single upper extremity, whereas cervical cord neuropraxias typically present with transient quadriplegia and either loss of sensation in all four extremities or a burning or tingling sensation. Motor function usually recovers within minutes, but sensory changes can last longer. Athletes with a congenital narrowing or stenosis are thought to be at increased risk of cervical cord neuropraxias. Although the determination of cervical stenosis is an area of some controversy, general consensus holds that between C3 and C7 the anteroposterior (AP) spinal canal heights in adolescents and adults are normal above 15 mm and stenotic below 13 mm. Resnick et al. have stated that CT and myelography are more sensitive than plain X-rays in determining spinal stenosis [26]. They note that X-rays fail to appraise the width of the spinal cord and cannot detect when stenosis results from ligamentous hypertrophy or disc protrusion. Ladd and Scranton state that the AP diameter of the spinal canal is "unimportant" if there is total impedance of the contrast medium [27]. For all these reasons, spinal stenosis cannot be ruled out based only on bony measurements. "Functional" spinal stenosis, defined as the loss of the cerebrospinal fluid around the cord or in more extreme cases deformation of the spinal cord, whether documented by contrast CT, myelography, or MRI, is a more accurate measure of stenosis [28]. The term functional is taken from the radiographic term "functional reserve" as applied to the protective cushion of cerebrospinal fluid (CSF) around the spinal cord in a normal spinal canal.

Cervical spinal stenosis in the athlete may be a congenital/developmental condition or may be caused by acquired degenerative changes in the spine. For the athlete with severe stenosis and no CSF around the spinal cord on MRI, it is this author's opinion that collision sports should be avoided. The athlete with spinal stenosis is at risk for neurologic injury during hyperextension of the cervical spine [29]. When the neck is hyperextended, the sagittal diameter of the spinal canal is further compromised by as much as 30 % by infolding of the interlaminar ligaments. Matsuura et al. studied 42 athletes who sustained spinal cord injury and compared them to 100 controls [30]. They found that "the sagittal diameter of the spinal canals of the control group was significantly larger than those of the spinal cord injured group." Eismont et al. have stated that "the sagittal diameter of the spinal canal in some individuals may be inherently smaller than normal, and … this reduced size may be a predisposing risk factor for spinal cord injury" [29]. The idea that spinal stenosis predisposes to spinal cord injury is not new, with multiple authors as far back as the 1950s reaching the same conclusion including Wolfe et al. [31], Penning [32], Alexander et al. [33], Mayfield [34], Nugent [35], and Keenan et al. [15] who stated that "patients who have stenosis of the cervical spine should be advised to discontinue participation in contact sports." More recent support for this stand comes from the National Center for Catastrophic Sports Injury Research, where cases of quadriplegia have been seen in athletes with cervical stenosis but without fracture or dislocation. In athletes with a normal-size canal, quadriplegia has not been seen without fracture/dislocation of the spine. And most importantly, full neurologic recovery has been observed in 21 % of athletes who were rendered initially quadriplegic after fracture/dislocation with normal-size cervical canals, while complete neurologic recovery has not been seen in any athlete after fracture/dislocation and quadriplegia when spinal stenosis was documented by MRI.

Ligamentous Injury

Cervical instability due to ligamentous disruption may prove challenging to diagnose immediately after injury in the youth or adolescent athlete. As previously mentioned, some degree of laxity can be normal in children, and muscle spasm following injury may prevent initial subluxation of the cervical spine. Atlantooccipital dislocation is a serious injury in children with a mortality rate of approximately 50 % [36]. Fortunately this injury is quite rare in sports and typically results from distraction forces more typically seen in high-speed motor vehicle collisions (see Fig. 11.5). The atlantooccipital joint is less stable than the lower cervical joints, with the alar ligaments, joint capsule, and the tectorial membrane serving as the primary stabilizers. The basion-dental interval (BDI) or distance from the basion to the tip of the odontoid as seen on a lateral radiograph can be used to assess for atlantooccipital dislocation (see Fig. 11.6). A BDI >12.5 mm is indicative of injury, although this measurement is not as reliable in children less than 5 years of age [37, 38]. Atlantoaxial injury can occur as the C1–C2 articulation is also relatively less stable than lower cervical joints. The transverse ligament runs posterior to the odontoid and limits anterior translation of C1. The apical and two alar ligaments serve to limit rotation around the odontoid. The atlantodens interval (ADI) or distance from the anterior aspect of the odontoid to the posterior cortex of the C1 anterior ring should measure <5 mm in children less than 8 years of age and <3 mm in older children and adolescents [39]. With injury to the transverse ligament, the ADI will increase, causing a decrease in the space available for the cord, but provided the apical and alar ligaments are intact, translation will usually be limited and spinal cord compression is rare.

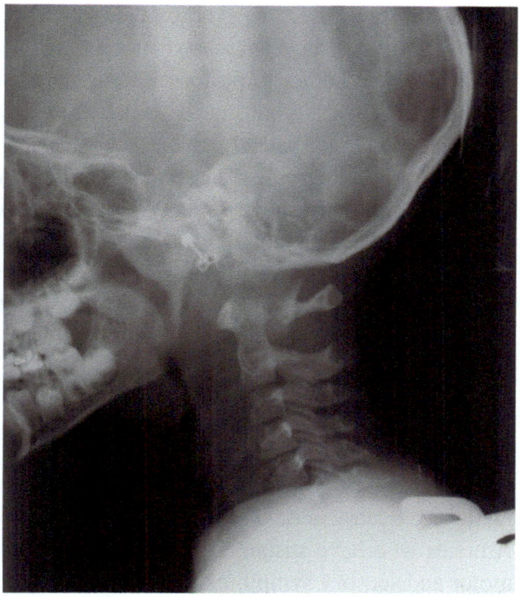

Fig. 11.5 Lateral c-spine X-ray showing atlantooccipital dislocation

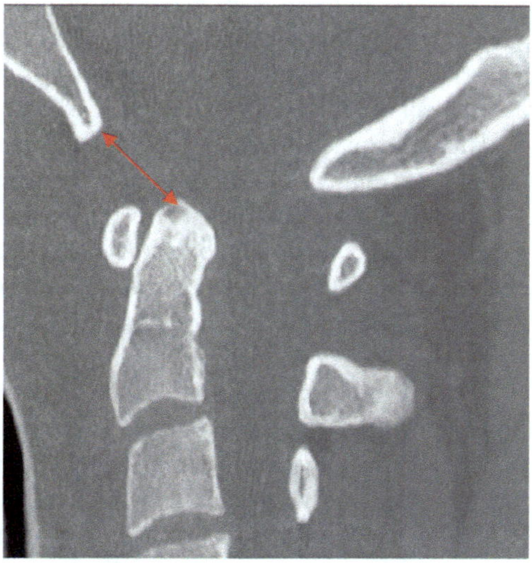

Fig. 11.6 Representation of abnormal basion-dental interval as seen on CT scan

Atlantoaxial rotatory subluxation involves a rotational deformity of C1 on C2. This condition can be seen with trauma or secondary to infection such as Grisel's syndrome. A young athlete with atlantoaxial subluxation will present with the neck flexed to one side and rotated toward the other. The odontoid-view X-ray will show asymmetry of the lateral masses; the lateral mass that is more anterior will appear wider and closer to midline. CT scan usually provides the most complete view of the injury, including the degree of facet subluxation.

The athlete with Down syndrome deserves special consideration. Individuals with Down syndrome have increased mobility at the occipitocervical and atlantoaxial articulations. Whether to perform radiographic screening of the child or adolescent athlete with Down syndrome is a matter of debate. Many of the Special Olympic organizations require lateral flexion and extension radiographs for athletes in high-risk sports such as diving, equestrian, and soccer [40]. Athletes with normal radiographs may participate without restrictions, but those with an increased atlantodens interval should avoid high-risk sports. For athletes in low-risk sports with normal neck and neurologic exam, radiographic screening is generally not recommended. As Herman has stated, "for many of these special athletes, the value of participation in safe and well-supervised sports and recreational programs outweighs the potential risks of injury related to cervical hypermobility" [40].

Treatment

Definitive treatment of cervical injuries depends on the type and level of involvement. Athletes who have sustained a stinger can generally return to competition when all motor and sensory symptoms have cleared and they have full painless cervical range of motion. In rare cases the motor and sensory symptoms of a stinger last more than a few minutes. In these cases magnetic resonance imaging of the spine should be considered to look for a herniated disc or other compressive pathology. If symptoms persist more than 2 weeks, then electromyography (EMG) can allow for an accurate assessment of the degree and extent of injury.

Transient quadriplegia or any bilateral motor or sensory symptoms after injury necessitates removal of the athlete from competition and further diagnostic evaluation. CT scanning can identify subtle fractures or malalignment, but may not show ongoing extrinsic cord compression or intrinsic cord abnormalities; MRI is the most sensitive study to evaluate for these conditions. Somatosensory-evoked potentials may prove useful in documenting physiological cord dysfunction. Definitive treatment depends on the pathology identified.

Treatment of cervical spine fractures also depends on the type and level of injury. Some bony injuries, such as spinous process fractures or unilateral laminar fractures, may require no treatment or only immobilization in a cervical collar. Others, such as the bilateral pars interarticularis fracture of C2 ("hangman's fracture"), may be treated with a cervical collar or halo vest immobilization. Unstable injuries such as fracture dislocations should initially be reduced and temporarily stabilized with cervical traction using Gardner-Wells tongs or a halo ring device. Surgical treatment may subsequently be required for severely comminuted vertebral body fractures, unstable posterior element fractures, type 2 odontoid fractures, incomplete spinal cord injuries with canal or cord compromise, and in those patients with progression of their neurologic deficit [41].

Treatment of the spinal cord-injured patient depends on the underlying injury. Injury to the spinal cord involves an initial mechanical disruption of axons, blood vessels, and cell membranes which is then followed by secondary injury involving further swelling and inflammation, ischemia, free radical production, and cell death. Only prevention can limit the initial injury and treatment is focused on preventing secondary damage. In a review of 57 rugby players who sustained an acute spinal cord injury, most commonly due to facet dislocations, five out of eight who underwent reduction of the injury within 4 h had compete neurologic recovery, whereas 0 out of 24 who were reduced beyond 4 h had complete recovery [42].

Return to Play

The return-to-play decision depends largely on the type and extent of injury. The athlete with a cervical ligament sprain or muscle strain/contusion with no neurologic or osseous injury can return to competition when he or she is free of neck pain with and without axial compression, has full range of motion, and neck strength is normal. Cervical radiographs should show no subluxation or abnormal curvature. It is preferable that the athlete is asymptomatic and can perform at his pre-injury ability prior to returning to competition.

The athlete who has sustained a stinger-type injury should be held out until motor and sensory symptoms have resolved and there is full and painless cervical range of motion. If residual symptoms are present or if there is concern for neck injury, return to play should be deferred. Athletes with brachial plexus injuries may be considered healed and safe for return to play when their neurologic examination returns to normal and they are symptom-free. An athlete with a permanent neurologic injury should be prohibited from further competition.

The athlete who has sustained transient motor or sensory symptoms (neuropraxia) bilaterally or in an arm and leg must have a cervical spine MRI to rule out a spinal cord injury or a condition that puts the spinal cord at risk. If the cervical MRI is normal, the athlete can return to competition when free of neurological symptoms, free of neck pain with and without axial compression, has full range of motion with normal neck strength, and the neurologic exam is normal. Even with complete resolution of symptoms and a normal exam, having had such an event would be considered by some a relative risk for return to play. For the athlete who has had three such events, most would agree this is an absolute contraindication to return.

For the athlete who has sustained a cervical spine fracture, return to play is deferred at least until the fracture has healed. Generally, stable fractures managed non-operatively, such as those involving a spinous process or a unilateral lamina that has healed completely, will allow the player to return to competition by the next season. Athletes with a healed fracture who have required halo vest or surgical stabilization as part of the treatment are considered to have insufficient spinal strength to safely return to contact sports, unless formal testing demonstrates it has returned to normal. Even after the fracture has healed and strength has returned, the altered biomechanics in surrounding spinal segments may produce an increased risk of further sports-related injury. If there is a one-level anterior or posterior fusion for a fracture, athletes are usually allowed to go back when neck pain is gone, the range of motion is complete, muscle strength of the neck is normal, and the fusion is solid.

It is the general opinion that when multilevel fusions or a fusion involving C1–C2 or C2–C3 are involved, return to contact or collision sports is contraindicated. The athlete could return to non-contact sports with low risk of neck injury, such as golf or tennis.

Conclusion

Cervical spine injuries in young athletes range from mild muscle contusions to severe fracture dislocations with neurologic compromise. Given the potential for serious injury, when in doubt it is better to hold the athlete out until all appropriate diagnostic testing is performed. Younger children have different anatomy than adults with unfused apophyses and generally more lax ligamentous structures which may make radiographic diagnosis more challenging. MRI can prove useful to rule out ligamentous injury when plain radiographs are equivocal and can also help to determine if there is any soft tissue compression of the spinal cord. Return to competition after an injury is an individual decision, but as a general guideline all symptoms should have resolved, neurologic exam should be normal, cervical motion and strength should be normal, and imaging of the cervical spine should not show any residual instability or functional stenosis.

References

1. Dompier TP, Powell JW, Barron MJ, Moore MT. Time-loss and non-time-loss injuries in youth football players. J Athl Train. 2007;42(3):395–402.
2. Meehan 3rd WP, Mannix R. A substantial proportion of life-threatening injuries are sports related. Pediatr Emerg Care. 2013;29(5):624–7.
3. Leonard JR, Jaffe DM, Kuppermann N, Olsen CS, Leonard JC, for the Pediatric Emergency Care Applied Research Network (PECARN) Cervical Spine Study Group. Cervical spine injury patterns in children. Pediatrics. 2014;133(5):e1179–88.
4. Swenson TM, Lauerman WC, Blanc RO, et al. Cervical spine alignment in the immobilized football player: radiographic analysis before and after helmet removal. Am J Sports Med. 1997;25:226–30.
5. Treme G, Diduch DR, Hart J, et al. Cervical spine alignment in the youth football athlete-recommendations for emergency transportation. Am J Sports Med. 2008;36(8):1582–6.
6. Swartz EE, Mihalik JP, Beltz NM, Day MA, Decoster LC. Face mask removal is safer than helmet removal for emergent airway access in American football. Spine J. 2014;14(6):996–1004.
7. Delaney JS, Al-Kashmiri A, Baylis P, et al. The assessment of airway maneuvers and interventions in university Canadian football, ice hockey, and soccer players. J Athl Train. 2011;46(2):117–25.
8. Shaw M, Burnett H, Wilson A, Chan O. Pseudosubluxation of C2 on C3 in polytraumatized children: prevalence and significance. Clin Radiol. 1999;54(6):377–80.
9. Eubanks JD, Gilmore A, Bess S, Cooperman DR. Clearing the pediatric cervical spine following injury. J Am Acad Orthop Surg. 2006;14(9):552–64.
10. Rana AR, Drongowski R, Breckner G, Ehrlich PF. Traumatic cervical spine injuries: characteristics of missed injuries. J Pediatr Surg. 2009;44:151–5.
11. Nunez D, Zuluaga A, Fuentes-Bernardo D, et al. Cervical spine trauma: how much more do we learn by routinely using helical CT. Radiographics. 1996;16:1307–18.
12. Hoffman JR, Mower WR, Wolfson AB, et al. Validity of a set of clinical criteria to rule out injury to the cervical spine in patients with blunt trauma. N Engl J Med. 2000;343:94–9.

13. Gale SC, Gracias VH, Reilly PM, et al. The inefficiency of plain radiography to evaluate the cervical spine after blunt trauma. J Trauma. 2005;59:1121–5.
14. Griffen MM, Frykberk ER, Kerwin AJ, et al. Radiographic clearance of blunt cervical spine injury: plain radiograph or computed tomography scan. J Trauma. 2003;55:222–7.
15. Keenan HT, Hollingshead MC, Chung CJ, et al. Using CT of the cervical spine for early evaluation of pediatric patients with head trauma. Am J Roentgenol. 2001;177:1405–9.
16. Flynn JM, Closkey RF, Mahboubi S, et al. Role of magnetic resonance imaging in the assessment of pediatric cervical spine injuries. J Pediatr Orthop. 2002;22(5):573–7.
17. Adelgais KM, Grossman DC, Langer SG, et al. Use of helical computed tomography for imaging the pediatric cervical spine. Acad Emerg Med. 2004;11:228–36.
18. Kamel IR, Hernandez RJ, Martin JE, et al. Radiation dose reduction in CT of the pediatric pelvis. Radiology. 1994;190:683–7.
19. Chan CY, Wong YC, Chau LF, et al. Radiation dose reduction in paediatric cranial CT. Pediatr Radiol. 1999;29:770–5.
20. Nigrovic LE, Rogers AJ, Adelgais KM, Olsen CS, Leonard JR, Jaffe DM, et al. Utility of plain radiographs in detecting traumatic injuries of the cervical spine in children. Pediatr Emerg Care. 2012;28(5):426–32.
21. Banerjee R, Palumbo MA, Fadale PD. Catastrophic cervical spine injuries in the collision sport athlete, Part 1. Am J Sports Med. 2004;32(4):1077–87.
22. Torg JS, Quedenfeld TC, Burstein A, et al. National football head and neck injury registry: report on cervical quadriplegia, 1971 to 1975. Am J Sports Med. 1979;7:127–32.
23. Cantu RC, Mueller FO. Catastrophic spine injuries in American football, 1977–2001. Neurosurgery. 2003;53:358–63.
24. Tator CH, Carson JD, Edmonds VE. Spinal injuries in hockey. Clin Sports Med. 1998;17:183–94.
25. Kelly 4th JD, Aliquo D, Sitler MR, et al. Association of burners with cervical canal and foraminal stenosis. Am J Sports Med. 2000;28:214–7.
26. Resnick D. Degenerative disease of the spine. In: Diagnosis of bone and joint disorders. Philadelphia: W.B. Saunders; 1981. p. 1408–15.
27. Al L, Scranton PE. Congenital cervical stenosis presenting as transient quadriplegia in athletes. J Bone Joint Surg. 1986;68:1371–4.
28. Cantu RC. Functional cervical spinal stenosis: a contraindication to participation in contact sports. Med Sci Sports Exerc. 1993;25:316–7.
29. Eismont FJ, Clifford S, Goldberg M, et al. Cervical sagittal spinal canal size in spinal injury. Spine. 1984;9:663–6.
30. Matsuura P, Waters RL, Adkins S, et al. Comparison of computed tomography parameters of the cervical spine in normal control subjects and spinal cord-injured patients. J Bone Joint Surg. 1989;71:183–8.
31. Wolfe BS, Khilnani M, Malis L. The sagittal diameter of the bony cervical spinal canal and its significance in cervical spondylosis. J Mt Sinai Hosp N Y. 1956;23:283–92.
32. Penning L. Some aspects of plain radiography of the cervical spine in chronic myelopathy. Neurology. 1962;12:513–9.
33. Alexander MM, Davis CH, Field CH. Hyerextension injuries of the cervical spine. Arch Neurol Psychiatry. 1958;79:146.
34. Mayfield FH. Neurosurgical aspects of cervical trauma, Clinical neurosurgery, vol. II. Baltimore: Williams and Wilkins; 1955.
35. Nugent GR. Clinicopathologic correlations in cervical spondylosis. Neurology. 1959;9:273–81.
36. McCall T, Fassett D, Brockmeyer D. Cervical spine trauma in children: a review. Neurosurg Focus. 2006;20(2), E5.
37. Bulas DI, Fitz CR, Johnson DL. Traumatic atlanto-occipital dislocation in children. Radiology. 1993;188(1):155–8.
38. Jarris Jr JH, Carson GC, Wagner LK. Radiologic diagnosis of traumatic occipitovertebral dissociation: 1. Normal occipitovertebral relationships on lateral radiographs of supine subjects. Am J Roentgenol. 1994;162(4):881–6.

39. Jones TM, Anderson PA, Noonan KJ. Pediatric cervical spine trauma. J Am Acad Orthop Surg. 2011;19:600–11.
40. Herman MJ. Cervical spine injuries in the pediatric and adolescent athlete. Instr Course Lect. 2006;55:641–6.
41. Maroon JC, Bailes JE. Athletes with cervical spine injury. Spine. 1996;21:19.
42. Newton D, England M, Doll H, et al. The case for early treatment of dislocations of the cervical spine with cord involvement sustained playing rugby. J Bone Joint Surg Br. 2011;93-B:1646–52.

Cervical Disc Disease

12

Pierre A. d'Hemecourt and Courtney Gleason

Introduction

A spectrum of cervical disc injuries and changes may occur in young athletes. This spectrum includes disc degeneration, annular tears, and disc herniation. These pathologic changes may affect neurologic integrity and be reflected with radicular (peripheral) or central (myelopathic) nerve injury. Due to the potential for devastating outcomes from cervical spine injuries, it is important to recognize symptoms associated with cervical spine compromise in the setting of athletics to minimize the risk of permanent neurologic sequela. This chapter will review disc pathology and its considerations in the athletic population.

Cervical Disc Disease and Biomechanics

In the human axial skeleton, there are 25 discs interposed between each vertebra from the cervical spine to the sacrum. The discs assist with motion and stability of the spine and act as shock absorbers to mechanical loads [1]. The intervertebral discs become progressively larger moving from the cervical, thoracic, and finally to the lumbar spine [2]. The discs are largely made up of three components: the annular ligaments on the outside, the nucleus pulposus on the inside, and the endplates

P.A. d'Hemecourt, M.D. (✉)
Division of Sports Medicine, Boston Children's Hospital, Boston, MA, USA
e-mail: Pierre.DHemecourt@childrens.harvard.edu

C. Gleason, M.D.
Division of Sports Medicine, Rhode Island Hospital, Warren Alpert School of Medicine, Brown University, Providence, RI, USA
e-mail: courtneyngleason@gmail.com

M. O'Brien, W.P. Meehan III (eds.), *Head and Neck Injuries in Young Athletes*, Contemporary Pediatric and Adolescent Sports Medicine,
DOI 10.1007/978-3-319-23549-3_12

at the cranial and caudal margins of the vertebrae [1]. The outer annulus fibrosis is composed of 15–25 layers of concentric lamellae arranged in parallel to collagen fibers [1]. The outer annulus fibrosis is 90 % type I collagen [1, 3]. There is a transition from a predominance of type I collagen to type II collagen moving from the outer to inner annulus fibrosis [1]. The annulus fibrosis encircles the central portion of the disc, referred to as the nucleus pulposus. The nucleus pulposus is composed of a random arrangement of type II collagen surrounding high levels of proteoglycans which gives the nucleus pulposus its soft cartilaginous or gelatinous properties [1]. The nucleus pulposus is particularly important for shock absorption to the spine and allows for motion [1]. The cartilaginous endplates are positioned at the cranial and caudad margins of the vertebral body and attach to the intervertebral discs. The endplates separate the annulus and nucleus pulposus from the vertebral body [2, 3]. There is no blood supply to the intervertebral discs; therefore, the endplate provides the nutrition to the disc from hydrostatic pressure during motion [2].

Because of unique biomechanical and anatomic factors, there is generally a different pattern of injury to the cervical spine in children when compared to adults [4, 5]. The majority of spinal injuries in the pediatric population occur in the cervical spine (60–80 %) [4, 5]. In children under 8 years of age, injuries frequently occur at the C3 level or above [4, 5]. In adults, the majority of injuries to the cervical spine involve C5 or below [4–6]. In the child and adolescent athlete, the endplates are composed of soft growth cartilage and are susceptible to injury [2]. The cartilaginous end plate is typically the first structure to fail with compressive loads in the adolescent athlete [3].

The orientation of the facet joints changes between the cervical and lumbar spine to allow for functional differences between the upper and lower spine. The cervical facets are aligned in an axial plane to allow for an increase in rotational motion. The lumbar facets are sagittally oriented for flexion and extension [7]. The most devastating injuries in sports often involve axial load with cervical flexion. These types of injuries are one of the main reasons that "spear tackling" in football was outlawed. These injuries have been associated with unstable fractures and dislocation, which can also involve the soft tissue disc and ligamentous structures [2, 7].

Degenerative Disc Disease

Intervertebral discs undergo a number of natural changes over time which may or may not be associated with pain or loss of function [2, 8, 9]. For example, many discs will undergo gradual disc desiccation and loss of hydration of the nucleus pulposus resulting in loss of disc height and a darker appearance on MRI images [2, 9]. Generally, these are benign normal findings as the spine ages and do not correlate with injury or pain [2]. In asymptomatic individuals in the general population younger than 40 years old, MRI changes suggestive of cervical disc degeneration is present in an estimated 25 % of people [8, 10]. Certain athletic endeavors may hasten the normal physiologic progression of disc disease or contribute to injury for the patient [8]. Repetitive axial compressive and torsional forces from sports place athletes at risk for disc degeneration [11]. For instance, cervical spine injuries are estimated to occur in 4–10 % of football players [3, 7, 10]. Conversely, non-contact sports may decrease the likelihood of disc disease due to better postural stability and control [12].

Degenerative disc disease is associated with loss of the annular ligament strength. This leads to instability with excessive motion and stress to the vertebrae above and below [2, 9, 13] the affected disc. In addition, disc desiccation and dehydration is associated with a loss of disc height, which may predispose to foraminal narrowing and/or spinous process abutment syndrome. The degenerative process of the cervical disc is a bit unique from the thoracic and lumbar spine due to the uncovertebral articulation of the cervical spine. Here, the posterolateral aspect of the vertebral body forms boney projection towards the adjacent vertebrae and forms a unique pseudarthrosis called an uncovertebral joint. The degenerative or spondylosis that occurs with the disc collapse causes protrusion of this pseudarthrosis posteriorly into the neuroforamina worsening the lateral stenosis. The neuroforamina is further compromised by the facet joint degeneration posteriorly in the foramina. As such, the nerve root becomes compressed from anterior and posterior degeneration. When this occurs, it is referred to as lateral or foraminal stenosis. When the disc degeneration protrudes centrally, it is referred to as central stenosis. When nerve roots are compressed, the patient will likely complain of radiating pain or paresthesias, and possibly weakness in the corresponding dermatome.

A variant of disc degeneration involves an isolated tear to the annulus. In an isolated annular ligament tear, the nucleus pulposus remains intact, but there is a tear in the outer annulus where there are pain fibers [2]. Therefore, a tear of the cervical annular ligament is commonly associated with neck pain. Annular tears may extend from the nucleus pulposus through the annulus to the periphery of the disc and may be either from an acute traumatic episode or from chronic overuse [2, 11].

The clinical presentation of disc degeneration is variable. Disc desiccation itself is typically not painful initially, but can become painful as disc degeneration progresses. Initially, athletes may have less pain with activity and more pain at rest. Athletes may also have radiating pain if the nerve roots are compressed as they exit through narrowed foramen. This is exacerbated during sports but also with daily activities such as working on a computer with a chin forward posture, which compresses the neuroforamina and facet joints.

With disc degeneration, the physical exam findings will often include pain with axial loading of the spine. The facet joints may also be tender if they are involved in the process of degenerative spondylosis. Most often the neurologic exam is normal unless there is significant stenosis with existing foraminal stenosis.

The clinical evaluation of these athletes will include with plain radiographs including an AP, lateral and open mouth odontoid views. These may demonstrate loss of disc height and vertebral osteophytes. At times there may even be a subluxation of one vertebra over the subjacent vertebrae. In this setting, flexion and extension views are helpful in detecting instability. The MRI findings in cervical disc degeneration will include at least one of the following: decrease in signal intensity of disc, anterior compression of dura and spinal cord, posterior disc protrusion, disc space narrowing, and/or foraminal stenosis [14].

The treatment of degenerative disc disease will often involve a conservative program of postural strengthening of the cervical spine and upper trunk. Biomechanics of the sport and classroom ergonomic factors are also addressed, as these are often instrumental in the exacerbation of the pain. Non-steroidal anti-inflammatory medications (NSAIDS) may be adjunctive. Significant stenosis with radicular or myelopathic symptoms are discussed below.

Disc Herniation

Cervical disc herniations occur when part of the nucleus pulposus extrudes beyond the confines of an intact annular ligament and into the spinal canal. Depending on the size, the position of the disc herniation within the spinal canal, and the vertebral level at which the herniation occurs, athletes may be asymptomatic, or may complain of a wide variety of pain and or weakness. Disc injuries in the cervical spine occur most frequently at C5-6 and C6-7 [2, 6]. If the herniated disc protrudes laterally and impinges upon a cervical nerve root as it exits the spinal canal through the spinal foramen, an athlete will complain of radicular symptoms into the shoulder, arm, or hand [13, 15]. The radiation of pain will follow a specific pattern determined by the level of disc herniation and nerve root affected (Table 12.1). If the disc herniation or protrusion is more centralized and does not affect the nerve roots, there may be axial pain associated with neck or upper back pain [2, 15]. In more extreme instances of centralized cervical disc herniation, myelopathy can result. Cervical disc herniation in athletes is one of a number of possible causes for cervical radiculopathy and myelopathy. Radiculopathy and myelopathy are discussed in the next sections.

Typically, treatment for cervical disc herniation is conservative and includes a combination of rest, anti-inflammatories, and activity modification [13]. In any case of suspected disc herniation, it is important to assess for neurological deficits including persistent pain, paresthesias, or progressive weakness. Imaging should be performed if there are persistent symptoms lasting longer than 6 weeks in the adult or 3 weeks in a child [2], or earlier if there are progressive or severe neurological symptoms. An MRI is usually the most appropriate imaging tool, but a CT scan can be done if an MRI cannot be performed [2].

Table 12.1 Radicular patterns

Nerve root	Sensation	Motor	Reflex
C5	Lateral aspect of upper arm	Deltoid and biceps muscles	Biceps
C6	Thumb, index finger, lateral forearm	Biceps, wrist extensors, brachioradialis	Brachioradialis
C7	Middle finger	Triceps, wrist flexors	Triceps
C8	Little finger	Finger flexion	None
T1	Medial aspect upper arm	Finger adduction and abduction	None

Radiculopathy

Radiculopathy is defined as pain and peripheral neurological deficits within a specific nerve root distribution [16]. In radiculopathy, peripheral symptoms of arm pain, numbness/tingling, and/or weakness generally exceed symptoms of neck pain [16]. Radicular symptoms are expected to be reproducible, and may be acute or chronic. They can present as isolated pain, numbness, or weakness or a combination of these symptoms [16]. Depending on the etiology of cervical radiculopathy, patients may present with a single nerve root affected, multiple levels affected, or bilateral symptoms [16]. Radicular symptoms are typically affected by neck position. Commonly, athletes will report exacerbation of symptoms with lateral rotation of the neck, lateral flexion/bend, and neck extension [16].

Vascular connective tissue surrounds cervical nerve roots and protects the nerve roots from injury [5]. Cervical radiculopathy results from compression or injury to the cervical nerve roots as they exit the cervical foramen. Compression can be caused by multiple etiologies including disc herniation, cervical foraminal stenosis from degenerative arthritis, or from other less common etiologies such as infection, tumor, or fracture [17]. In contrast to these compressive etiologies, there are occasions in sports where radiculopathy may occur from excessive traction forces applied along the length of the nerve root [5]. Some of these peripheral nerve traction injuries are described as "stinger" or "burners" and are described in more detail in other parts of this book.

On physical exam, a positive Spurling's test is described as reproduction of symptoms with axial loading of the cervical spine with the neck in hyperextension and ipsilateral rotation [16]. Spurling's maneuver consists of two steps: it begins with axial loading with the neck in extension. If radicular symptoms are not reproduced with neck extension, the second part of the test is performed and consists of rotation of the extended neck toward the symptomatic arm. The test is positive if radicular symptoms are elicited [17]. Spurling's maneuver is positive in 25–50 % of patients with discogenic radiculopathy [16]. The head compression test can also be helpful in diagnosing radiculopathy. Symptoms may improve with axial traction (10–15 lb) or elevation of the hands above the head [15, 16, 18]. The shoulder abduction test involves abducting the arm and putting the patient's hand behind their head. This test is considered positive confirmation of cervical radiculopathy if this maneuver relieves the patient's radicular pain or numbness (Bakody's sign) [17, 18].

Clinical evaluation of radiculopathy includes evaluation of cervical nerve roots to identify which levels are affected. A brief review of cervical nerve root distributions is given in Table 12.1 [15–18].

The work-up of radiculopathy includes plain radiographs and an MRI. Electromyography (EMG) may be helpful when multiple disc levels or dermatomes are affected. It may also be helpful when a coexisting peripheral nerve impingent is involved such as a carpal tunnel syndrome with a C-6 radiculopathy. This situation, where nerve symptoms are potentiated by a more proximal nerve compromise is often called a double crush syndrome.

After confirming the diagnosis with an MRI, athletes with herniated discs frequently respond to conservative, nonoperative treatment including relative rest, NSAIDs, and physical therapy. For severe or refractory symptoms sometimes oral or injectable corticosteroids are considered [10]. If conservative measures fail or if neurologic symptoms progress, surgical decompression may be needed. In the setting of radiculopathy, three clinical situations warrant surgical consideration: progressive motor weakness, loss of bowel or bladder control (extremely rage, but emergent), and refractory symptoms. The latter situation is somewhat subjective. In severe pain, this may be as early as 6–8 weeks. In moderate cases, it may be months before surgery is considered [2]. In most instances of cervical disc herniation, surgery to include an anterior cervical discectomy and fusion is the standard of care [10]. Surgical management of far lateral cervical disc herniations that do not respond to conservative treatment usually includes minimally invasive posterior foraminotomy and nerve root decompression [10].

Return to Play Criteria

Return to play decisions in the athlete with radiculopathy should be made with care. Typically, one must rule out any instability from associated fractures or ligamentous instability. The athlete should attain a full range of motion with full strength and resolution of numbness. A multi-level fusion is an absolute contraindication to contact sports, while a single level is a relative contraindication.

Myelopathy

Cervical myelopathy involves compromise of the spinal cord secondary to spinal stenosis. Etiologies of spinal stenosis range from centralized disc herniation, spondylotic spurs, congenitally narrow spinal canal, tumor, or cervical spine fracture or dislocation [17]. Myelopathy is less common than radiculopathy. The sequelae seen in cervical myelopathy results from the interplay of multiple factors including canal narrowing, vascular compromise, and intermittent mechanical compression from repetitive motions [16].

The most common presentation of myelopathy is central cord syndrome [17]. Athletes should be asked about gait disturbances, stumbling, widely based gait, loss of balance, loss of manual dexterity (for example, difficulty with buttoning their shirt, or change in handwriting), problems with bowel and bladder control, and the presence of numbness, weakness, or pain in their upper or lower extremities [17]. On exam, pain and reproduction of neurologic symptoms are typically reproduced with axial compression of the flexed head and cervical spine, called L'hermitte's sign. A positive Hoffman's sign or Babinski sign indicates upper motor neuron findings and spinal cord compromise. Strength in the muscle groups of the bilateral upper extremities including intrinsic hand muscles should be precisely assessed. A positive Froment's sign is an indication of intrinsic weakness and is evaluated by adduction strength of the thumb and first digit. A positive test (intrinsic weakness) is typically seen with obligatory flexion of the thumb IP joint when attempting to tightly grasp a sheet of paper. In cases of prolonged cervical myelopathy, decreased muscle bulk and atrophy of the intrinsic muscles of the hands may also be seen. It should be noted that coexisting radiculopathy and myelopathy may occur.

If cervical myelopathy is suspected, the imaging modality of choice is magnetic resonance imaging (MRI). Changes in signal intensity will be seen in the spinal cord with cervical myelopathy. If an MRI cannot be obtained, a contrast CT scan is indicated. Obtaining an EMG may help differentiate the radiculopathic component. Medical evaluation may also be done concomitantly to rule out other potential etiologies of neurologic signs and symptoms such as diabetes, demyelinating disorders, and other systemic neurologic disorders.

The treatment for myelopathy will most often involve a cervical decompression and fusion. The presence of myelopathy usually excludes the athlete from collision sports.

Rehabilitation Considerations for Cervical Disc Disease

The considerations for cervical disc rehabilitation should follow a stepwise sequence. The cervical spine can be very sensitive to an initial intense program that involves aggressive motion. The stages are often divided into the acute, sub-acute, progressive, and sport specific phases. Initially, in the more acute phase, analgesics and NSAIDS and traction may be used to quiet the inflammation. Once the acute inflammation is improved, isometric strengthening is started. This involves the core, upper trunk and cervical muscles. Once this is well tolerated, low resistance exercises with progressive range of motion are started. The next step involves gradual progression towards increased resistance in both open and closed chain involvement. Finally, the sport specific phase is initiated.

Since the disc involves inflammatory components, an anti-inflammatory medication is very useful, along with analgesics. Oral corticosteroids or epidural corticosteroid injections may be very useful in accelerating the recovery phase. Intermittent traction has been found to be quite helpful in some cases. Acupuncture has also been used as an adjunct for treating the pain component and accelerating rehabilitation.

Critical Relationship to Stingers and Transient Quadriparesis

Stingers and transient quadriparesis are discussed in subsequent chapters. However, it is important to recognize that disc disease may play a role in these clinical entities. Stingers are common injuries in collision sports such as football. Players typically complain of searing or burning pain and/or numbness or tingling starting in the area of the trapezoid. The symptoms typically course down into the arm with transient loss of function and, occasionally, temporary paralysis in the affected arm [5, 7, 17]. There are two common patterns of injury resulting in stingers. Stingers caused by forced extension and ipsilateral rotation produce radicular symptoms felt in shoulder and arm of the ipsilateral side head motion. This results in compression of the nerve root(s) as it exits the foramina and is most common in the older athlete [17]. Degenerative disc processes described above may contribute to this compression in adult athletes. However, in contrast to the compression seen in older athletes, the mechanism most common in younger adolescents involves a set of circumstances that creates a traction effect. Typically, a contralateral neck flexion with ipsilateral shoulder depression results in a stretch to the nerve roots and brachial plexus. The symptoms occur on the ipsilateral side to the shoulder depression [7] and are not usually related to disc degeneration.

Transient quadriparesis, also called cervical cord neuropraxia (CCN), involves transient functional disruption of the spinal cord [7]. In contrast to a stinger that causes unilateral symptoms in an extremity as a result of injury to nerve roots, transient quadriparesis results in bilateral symptoms below the level of involvement as a result of direct spinal cord injury [7]. The mechanism of injury of transient quadriparesis involves hyperextension of the cervical spine resulting in transiently decreased diameter of the spinal canal and compression of the spinal cord [7]. Cervical disc disease can certainly play a role in some cases when the central canal is diminished due to disc protrusion.

References

1. Chan WC, Sze KL, Samartzis D, Leung VY, Chan D. Structure and biology of the intervertebral disk in health and disease. Orthop Clin North Am. 2011;42(4):447–64, vii.
2. D'Hemecourt PA. Intervertebral disk disease. In: Micheli LJ, editor. Encyclopedia of sports medicine. Thousand Oaks: Sage; 2011. p. 719–22.
3. Micheli L, Young S, D'Hemecourt P. Lumbar spine injuries. In: Garrick JG, editor. OKU orthopaedic knowledge update: sports medicine 3. 3rd ed. Rosemont: American Academy of Orthopaedic Surgeons; 2004. p. 19–27.
4. Kelly B, Snyder B. Anatomy and development of the young spine. In: Micheli LJ, Stein CJ, O'Brien M, D'Hemecourt P, editors. Spinal injuries and conditions in young athletes. New York: Springer; 2014. p. 1–15.
5. Jagannathan J, Dumont AS, Prevedello DM, Shaffrey CI, Jane Jr JA. Cervical spine injuries in pediatric athletes: mechanisms and management. Neurosurg Focus. 2006;21(4):E6.
6. Krabak BJ, Kanarek SL. Cervical spine pain in the competitive athlete. Phys Med Rehabil Clin N Am. 2011;22(3):459–71, viii.
7. Light D, Kerr H. Spinal injuries in collision/heavy contact sports. In: Micheli LJ, Stein CJ, O'Brien M, D'Hemecourt P, editors. Spinal injuries and conditions in young athletes. New York: Springer; 2014. p. 75–87.
8. Triantafillou KM, Lauerman W, Kalantar SB. Degenerative disease of the cervical spine and its relationship to athletes. Clin Sports Med. 2012;31(3):509–20.
9. Ferrara LA. The biomechanics of cervical spondylosis. Adv Orthop. 2012;2012:493605.
10. Boden BP, Jarvis CG. Spinal injuries in sports. Phys Med Rehabil Clin N Am. 2009;20(1):55–68, vii.
11. Cooke PM, Lutz GE. Internal disc disruption and axial back pain in the athlete. Phys Med Rehabil Clin N Am. 2000;11(4):837–65.
12. Mundt DJ, Kelsey JL, Golden AL, Panjabi MM, Pastides H, Berg AT, et al. An epidemiologic study of sports and weight lifting as possible risk factors for herniated lumbar and cervical discs. The Northeast Collaborative Group on Low Back Pain. Am J Sports Med. 1993;21(6):854–60.

13. Zmurko MG, Tannoury TY, Tannoury CA, Anderson DG. Cervical sprains, disc herniations, minor fractures, and other cervical injuries in the athlete. Clin Sports Med. 2003;22(3): 513–21.
14. Okada E, Matsumoto M, Ichihara D, Chiba K, Toyama Y, Fujiwara H, et al. Aging of the cervical spine in healthy volunteers: a 10-year longitudinal magnetic resonance imaging study. Spine (Phila Pa 1976). 2009;34(7):706–12.
15. Hoppenfeld S. Evaluation of nerve root lesions involving the upper extremity. In: Hoppenfeld S, Hutton R, editors. Orthopaedic neurology: a diagnostic guide to neurologic levels. Philadelphia: Lippincott; 1977. p. 7–44.
16. Zeidman S, Ducker T. Evaluation of patients with cervical spine lesions. In: Clark CR, Ducker TB, Dvorak J, Garfin SR, Herkowitz HN, Levine AM, et al., editors. The cervical spine. 3rd ed. Philadelphia: Lippincott-Raven; 1998. p. 143–61.
17. Bradley J, Tibone J, Watkins R. History, physical examination, and diagnostic tests for neck and upper extremity problems. In: Watkins RG, Williams L, Lin P, Elrod B, Kahanovitz N, editors. The spine in sports. St. Louis: Mosby; 1996. p. 71–81.
18. Van Zundert J, Huntoon M, Patijn J, Lataster A, Mekhail N, van Kleef M, et al. Cervical radicular pain. Pain Pract. 2010;10(1):1–17.

Facial Fractures and Epistaxis

13

James P. MacDonald and Jane P. Sando

Overview

Facial injuries are commonly seen in youth athletes. Overall, the incidence of facial bone fractures is lower in the pediatric than in the adult population, with one large, national series showing that pediatric patients make up only 14.7 % of all facial fractures [1]. The frequency of facial fractures increases with age: only 5.6 % occur in youth younger than 5, while 55.9 % of all pediatric facial fractures occur in the 15- to 17-year age group [1].

There are a number of reasons that are thought to contribute to these differences, including a larger cranium-to-face ratio in children, underdeveloped paranasal sinuses, unerupted secondary teeth which provide stability to the mandible and maxilla, comparatively more compliant bones than seen in adults, and relatively thicker adipose and muscle tissue in the face of children [2].

Despite these protective factors, sports commonly cause facial fractures and epistaxis in youth. The incidence of such athletic injuries in adolescents approaches that seen in adults. One study found that 42 % of all facial fractures in youth were sports related [3]. The incidence of such injuries is much greater in males than in females, with upwards of 88 % of all youth sports-related facial fractures occurring in boys [3]. Common sports resulting in pediatric facial injuries often involve either a ball acting as a projectile or are collision sports, for example, baseball, basketball, football, martial arts, racquetball, rugby, skiing/snowboarding, soccer, and softball [3–5].

J.P. MacDonald, MD, MPH (✉)
Division of Sports Medicine, Department of Pediatrics, Nationwide Children's Hospital, 5680 Venture Drive, Dublin, OH 43017, USA
e-mail: jmacdmd@gmail.com; james.macdonald@nationwidechildrens.org

J.P. Sando, MD
Department of Pediatric Emergency Medicine, Johns Hopkins Hospital, Baltimore, MD, USA
e-mail: jane.hee.park@gmail.com; jamepark@post.harvard.edu

M. O'Brien, W.P. Meehan III (eds.), *Head and Neck Injuries in Young Athletes*, Contemporary Pediatric and Adolescent Sports Medicine,
DOI 10.1007/978-3-319-23549-3_13

Fractures of the nose are the third most commonly fractured bone in the entire body, and the nose is the most commonly fractured bone in the face [6]. The most common traumatic high school sport injury of the nose is a fracture: in one series, 77 % of all nasal injuries were fractures and over 7 % of fractures of all types seen in this group occurred in the nose [7]. Softball is the most common cause of sports-related nasal fracture in youth athletes [6]. The mandible is the second most commonly fractured facial bone [8, 9]. It is the body site most often requiring surgical treatment for fracture in high school athletes: 65 % of such fractures require surgery [7]. The orbit is not uncommonly injured in sports and there may be associated injury to the eye. Up to 600,000 sports-related eye injuries are reported in the United States every year [4]. Though seen less commonly than other maxillofacial fractures, frontal bone fractures can be a serious injury with sports second only to motor vehicle accidents as a cause [10]. Epistaxis, or nosebleeds, is a common, non-bony injury of the nose especially seen in contact sports.

Assessment begins with a history. The sport involved, the details of the injury, the time interval between injury and assessment, and associated signs and symptoms should be ascertained. Though the history is often straightforward, when youth sustain facial injuries, consideration should be given to the possibility of assault or abuse. A relevant inquiry should be initiated if indicated.

The general management of such diverse injuries begins with a primary survey, as the airway can be compromised with nasal or oral trauma [11]. The fundamental "ABCs" of trauma management should be conducted: establishing a patent *a*irway, verifying a stable *b*reathing and *c*irculatory status, and making appropriate interventions as indicated. After determining that airway, breathing and circulation are not compromised, a secondary survey should be initiated. Nearly a third of pediatric patients with a facial fracture sustain a concussion, and so a high index of suspicion should be maintained when a young athlete sustains a facial fracture [12]. When indicated, the Standardized Concussion Assessment Tool 3 (SCAT3) should be administered, and appropriate management instituted [13]. Cervical spine precautions should be instituted for any athlete who is unconscious, complaining of persistent neurological symptoms in the extremities or is complaining of bony tenderness of the cervical spine. The eyes may have been injured, and so consideration should be given to performing a basic ophthalmological examination, including visual acuity and pupillary reaction at a minimum. Formal ophthalmological consultation may be necessary.

It should be remembered that individual facial fractures often do not occur in isolation [5]. Thus, when assessing a youth athlete for one of the injuries discussed in this chapter, the entire maxillofacial region should be examined thoroughly [10]. Maxillofacial fractures should also prompt a clinician to inquire about an individual's tetanus status. Tetanus toxoid should be given if previous immunization was last given more than 5 years ago (for deep and/or contaminated wounds) or 10 years ago (for all other wounds) [14].

When discussing return-to-play decisions in young athletes with these injuries, it should be noted that there is a lack of evidence, and no specific consensus guidelines exist. One set of recommendations is based on the known biology of facial bony healing [15] and is found in Table 13.1. Athletes have been returned to sport more quickly than indicated by these guidelines when using protective equipment

Table 13.1 General return-to-play criteria for adolescent athletes recovering from a facial fracture

Step	Duration	Activity allowed
1	Day 0–20	Activities of daily living
2	Day 21–30	Aerobic activity
3	Day 31–40	Noncontact, sport-specific drills
4	Day 41–on	Full-contact practice and game play may be considered[a]

[a]Martial artists should avoid their sport for 3 months

n.b. Athlete must remain asymptomatic at each step prior to progressing to next step

such as face shields, but no evidence-based standards exist for this practice, most especially in youth athletes [16].

Nasal Bone Fractures

Anatomically, the nose is a structure with two nasal passages separated by a midline septum comprised primarily of cartilage. The lower two-thirds of the nose is soft tissue, and the upper third is supported by the nasal bones, which articulate in the midline. Superiorly, these bones are attached to the frontal bone of the face, and laterally, they are attached to the maxilla [17]. Children's noses are structurally different than adults' noses, with the former being comprised predominantly of compliant cartilage; consequently, in young children, nasal fractures are uncommon [17]. As the bony anatomy of the adolescent nose more closely resembles that of the adult, the incidence of nasal bone fractures rises.

The history is typically straightforward, with an obvious mechanism such as a ball or blow from another athlete striking the nose either directly or tangentially. As discussed elsewhere, one must always begin an examination with a primary survey emphasizing the ABCs of trauma, ensuring there is an adequate airway, and controlling the possible bleeding. On inspection, there is usually an obvious deformity and, often, associated epistaxis. Palpation of the nose and maxillofacial structures is done to assess crepitus or deformity of the nasal bone. Uncommon findings include evidence of cerebrospinal fluid (CSF) leakage and potential signs and symptoms of concomitant injury, such as diplopia (seen with orbital fractures), mental status changes (seen with intracranial pathology), or malocclusion (seen with other maxillofacial injuries) [18]. If the presence of CSF is suspected, the confirmatory laboratory analysis is the beta-2 transferrin test [19].

Crucial to the examination of a nasal fracture is an internal assessment of the nasal septum to rule out a septal hematoma, a condition which should not be missed. On direct visualization, such hematomas appear as bulging, bluish masses in the nasal septum [11]. Following nasal trauma, with or without a bony fracture, children are especially susceptible to septal hematoma and its complications [6]. The flexible nasal cartilage of youth athletes can buckle under deforming forces, producing a separation between the perichondrium and the cartilage, and a hematoma can form in this potential space [6]. Separated from its overlying nutrition, the septal cartilage can necrose and perforate; eventually, a patient may develop the dreaded complication of a saddle nose deformity [17]. If a septal hematoma is identified, it should be aspirated or incised immediately using local anesthesia [20].

There is a limited role for imaging in such injuries. Despite a lack of sensitivity and specificity of plain films for this condition, X-rays are frequently obtained and rarely alter management (Fig. 13.1). Computerized tomography (CT) scans have much greater sensitivity and specificity, but are not justified in isolated nasal fractures given the associated cost and radiation exposure; CT scans do, however, play a role in the patient who has sustained extensive maxillofacial trauma (Fig. 13.2) [6].

Treatment of nasal bone fractures begins with controlling bleeding (see section on epistaxis), treating associated soft tissue injuries, and achieving adequate analgesia. Non-displaced nasal fractures may require no further treatment, whereas significantly displaced fractures typically will undergo closed or open reduction with the goals being realignment of the cartilaginous and bony structures to decrease discomfort and maximize airway patency [20]. In pediatric patients specifically, fractures should be reduced within 3–5 days, as later reduction may be more challenging [17]. Closed reductions are occasionally performed by primary care clinicians as well as specialists; the details of the procedure are beyond the scope of this book [18]. When aesthetic concerns are paramount, either (1) an open reduction or (2) a closed reduction followed by expected rhinoplasty should be chosen [17].

Prompt attention is needed for nasal bone fractures, but with adequate treatment and protection, such injuries do not always require immediate or extended removal from sports. Table 13.2 describes return-to-play conditions for the youth athlete pre- or post-definitive management [11].

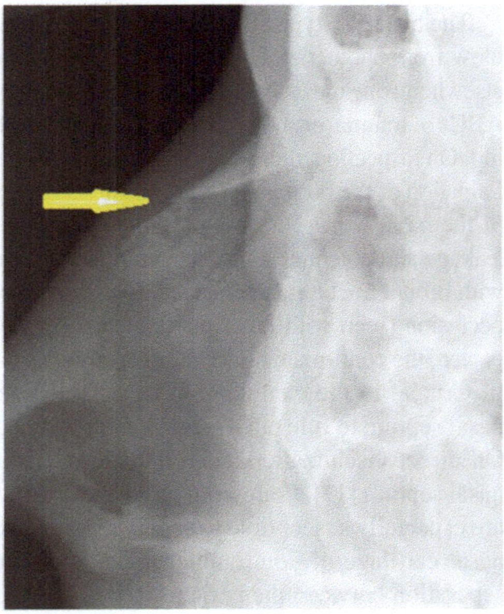

Fig. 13.1 Plain film of nasal fracture in a 16-year-old boy who was punched

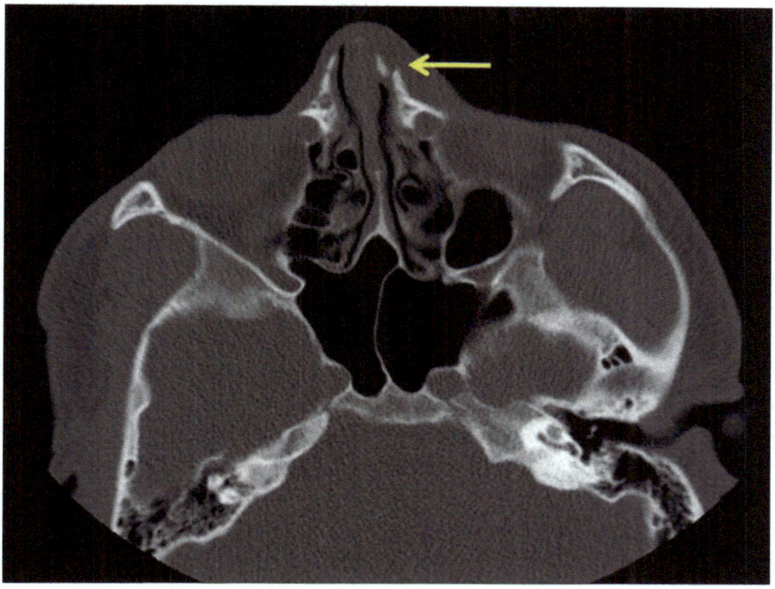

Fig. 13.2 CT scan of nasal fracture in a 13-year-old boy injured while playing basketball

Table 13.2 Return-to-play criteria for adolescent athletes with a nasal fracture

1	Fracture should be closed (no associated laceration)
2	Adequate hemostasis has been achieved and a septal hematoma has been ruled out
3	The athlete and his/her parents understand the risk for worsening injury and adequate assent/consent have been obtained
4	The athlete wants to return to play
5	Adequate analgesia has been achieved
6	There exist no visual concerns: visual acuity is baseline; visual fields are full; there is no diplopia
7	Protective headgear/face mask is recommended

Mandible Fractures

The mandible has six defined anatomic regions including the symphysis or parasymphyseal region, body, ramus, angle, the coronoid process, and the condyles. Mandible fractures are categorized based on which of these regions are affected. More than 50 % of patients with trauma to the mandible will have fractures in more than one area [21]. Fractures of the condyle are more common in children less than 10 years old, whereas fractures of the symphysis, body, and ramus increase in frequency with age [22].

The history usually involves a forced occlusion: a fall with the chin striking a surface or a blow, from an object or another player, from the lateral or frontolateral direction. After assessing and addressing the ABCs of trauma, physical examination should begin with inspection of the soft tissues. The clinician should note the presence of edema, ecchymosis, hematoma, and lacerations (especially at the chin) and should inspect the oral cavity for the presence of dental injuries/avulsion of the teeth, ecchymosis of the floor of the mouth, lacerations of the mucosa, and integrity of the gingiva. This should be followed by palpation of the entire mandible, intraorally and extraorally, and the temporomandibular joints (TMJ) while the patient opens and closes the mouth to assess the condyles. The examiner should also evaluate occlusion as well as voluntary mandibular mobility, noting deviations on mouth opening and pain and/or difficulty with opening. Sensation should be tested as patients may have numbness of the lip, teeth, and chin (associated with injury to the inferior alveolar nerve) or of the anterior tongue, lip, and cheek mucosa (associated with injury to the lingual or long buccal nerves) [23]. Patients may also present with drooling. Malocclusion may not be obvious on exam; thus, asking a patient about subjective perception of malocclusion may be useful [24]. Patients may be unable to bite down and hold a tongue depressor between their teeth if there is malocclusion [24, 25]. It must be remembered that a force great enough to fracture the mandible is capable of causing injury to other organ systems, and so a thorough secondary examination of the face and body should be done [26].

Diagnosis can be made with plain film radiographs and CTs. Radiographs have been advocated as the study of choice in isolated mandible fractures [23]. Panoramic radiographs are desirable because they provide an excellent image of the entire mandible; however, they are not always available in emergency departments. Panoramic radiographs also require the patient to sit upright in a steady position. If a patient is unable to sit for this study or if it is unavailable, alternate views can be utilized. These include the Towne's (anterior/posterior projection to look at the condyles) posteroanterior, bilateral oblique, lateral, and submentovertex views [23]. CT with axial and coronal cuts allows for accurate visualization of the injury (Fig. 13.3), and three-dimensional (3D) reconstruction can be valuable for preoperative assessment and surgical planning [8]. CT should be done for patients with significant trauma and suspicion of fractures of other facial bones.

The management of mandible fractures will differ based on multiple variables. These include fracture location, complexity (e.g., displacement, comminution, number of sites), the presence of malocclusion, and the patient's age and stage of skeletal and dental development [27]. The primary goal of treatment is reestablishment of occlusion. Children with primary or mixed dentition are often treated more conservatively as surgical repair can damage tooth buds and result in maldevelopment of permanent teeth [28]. In adolescent patients, the treatment objective is to establish the best alignment of bony fragments with the least invasive technique [21]. Mandible fractures may be treated with closed reduction and maxillomandibular fixation, which is when the upper and lower jaws are temporarily connected by wires, elastic bands, or metal splints. Fractures with greater degrees of displacement may require surgical correction with open reduction and internal fixation (ORIF)

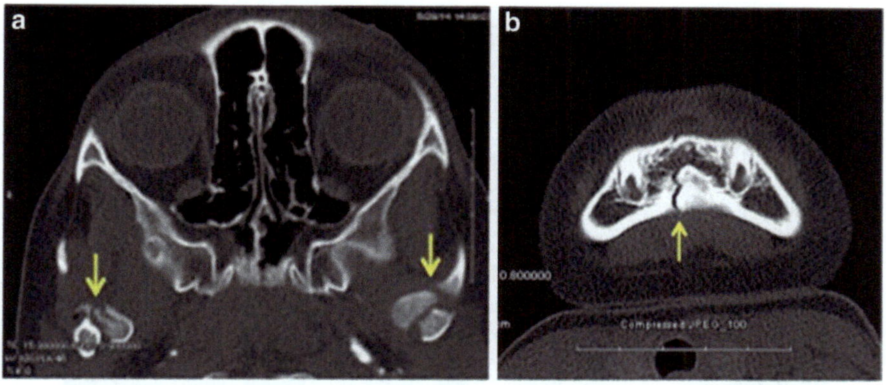

Fig. 13.3 6-year-old female who fell off a bicycle and struck her chin on the ground. (**a**) CT scan showing bilateral mandible condylar fractures. (**b**) CT scan showing an additional parasymphyseal fracture

[21]. Adolescents have a greater potential for regeneration and remodeling compared to adults, and so fixation duration may be shorter [26]. Antibiotics that cover oral flora are recommended for open fractures, such as those with intraoral lacerations, disruption of gingiva, or dislodgement of teeth [23].

Nutritional intake must be monitored and optimized during healing as oral intake may be anatomically compromised and poor nutritional status could hinder the healing process [26]. Frequent postoperative follow-up is recommended to detect and treat complications such as infection, malocclusion, malunion, or nonunion. Patients must also be monitored for long-term complications such as damage to permanent teeth, growth disturbance, mandibular hypoplasia, neurosensory changes, TMJ dysfunction, and ankylosis in condylar fractures (the inability to open the jaw more than 5 mm) [21, 26, 27]. Return-to-play guidelines in this chapter's Overview section may be followed.

Orbital Fractures

The orbit is the bony cavity that holds the eyeball and its associated tissues and appendages. Orbital fractures occur with direct blunt trauma to the globe and orbital rim. Fractures of the orbit may involve the bony structures making up the rim or the orbital walls. Orbital fractures may occur as isolated injuries, though they are often associated with more complex fractures including those involving the anterior cranial vault, naso-orbitoethmoid, or zygomatic complex and Le Fort injuries [9, 29]. The orbital rim is composed of three bony regions: frontal, zygomatic, and nasoethmoidal maxillary. The walls that make up the orbital cavity are the superior (or roof), inferior (or floor), medial, and lateral. The orbital floor is the most frequently fractured (Fig. 13.4) [30, 31] followed by the medial wall [9]. Orbital roof fractures occur in younger children who lack frontal sinus pneumatization and have larger craniofacial ratios; these fractures have a higher likelihood of associated neurocranial injuries [29, 32]. Pressure to the orbital rim may fracture just the orbital walls, which is called a

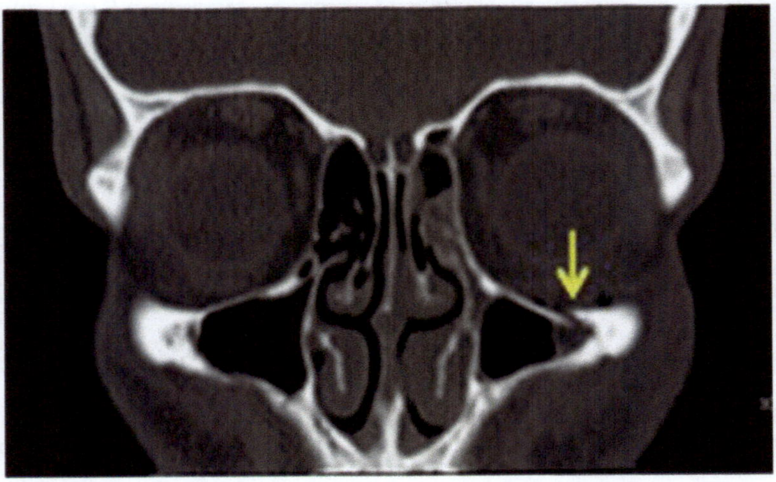

Fig. 13.4 CT scan of an orbital floor fracture in a 16-year-old male struck by a baseball

"blowout fracture." Blowout fractures can result in entrapment of one or more soft tissue structures, which limits vertical motility and causes diplopia and enophthalmos (posterior displacement of the globe resulting in a sunken appearance). Blowout fractures with minimal displacement of the bone fragment are more common in the pediatric population [30] and are termed "trapdoor fractures." These occur when a circular segment of the orbital wall may fracture and become displaced but remain attached on one side. Entrapment of orbital contents can occur in these injuries.

The typical history includes an object, such as a baseball or elbow, striking the periorbital region. Physical examination should begin with inspection noting ecchymosis, edema, and globe position and then follow with palpation of the periorbital rim. A detailed sensory exam including visual acuity testing should be performed and patients should be asked if they have double vision. Signs and symptoms of orbital fractures can be quite varied, and there can be a range of patient presentations, from asymptomatic with minimal bruising and swelling to diplopia, enophthalmos, hypoglobus (downward globe displacement), and hypoesthesia along the maxillary nerve (numbness of the cheek, upper lip, and upper gingiva) [33]. With 14–40 % of patients reportedly suffering from intraocular complications, patients with orbital fractures must receive a complete ophthalmic evaluation to rule out concurrent ocular injury [31, 34, 35] (see chapter on "Eye Injuries"). The "white-eyed blowout" fracture is a pattern seen in pediatric patients. It was first described in 1998 as an orbital floor fracture that has minimal soft tissue signs of trauma (edema, ecchymosis), lacks enophthalmos, and has minimal evidence of floor disruption on imaging exams, but results in marked motility restrictions in vertical gaze suggesting entrapment of the inferior rectus muscle [36]. Nausea and vomiting have been described as another sign of inferior rectus entrapment with some patients exhibiting the oculocardiac reflex (triad of nausea/vomiting, bradycardia, and syncope) [30, 37]. This injury should be considered in children and adolescents with vertical diplopia, gaze restriction, and nausea/vomiting in the setting of periorbital trauma.

CT with thin-cut high-resolution coronal, axial, and sagittal views of the orbits with 3D reconstructions is the most efficacious imaging modality [29]. Plain radiographs are not recommended as they result in a high number of false negatives and nondiagnostic results [33]. MRI is inferior to CT in the evaluation of these injuries, as MRI provides poor visualization of bone. MRI may be useful if a vascular injury is being considered [38].

Orbital fractures are managed both surgically and nonsurgically. Initial management includes cold packs to the site for the first 48 h, use of nasal decongestants, elevation of the head of the bed, avoidance of aspirin, and avoidance of nose blowing. Steroids should be considered as well as antibiotics covering sinus pathogens, such as amoxicillin/clavulanate [33]. Isolated floor fractures that require urgent (within 48 h) repair include (1) diplopia present with radiological evidence of an entrapped muscle or periorbital tissue and nausea/vomiting with or without oculocardiac reflex or (2) the "white-eyed" fracture in a patient less than 18 years old with vertical limitation in eye movement and corresponding radiological evidence of an entrapped inferior rectus muscle or perimuscular soft tissue [30, 36] and early enophthalmos or hypoglobus [37]. It is generally thought that surgery is indicated within two weeks for patients with persistent diplopia, persistent enophthalmos, significant hypo-ophthalmos, and large fractures [37]. Complications include extraocular muscle entrapment, resulting in permanent limitation of eye movements, persistent diplopia, enophthalmos, and impaired binocular vision. All such complications can be difficult to treat later on [9]. There are no set guidelines for return to play after an orbital fracture. Guidelines in the Overview section may be followed if there is no functional or binocular vision loss and the athlete has been cleared by an ophthalmologist.

Zygoma and Maxilla Fractures

Fractures involving the zygomatic and maxillary bones, or "midface" fractures, are much less common in children than adults [8]. In the pediatric population, fractures of the midface region typically do not occur before pneumatization of the maxillary sinus around 5 years of age and are most common in adolescent patients, after pneumatization and growth of the paranasal sinuses have occurred; this is especially true of Le Fort fractures [8, 39].

The zygoma is composed of the malar eminence, or body, and the arch. It attaches to the maxillary, frontal, and temporal bones and forms the infraorbital rim. A zygomaticomaxillary complex (ZMC, tripod, malar) fracture describes a fracture through the frontozygomatic suture, zygomatic arch, infraorbital rim, and zygomatic buttress.

Maxillary fractures have classically been categorized by three fracture patterns described by Rene Le Fort in 1901. In Le Fort Type I, the maxilla is separated from its attachments above the teeth roots; in Type II (pyramidal), the fracture extends superiorly in the midface to include the nasal bridge, maxilla, lacrimal bones, orbital

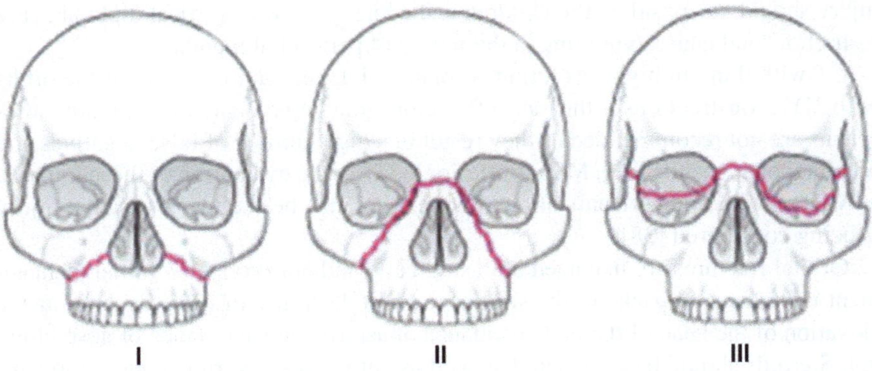

Fig. 13.5 Le Fort classification of midface fractures. **I** Only the lower maxilla; **II** the infraorbital rim; **III** complete detachment of the midface from the skull (craniofacial dissociation). *Source*: Reprinted with permission from the Merck Manual of Diagnosis and Therapy, edited by Robert Porter. Copyright 2013 by Merck Sharp & Dohme Corp., a subsidiary of Merck & Co, Inc., Whitehouse Station, NJ. Available at http://www.merckmanuals.com/professional/. Accessed date 8/26/14

floor, and rim; in Type III (craniofacial dissociation), all attachments of the midface to the skull have been separated (Fig. 13.5). Le Fort maxillary fractures are seen in 5–10 % of pediatric facial fractures [8, 39]. These fractures generally occur as part of a complex facial fracture pattern [9].

Patients with midface fractures incur blunt trauma to the region. Assessment of a patient with midface trauma includes inspection from all vantages, palpation, and manipulation to assess midface instability [40]. Most fractures are associated with overlying soft tissue trauma including laceration, abrasion, and edema. There may be palatal, vestibular, and periorbital ecchymosis and oral mucosa and conjunctival hemorrhage. The midface should be inspected for asymmetry, facial flattening over the malar prominence or zygomatic arch, and elongation of the middle third of the face, a finding associated with Le Fort fractures. Assessment of the eyes may reveal ocular dystopia (uneven pupillary levels). Patients with zygoma fractures may also exhibit painful limitation of mouth opening and pain with forced occlusion as well as malocclusion. Common problems that may be associated with zygomatic complex fractures are similar to those described in the Orbital Fractures section of this chapter. There should be a low threshold for consulting ophthalmology [40]. Mobility of the midface can be assessed by grasping the upper incisor teeth with the index finger and thumb while the forehead and nasal bridge are stabilized with the opposite hand [27].

When a midface fracture is suspected and after the ABCs of trauma are addressed, CT should be done as it provides the detail necessary for accurate diagnosis and surgical planning (Fig. 13.6) [8].

Management of midface fractures is dictated by the severity of the injury and can vary from simple observation to extensive craniofacial reconstruction with bone

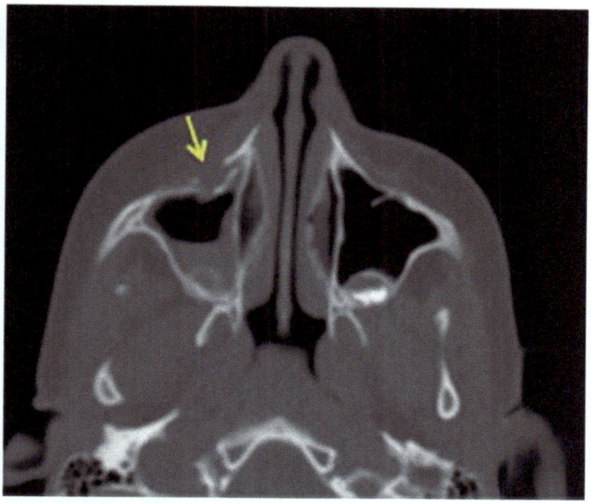

Fig. 13.6 CT scan of a patient struck in the face by another player's knee showing a right maxillary fracture

grafting and rigid fixation [2]. Midface fractures that are not comminuted and are without displacement, disfiguring facial contours, or functional deficits (such as nasolacrimal duct obstruction, vision disturbance from eye muscle entrapment, trismus) may be treated conservatively with observation [2, 37]. There are no specific return-to-play guidelines for midface fractures; thus the guidelines in the Overview section may be followed.

Frontal Bone Fractures

The frontal bone, located above the orbits, contains paired pneumatized cavities, the frontal sinuses. The bone is stronger than the other facial bones and is less apt to fracture [10]. Both the anterior and posterior wall of the sinuses may be damaged. Because of the posterior wall's proximity to the dura mater and frontal lobes of the brain, frontal bone fractures can be quite serious and may result in central nervous system (CNS) complications such as a CSF leak or meningitis. The bone also contains the important frontonasal ducts, which drain each frontal sinus into the middle meatus of the nose [41]. Integrity of this duct is vital for proper functioning of the sinus.

The patient will typically present with focal pain in the frontal bone after a direct hit from a projectile (e.g., baseball) or another player (e.g., elbow or head to face in soccer). On examination, the most common finding is a focal laceration; any ecchymosis in the area should raise clinical suspicion of a frontal bone or sinus injury [10]. The entire forehead should be assessed for the possibility of crepitus or depression of the bony anatomy. As discussed in the section on nasal fractures, with frontal bone fractures, nasal secretions should be examined for the possibility of a CSF leak.

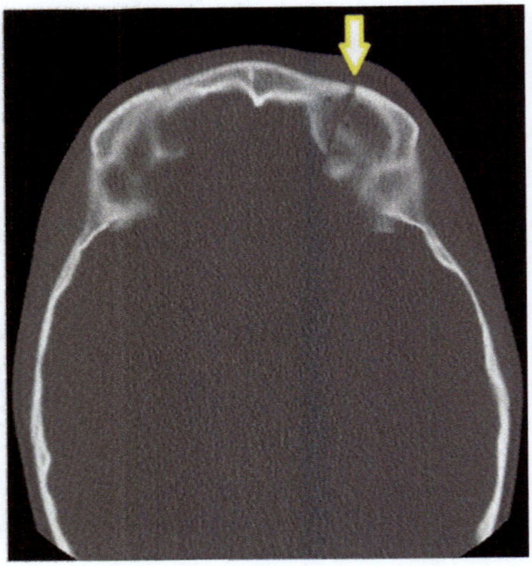

Fig. 13.7 CT scan of frontal bone, demonstrating fracture involvement of both anterior and posterior walls, in an 11-year-old who fell from a height

The clinical examination alone is insufficient to determine the extent of the injury and radiographs are not sufficiently sensitive. Thin-section axial and coronal CT scans are imperative to determine if there has been damage to the posterior wall of the frontal sinus or damage to the frontonasal duct; both findings significantly alter management (Fig. 13.7) [10].

There are limited case reports in the literature for managing young athletes with this injury [41]. Treatment of a frontal bone fracture may be conservative if the anterior wall alone is affected. Specialty referral and/or surgery is mandatory for the following: (1) fracture of the posterior wall, as seen on CT scan; (2) presence of CSF fluid; (3) damage to the frontonasal duct (defect noted on CT imaging and/or retention of mucus or blood in the sinus); and (4) presence of an overlying laceration signifying an open fracture [41]. Inappropriate recognition of these issues may lead to late and serious complications, including mucopyocele, meningitis, and brain abscess [10].

Conservative treatment includes initially ice and rest, and the return-to-play guidelines in this chapter's Overview section may be followed.

Epistaxis

Epistaxis (nosebleeds) is frequently encountered in pediatric athletes, especially athletes who participate in contact or collision sports such as wrestling, basketball, and football [42]. Youth athletes can present with both traumatic and atraumatic epistaxis; the condition may be isolated or recurrent [43]. The focus in this section will be on the management of episodic, traumatic epistaxis. Epistaxis can also be classified by posterior or anterior vascular origins. Posterior epistaxis accounts for only 5–10 % of all nosebleeds and is uncommonly seen in athletes but can be a true emergency [42]. Traumatic, anterior epistaxis accounts for the vast majority of nosebleeds seen in the youth athlete, as the location of the involved arteries makes them particularly vulnerable to direct blows to the nose.

The bony anatomy of the nose has been previously described in this chapter (see Nasal Fractures). The vascular anatomy of the nose is quite complex. Kiesselbach's plexus, an area of the anteroinferior part of the nasal septum where four arteries anastomose, gives rise to the majority of normal epistaxis episodes. Nasal bleeding from trauma can arise from other locations such as the anterior ethmoid artery (a cause of anterior bleeding) and a branch of the sphenopalatine artery (a cause of posterior bleeding) [18]. The highly vascular soft tissue of the nose explains how relatively minor trauma may lead to quite dramatic bleeding.

The evaluation of a youth athlete with an acute episode of epistaxis resembles that described previously in the section on nasal fractures. Assessing for airway compromise and concomitant injuries is imperative. Once hemostasis has been achieved, one must rule out a septal hematoma. If hemostasis is difficult to achieve, consideration should be given to the presence of a posterior bleed, as injury to the sphenopalatine artery can cause more severe, recalcitrant bleeding [42]. Imaging is not indicated for isolated epistaxis.

Management consists primarily of achieving hemostasis, which begins with having the athlete tilt his head forward while applying direct compression to the nostril with or without the use of ice. Patience is advised, as this may require 10–15 min of treatment. Ice may also be applied to the back of the neck, as this causes a reflex vasoconstriction of the nasal vasculature [20]. Nasal decongestant and packing of

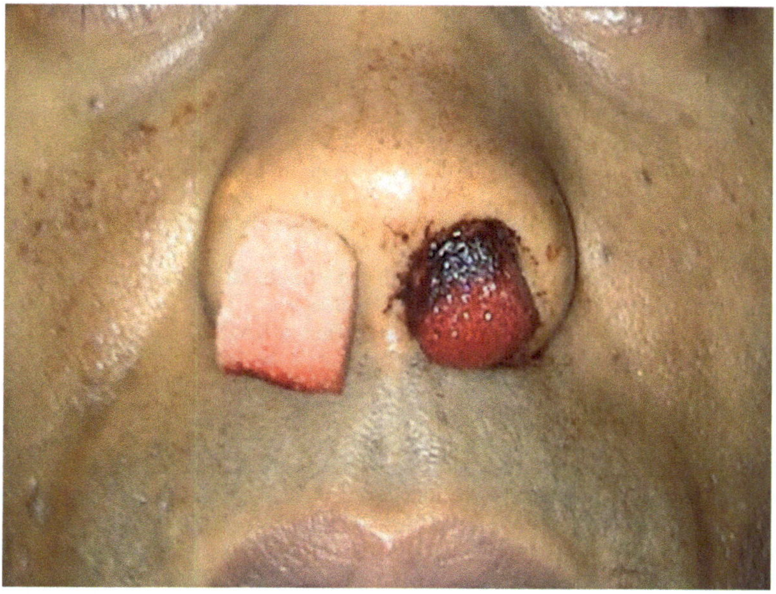

Fig. 13.8 Nasal packing demonstrating recommended positioning both for achieving hemostasis and ease of removal

the affected nostril may be considered for recalcitrant bleeding. Recommended vasoconstrictive decongestants include oxymetazoline and phenylephrine hydrochloride [18]. Although rare, nasal packing has been associated with toxic shock syndrome; therefore it is recommended that packing be covered in a topical antibiotic such as mupirocin and changed regularly [11]. The packing should be left exposed 1.25 cm outside the nostril for ease of removal (Fig. 13.8) [42]. If hemostasis cannot be achieved despite the above measures, a posterior bleed may be present, and specialty referral for arterial ligation or embolization should be considered while continuing to monitor the patient and ensure an adequate airway [20].

Return to play can be considered once adequate hemostasis has been achieved. Given existing concerns and regulations pertaining to the handling of blood-borne pathogens, hemostasis is important not only for a player's own safety but for others as well.

References

1. Vyas RM, Dickinson BP, Wasson KL, Roostaeian J, Bradley JP. Pediatric facial fractures: current national incidence, distribution, and health care resource use. J Craniofac Surg. 2008;19(2):339–49.
2. Krakovitz PR, Koltai PJ. Pediatric facial fractures. In: Bailey BJ, Johnson JT, Newlands SD, editors. Head and neck surgery—otolaryngology. Philadelphia: Lippincott Williams & Wilkins; 2006. p. 1338–48.
3. Perkins SW, Dayan SH, Sklarew EC, Hamilton M, Bussell GS. The incidence of sports-related facial trauma in children. Ear Nose Throat J. 2000;79(8):632–8.
4. Goldstein MG, Wee D. Sports injuries: an ounce of prevention and a pound of cure. Eye Contact Lens. 2011;37(3):160–3.
5. Hwang K, You SH, Lee HS. Outcome analysis of sports-related multiple facial fractures. J Craniofac Surg. 2009;20(3):825–9.
6. Perkins SW, Dayan SH. Management of nasal trauma. Aesthetic Plast Surg. 2002;26 Suppl 1:S3.
7. Swenson DM, Yard EE, Collins CL, Fields SK, Comstock RD. Epidemiology of US high school sports-related fractures, 2005–2009. Clin J Sport Med. 2010;20(4):293–9.
8. Koltai PJ, Rabkin D. Management of facial trauma in children. Pediatr Clin North Am. 1996;43(6):1253–75.
9. Posnick JC, Wells M, Pron G. Pediatric facial fractures: evolving patterns of treatment. J Oral Maxillofac Surg. 1993;51(8):836–44.
10. Yavuzer R, Sari A, Kelly CP, Tuncer S, Latifoglu O, Celebi MC, et al. Management of frontal sinus fractures. Plast Reconstr Surg. 2005;115(6):79e–93e.
11. Romeo SJ, Hawley CJ, Romeo MW, Romeo JP, Honsik KA. Sideline management of facial injuries. Curr Sports Med Rep. 2007;6(3):155–61.
12. Afrooz PN, Grunwalkdt LJ, Zanoun RR, Grubbs RK, Saladino RA, Losee JE, et al. Pediatric facial fractures: occurrence of concussion and relation to fracture patterns. J Craniofac Surg. 2012;23(5):1270–3.
13. McCrory P, Meeuwisse W, Aubry M, Cantu B, Dvorak J, Echemendia RJ, et al. Consensus statement on concussion in sport—the 4th international conference on concussion in sport held in Zurich, November 2012. Clin J Sport Med. 2013;23(2):89–117.
14. Grindel SH. Head and neck. In: McKeag DB, Moeller JL, editors. ACSM's primary care sports medicine. 2nd ed. Philadelphia: Wolters Kluwer; 2007. p. 323.
15. Roccia F, Diaspro A, Nasi A, Berrone S. Management of sport-related maxillofacial injuries. J Craniofac Surg. 2008;19(2):377–82.

16. Reehal P. Facial injury in sport. Curr Sports Med Rep. 2010;9(1):27–34.
17. Desrosiers 3rd AE, Thaller SR. Pediatric nasal fractures: evaluation and management. J Craniofac Surg. 2011;22:1327–9.
18. Kucik CJ, Clenney T, Phelan J. Management of acute nasal fractures. Am Fam Physician. 2004;70(7):1315–20.
19. Prosser JD, Vender JR, Solares CA. Traumatic cerebrospinal fluid leaks. Otolaryngol Clin North Am. 2011;44(4):857–73.
20. Navarro RR, Romero L, Williams K. Nasal issues in athletes. Curr Sports Med Rep. 2013;12(1):22–7.
21. Goodday RH. Management of fractures of the mandibular body and symphysis. Oral Maxillofac Surg Clin North Am. 2013;25(4):601–16.
22. Thoren H, Iizuka T, Hallikainen D, Lindqvist C. Different patterns of mandibular fractures in children. An analysis of 220 fractures in 157 patients. J Craniomaxillofac Surg. 1992;20(7):292–6.
23. Ellis 3rd E, Miles BA. Fractures of the mandible: a technical prospective. Plast Reconstr Surg. 2007;120(7 Suppl 2):76S–89.
24. Schwab RA, Genners K, Robinson WA. Clinical predictors of mandibular fractures. Am J Emerg Med. 1998;16(3):304–5.
25. Alonso LL, Purcell TB. Accuracy of the tongue blade test in patients with suspected mandibular fracture. J Emerg Med. 1995;13(3):297–304.
26. Kademani D, Rombach DM, Quinn PD. Trauma to the temporomandibular joint region. In: Fonseca RJ, Barber HD, Walker RV, Powers MP, Betts NJ, editors. Oral and maxillofacial trauma. 3rd ed. St. Louis: Elsevier Saunders; 2005. p. 523–62.
27. Zimmermann CE, Troulis MJ, Kaban LB. Pediatric facial fractures: recent advances in prevention, diagnosis and management. Int J Oral Maxillofac Surg. 2006;35(1):2–13.
28. Shi J, Chen Z, Xu B. Causes and treatment of mandibular and condylar fractures in children and adolescents: a review of 104 cases. JAMA Otolaryngol Head Neck Surg. 2014;140(3):203–7.
29. Messinger A, Radkowski MA, Greenwald MJ, Pensler JM. Orbital roof fractures in the pediatric population. Plast Reconstr Surg. 1989;84(2):213–6.
30. Bansagi ZC, Meyer DR. Internal orbital fractures in the pediatric age group: characterization and management. Ophthalmology. 2000;107(5):829–36.
31. Manolidis S, Weeks BH, Kirby M, Scarlett M, Hollier L. Classification and surgical management of orbital fractures: experience with 111 orbital reconstructions. J Craniofac Surg. 2002;13(6):726–37.
32. Koltai PJ, Amjad I, Meyer D, Feustel PJ. Orbital fractures in children. Arch Otolaryngol Head Neck Surg. 1995;121(12):1375–9.
33. Brady SM, McMann MA, Mazzoli RA, Bushley DM, Ainbinder DJ, Carroll RB. The diagnosis and management of orbital blowout fractures: update 2001. Am J Emerg Med. 2001;19(2):147–54.
34. Converse JM, Smith B, Obear MF, Wood-Smith D. Orbital blow-out fractures: a ten year survey. Plast Reconstr Surg. 1967;39(1):20–36.
35. Kreidl KO, Kim DY, Mansour SE. Prevalence of significant intraocular sequelae in blunt orbital trauma. Am J Emerg Med. 2003;21(7):525–8.
36. Jordan DR, Allen LH, White J, Harvey J, Pashby R, Esmaeli B. Intervention within days for some orbital floor fractures: the white-eyed blowout. Ophthal Plast Reconstr Surg. 1998;14(6):379–90.
37. Burnstine MA. Clinical recommendations for repair of orbital facial fractures. Curr Opin Ophthalmol. 2003;14(5):236–40.
38. Lelli Jr GJ, Milite J, Maher E. Orbital floor fractures: evaluation, indications, approach, and pearls from an ophthalmologist's perspective. Facial Plast Surg. 2007;23(3):190–9.
39. McGraw BL, Cole RR. Pediatric maxillofacial trauma: age-related variations in injury. Arch Otolaryngol Head Neck Surg. 1990;116(1):41–5.
40. Salin MB, Smith BM. Diagnosis and treatment of midface fractures. In: Fonseca RJ, Barber HD, Walker RV, Powers MP, Betts NJ, editors. Oral and maxillofacial trauma. 3rd ed. St. Louis: Elsevier Saunders; 2005. p. 643–87.

41. Eirale C, Lockhart R, Chalabi H. Conservative treatment in an isolated anterior wall frontal bone fracture in an elite soccer player. Clin J Sport Med. 2010;20:125–7.
42. Weir JD. Effective management of epistaxis in athletes. J Athl Train. 1997;32(3):254–5.
43. Mulbury P. Recurrent epistaxis. Pediatr Rev. 1991;12(7):213–6.
44. Murray JM. Mandible fractures and dental trauma. Emerg Med Clin North Am. 2013;31(2):553–73.

Visual Dysfunction in Concussion

14

Aparna Raghuram and Ankoor S. Shah

Introduction

The last decade has seen a 60 % rise in sport-related brain trauma in emergency departments across the country [1]. Although prima facie disturbing, the steep rise can be attributed to increased awareness of deficits that can occur from concussion. The intent is not to discourage play but rather to enable people to engage in sport and recreational activity armed with knowledge to keep them playing longer, smarter, and safer.

Concussion is defined quite clearly across the literature. The Center for Disease Control and Prevention (CDC) describes it as a "Mild traumatic brain injury (mTBI) caused by a sudden jolt, bump or blow to the head that can change the way the brain normally works" [2]. However, since every concussion (mTBI) is different and cannot be diagnosed by brain imaging alone, identification and treatment require awareness of the full gamut of symptoms. The most common initial symptoms are headache, fatigue, dizziness, taking longer to think, nausea, emesis, and, occasionally, loss of consciousness. Later symptoms include sleep disturbances, frustration, and forgetfulness [3]. Another major indicator of concussion is vision-related irregularities.

About 50 % of brain areas are involved in visual information processing, and the visual cortex is a complex network within the central nervous system [4, 5]. This makes the visual system susceptible to many functional deficits from mTBI. A myriad of vision and ocular deficits post-concussion have been reported in the literature during the acute, subacute, and chronic phase of the injury with an incidence that varies

A. Raghuram, OD, PhD (✉)
Boston Children's Hospital and Harvard Medical School, Boston, MA, USA
e-mail: aparna.raghuram@childrens.harvard.edu

A.S. Shah, MD, PhD
Department of Ophthalmology, Boston Children's Hospital and Harvard Medical School, 300 Longwood Avenue, Fegan 4, Boston, MA 02115, USA
e-mail: ankoor.shah@childrens.harvard.edu

M. O'Brien, W.P. Meehan III (eds.), *Head and Neck Injuries in Young Athletes*, Contemporary Pediatric and Adolescent Sports Medicine,
DOI 10.1007/978-3-319-23549-3_14

between 30 and 90 % [6–8]. Left untreated, this visual dysfunction affects rehabilitative therapies [9] and delays recovery [10]. In evaluating mTBI in war veterans returning from Iraq and Afghanistan, vision-related deficits, particularly from a blast-related injury [11–16], have been better characterized, helped establish diagnostic protocols, and allowed targeted treatment. We can apply these lessons to the young athlete. This chapter provides an overview of the typical visual deficits and discusses diagnostic testing and treatment modalities for the visual sequelae of mTBI.

Mechanism of Injury

Cerebral dysfunction from TBI occurs in two categories. The primary effect manifests within minutes to hours and is due to direct trauma to the neurons. This direct trauma causes diffuse axonal injury. The secondary effect, which appears hours to days following the injury, results from nerve edema, inflammation, and/or compression from surrounding swollen areas. The damage from the secondary effect can be more pronounced and long standing than the primary effect and may cause the many symptoms in mTBI [17–19]. The neural injury from mTBI is transient, though recovery from symptoms can take a few days to 6 months, and in some cases, a year or longer [20–22].

Brief Overview of Brain Centers Involved in Processing Visual Information

The image of the visual world is transmitted from the retina through the optic nerve to the occipital lobe in the cerebral cortex. Most connections are directed toward area V1, which is the primary visual cortex of the brain. Information is then relayed to higher visual cortical pathways ultimately splitting into one directed to the temporal lobe ("what" pathway) and the other directed to the parietal lobe ("where" pathway). The "what" pathway, also called the ventral stream, processes information regarding object recognition (i.e., form, shape, and color). The "where" pathway, also called the dorsal stream, processes information regarding visual action (i.e., motion, eye movements, visual attention, and spatial localization). A separate subcortical pathway communicates information from the eye to the midbrain (superior colliculus), and this processing stream relays information on eye movement, pupil control, and accommodation (eye's ability to focus). Finally, the frontal cortex integrates information from the superior colliculus as well as the parietal, temporal, and occipital cortices. Visual information is processed by these centers in the human brain, and proper function is critical to integration of information; hence, disturbances across several cortical and subcortical regions lend individuals vulnerable to visual dysfunction after mTBI.

Since the effect of mTBI on the visual system is varied, tests incorporating multiple measures of visual function are necessary. Many of these tests can be excellent predictors of subtle cortical and subcortical changes in the brain from injury. Recently, a test incorporating eye movements, the King–Devick test (K–D), may be useful as a rapid screening tool in determining whether an athlete has suffered a concussion [23].

Vision-Related Symptoms

Visual complaints following concussion include blurry vision, difficulty focusing, light sensitivity, double vision, eyestrain, headache when reading, and difficulty reading. In addition, interactions between the visual and vestibular systems cause dizziness and motion sickness, especially in crowded environments. When these symptoms manifest, daily activities such as performance in sport and in school can be affected.

Etiologies for Visual Symptoms

Refractive Error

Symptom: blurred vision—intermittent or consistent at distance or at near.

Refractive error (the amount that the eye is out of focus) can account for blurred vision. Under normal circumstances, the visual system has the ability to compensate for small refractive errors, but if the focusing system (accommodation) is affected by concussion, the ability to compensate can be weak to nonexistent, making the patient symptomatic [6]. In these instances, correction of small magnitude of refractive error can provide better visual clarity post-concussion [6, 10, 24].

Treatment: An eye-care provider is needed to perform a full and dilated eye exam. Once this is done, a measure of the refractive state of the eye under cycloplegic conditions is necessary in young individuals. The cycloplegia (a paralysis of the ability to focus) is necessary since young individuals can change their focus easily. Once refractive error is determined, prescribing a pair of glasses with the appropriate correction can improve symptoms.

Accommodation (Eye Focusing Skill)

Symptoms: blurred vision, focusing difficulties, eyestrain, double vision, difficulty reading, fatigue with prolonged close work, difficulty concentrating and staying focused, and headaches.

A common cause for intermittent blurred vision is deficits in accommodation. Accommodation is defined as the ability of the eye to focus from distance to near and to maintain clarity of the target image. Multiple brain centers including the midbrain, cerebellum, and cortex control accommodation, and it can be easily affected by mTBI [25]. Loss of accommodation (accommodative insufficiency) is common after mTBI [6, 13, 25]. The incidence varies from 10 to 40 % [6, 8, 26]. This causes fluctuation in near vision affecting reading by causing fatigue with close work and inability to sustain reading for long periods of time.

Treatment: Near-vision spectacles (low-powered plus lenses) can be helpful when there is loss of accommodation. This is akin to reading glasses used by older individuals. Appropriate correction of distance farsightedness and astigmatism can also help the accommodative system function efficiently. Optometric vision rehabilitation measures are the treatment of choice to help normalize function of the accommodative system [27, 28].

Convergence Insufficiency (Eye Teaming Skill)

Symptoms: double vision, difficulty reading, skipping lines, skipping words, words moving on the page, intermittent blurry vision, eyestrain, visual fatigue, re-reading lines, and headache.

Vergence or eye teaming is the ability of the eyes to work together. This involves disconjugate eye movements where the eyes move in opposite directions while trying to focus on an object at near. The most common cause of visual symptoms post-mTBI is convergence insufficiency [6, 11–14, 29–32]. This deficit can also be caused by deficits in accommodation, which makes the convergence appear weak.

Treatment: Prism glasses can compensate for a difficulty in convergence and can be prescribed. Optometric vision rehabilitation measures are most effective in improving convergence insufficiency, overall symptoms, and quality of life related to this deficit [33].

Ocular Motility (Eye Tracking Skill)

Symptoms: difficulty following lines when reading, skipping lines, words, re-reading lines, words appearing to move or jump on a page, dizziness, and motion sensitivity.

Version or eye tracking is the ability of the eyes to follow objects conjugately. In this case, both eyes move in the same direction. This includes fixation, saccades, and pursuits. Fixation is the ability of the eyes to hold gaze in a particular position. Saccades are the ability of the eyes to fixate quickly between one target and another. Pursuits are the ability of the eye to follow or track a moving target. Areas of the midbrain, frontal cortex, and parietal cortex control the eye tracking ability [6, 34], and these areas are susceptible to injury from concussion. Studies suggest that eye movement deficits may be more sensitive than neuropsychological testing for persisting neurological anomalies [35, 36] after mTBI. The symptoms reported from eye focusing, eye teaming, and eye tracking skills affect daily activities like reading in school-aged children to employment tasks in teens and adults. They also affect overall performance in sports in an athlete.

Treatment: Optometric vision rehabilitation measures are the most effective in improving the eye tracking skills [37].

In this chapter, eye teaming (vergence), eye focusing (accommodation), and eye tracking (ocular motility) deficits have been discussed separately to highlight symptoms related to each system for ease of comprehension. In true essence, these deficits are rarely isolated, and there is substantial interaction between these visual systems. The goal of optometric vision rehabilitation is to normalize each of these systems to optimal levels with the aim of reducing or eliminating symptoms [10, 32, 38].

Light Sensitivity (Photophobia)

Symptom: Sensitivity to light indoors and outdoors.

Light sensitivity is a very common symptom post-concussion though the exact etiology is not known [10, 39]. It is common during the subacute stage of the injury. Improvement of symptoms occurs by 6 months, but some can remain for longer [40–42]. Patients have trouble with indoor and outdoor lighting; even back-illuminated light sources like televisions, computer screens, smartboards, iPads, and e-readers are overly bright.

Treatment: Indoors: Decreasing the brightness of electronic screens helps with function. Low-grade, tinted glasses of 20–30 % brown, rose, or gray alleviate symptoms; these are typically fit based on patient trial. Natural recovery occurs though a variable time course. Outdoors: Tinted lenses from 60 to 90 % gray and brown provide relief and are again chosen based on patient trial. Tinted lenses have to be used cautiously as there are reports that these lenses may cause symptoms to linger and psychological adaptation, which can cause difficulty weaning wear of these lenses [43].

Visual–Vestibular Deficits

Symptoms: dizziness, nausea, imbalance, vertigo, motion sickness, feeling overwhelmed in a crowded environment, reading in the car, and dynamic environments can be hard to handle [44, 45].

The vestibulo-ocular reflex helps in stabilizing the vision as the head moves. The control for this reflex comes from the semicircular canals in the inner ear. Vision provides indirect control for this reflex [45, 46].

Treatment: A comprehensive vestibular evaluation is important. Visual-motor rehabilitation including ocular motor control (fixation and pursuits) can help improve symptoms and function. Combined rehabilitative modalities with physical and occupational therapy are most effective.

Diagnostic Protocol

Early and accurate diagnosis is crucial as one of the current recommendations for concussion management is cognitive rest [3, 47–49]. Patients suspected of having concussion should undergo a standard battery of tests of the visual system, especially those with prolonged visual symptoms after the first 3–6 weeks.

This evaluation is necessary as part of the diagnostic work-up but also as part of the approach to treatment. The visual exam needs to include tests that assess eye teaming, eye focusing, and eye tracking skills. Specifically, recent evidence suggests that near point of convergence, accommodative amplitude, and vergence and accommodative peak velocity yield the highest sensitivity in identifying vision-related deficits post-concussion [50]. This diagnostic evaluation needs to be performed by an eye-care provider versed in addressing binocular visual function. Pediatric optometrists and optometrists specializing in binocular vision eye exam are typically the most proficient in performing these exams, and they should be sought out to appropriately diagnose and manage these patients.

While vision-specific complaints may arise after concussion, the post-concussive symptoms are likely multifactorial in nature. In other words, visual, vestibular, physical, and psychological dysfunctions may be contributing to the overall patient profile, and these various systems need to be evaluated thoroughly. Debilitating symptoms in athletes such as loss of balance, headache, dizziness, vertigo, weakened eye-motor coordination, decreased processing speed, and other cognitive difficulties like working memory and concentration may be attributed to all of these systems. Thus, we recommend a multidisciplinary approach with providers from each specialty. The combination of treatment modalities and the communication among the specialists are necessary to improve the quality of life and speed the recovery post-concussion.

Eye Movement Test for Diagnosing Concussion

The King–Devick (K–D) test [23], a rapid number naming test, is gaining popularity as a fast predictor of deficits post-concussion. Although the K–D test cannot replace the more thorough assessments of concussion such as the Sports Concussion Assessment Tool (SCAT)-3 [51] or computerized neurocognitive testing, it may be valuable in rapid assessments such as those necessary on the sidelines of sporting events. The K–D test hence has potential, being a quick test capable of being administered by any personnel and hence reducing return to play of athletes with potential impact from collisions and injuries. Recent study has also shown that adding the K–D test to cognitive (SAC) and balance (timed tandem gait test) assessment enhances the capacity of detecting concussion when administered on the sideline [52].

The K–D test was initially designed to assess eye movement behavior in patients with visual tracking deficits (deficits in saccades), and it captures impairment of eye movements, visual attention, language, concentration, and areas that correlate with suboptimal brain function. Baseline measures are necessary, and these can be compared to post-injury measures to relay deficits [53, 54]. Unfortunately, age-related baseline reference ranges are still needed for adolescent athletes, but the utility of this test may suggest that all young athletes be administered the K–D test along with their pre-sport physical examination. This baseline measure would then be filed for comparison to on-field or post-injury re-testing as needed [52].

Future Research

In the last decade, there has been significant research in the area of visual deficits related to TBI. These studies have focused on treatment of chronic symptoms, and they provide evidence for appropriate testing protocols, treatment, and management of symptoms. They do not address the time course of the acute, subacute, and chronic phases of visual symptoms post-concussion, and they do not address the appropriate timing of intervention. Moreover, we need a clearer understanding of the incidence of these vision problems and the natural recovery of symptoms without any intervention. There may be a subset that does not need treatment. It is important to identify these individuals as the process of oculomotor system rehabilitation is time-consuming and expensive, and it should be used judiciously. Finally, the impetus is starting to shift to appropriate training measures to help young athletes prevent sport-related head injuries. This can help reduce the overall incidence of concussion and help athletes and their families enjoy sport without trepidation over potential impact on quality of life.

Summary

1. Concussion affects multiple brain areas, and more than 50 % of the brain is involved in processing visual information. Hence, visual dysfunction is common after concussion.
2. The King–Devick (K–D) test is a rapid, objective screening test that has diagnostic implications for concussion. Its implementation immediately after head injury may add to the accurate diagnosis of a concussion.
3. Concussion patients with persistent visual symptoms beyond 3–6 weeks typically have blurry vision, difficulty focusing, light sensitivity, eyestrain, headache when reading, and difficulty reading.
4. Visual deficits after concussion involve eye focusing, eye teaming, eye tracking, and visual–vestibular interaction deficits. Each of these modalities can be measured objectively and may be rehabilitated effectively with optometric therapies. Thus, patients should be evaluated by a pediatric optometrist or eye-care provider trained in functional vision assessment and therapies.

References

1. Gilchrish JTK, Xu L, McGuire LC, Coronado VG. Nonfatal sports and recreation related traumatic brain injuries among children and adolescents treated in emergence departments in United States, 2001–2009. MMWR. 2011;60:1337–42.
2. Centers for Disease Control and Prevention. Traumatic brain injury. [updated 2014 Feb 24]. 2014. http://www.cdc.gov/TraumaticBrainInjury/get_the_facts.html
3. Eisenberg MA, Meehan 3rd WP, Mannix R. Duration and course of post-concussive symptoms. Pediatrics. 2014;133:999–1006.

4. Alvarez TL, Kim EH, Vicci VR, Dhar SK, Biswal BB, Barrett AM. Concurrent vision dysfunctions in convergence insufficiency with traumatic brain injury. Optom Vis Sci. 2012;89:1740–51.
5. Kaas JH. The evolution of the complex sensory and motor systems of the human brain. Brain Res Bull. 2008;75:384–90.
6. Ciuffreda KJ, Kapoor N, Rutner D, Suchoff IB, Han ME, Craig S. Occurrence of oculomotor dysfunctions in acquired brain injury: a retrospective analysis. Optometry. 2007;78:155–61.
7. Schlageter K, Gray B, Hall K, Shaw R, Sammet R. Incidence and treatment of visual dysfunction in traumatic brain injury. Brain Inj. 1993;7:439–48.
8. Suchoff IB, Kapoor N, Waxman R, Ference W. The occurrence of ocular and visual dysfunctions in an acquired brain-injured patient sample. J Am Optom Assoc. 1999;70:301–8.
9. Greenwald BD, Kapoor N, Singh AD. Visual impairments in the first year after traumatic brain injury. Brain Inj. 2012;26:1338–59.
10. Kapoor N, Ciuffreda KJ. Vision disturbances following traumatic brain injury. Curr Treat Options Neurol. 2002;4:271–80.
11. Brahm KD, Wilgenburg HM, Kirby J, Ingalla S, Chang CY, Goodrich GL. Visual impairment and dysfunction in combat-injured servicemembers with traumatic brain injury. Optom Vis Sci. 2009;86:817–25.
12. Capo-Aponte JE, Urosevich TG, Temme LA, Tarbett AK, Sanghera NK. Visual dysfunctions and symptoms during the subacute stage of blast-induced mild traumatic brain injury. Mil Med. 2012;177:804–13.
13. Goodrich GL, Flyg HM, Kirby JE, Chang CY, Martinsen GL. Mechanisms of TBI and visual consequences in military and veteran populations. Optom Vis Sci. 2013;90:105–12.
14. Stelmack JA, Frith T, Van Koevering D, Rinne S, Stelmack TR. Visual function in patients followed at a Veterans Affairs polytrauma network site: an electronic medical record review. Optometry. 2009;80:419–24.
15. Bulson R, Jun W, Hayes J. Visual symptomatology and referral patterns for Operation Iraqi Freedom and Operation Enduring Freedom veterans with traumatic brain injury. J Rehabil Res Dev. 2012;49:1075–82.
16. Cockerham GC, Goodrich GL, Weichel ED, et al. Eye and visual function in traumatic brain injury. J Rehabil Res Dev. 2009;46:811–8.
17. Greve MW, Zink BJ. Pathophysiology of traumatic brain injury. Mt Sinai J Med. 2009;76:97–104.
18. Kelts EA. Traumatic brain injury and visual dysfunction: a limited overview. NeuroRehabilitation. 2010;27:223–9.
19. Werner C, Engelhard K. Pathophysiology of traumatic brain injury. Br J Anaesth. 2007;99:4–9.
20. Alexander MP. Mild traumatic brain injury: pathophysiology, natural history, and clinical management. Neurology. 1995;45:1253–60.
21. Carroll LJ, Cassidy JD, Peloso PM, et al. Prognosis for mild traumatic brain injury: results of the WHO Collaborating Centre Task Force on Mild Traumatic Brain Injury. J Rehabil Med. 2004;43:84–105.
22. Hoge CW, McGurk D, Thomas JL, Cox AL, Engel CC, Castro CA. Mild traumatic brain injury in U.S. Soldiers returning from Iraq. N Engl J Med. 2008;358:453–63.
23. Galetta KM, Brandes LE, Maki K, et al. The King–Devick test and sports-related concussion: study of a rapid visual screening tool in a collegiate cohort. J Neurol Sci. 2011;309:34–9.
24. Hellerstein LF, Freed S, Maples WC. Vision profile of patients with mild brain injury. J Am Optom Assoc. 1995;66:634–9.
25. Green W, Ciuffreda KJ, Thiagarajan P, Szymanowicz D, Ludlam DP, Kapoor N. Accommodation in mild traumatic brain injury. J Rehabil Res Dev. 2010;47:183–99.
26. Al-Qurainy IA. Convergence insufficiency and failure of accommodation following midfacial trauma. Br J Oral Maxillofac Surg. 1995;33:71–5.
27. Thiagarajan P, Ciuffreda KJ. Effect of oculomotor rehabilitation on accommodative responsivity in mild traumatic brain injury. J Rehabil Res Dev. 2014;51:175–91.
28. Scheiman M, Wick B. Clinical management of binocular vision: heterophoric, accommodative, and eye movement disorders. 3rd ed. Philadelphia: Wolters Kluwer Health/Lippincott Williams & Wilkins; 2008. p. xii, 748.

29. Ciuffreda KJ, Rutner D, Kapoor N, Suchoff IB, Craig S, Han ME. Vision therapy for oculomotor dysfunctions in acquired brain injury: a retrospective analysis. Optometry. 2008;79:18–22.
30. Szymanowicz D, Ciuffreda KJ, Thiagarajan P, Ludlam DP, Green W, Kapoor N. Vergence in mild traumatic brain injury: a pilot study. J Rehabil Res Dev. 2012;49:1083–100.
31. Cohen M, Groswasser Z, Barchadski R, Appel A. Convergence insufficiency in brain-injured patients. Brain Inj. 1989;3:187–91.
32. Thiagarajan P, Ciuffreda KJ. Versional eye tracking in mild traumatic brain injury (mTBI): effects of oculomotor training (OMT). Brain Inj. 2014;28:930–43.
33. Thiagarajan P, Ciuffreda KJ. Effect of oculomotor rehabilitation on vergence responsivity in mild traumatic brain injury. J Rehabil Res Dev. 2013;50:1223–40.
34. Ventura RE, Balcer LJ, Galetta SL. The neuro-ophthalmology of head trauma. Lancet Neurol. 2014;13:1006–16.
35. Heitger MH, Jones RD, Macleod AD, Snell DL, Frampton CM, Anderson TJ. Impaired eye movements in post-concussion syndrome indicate suboptimal brain function beyond the influence of depression, malingering or intellectual ability. Brain. 2009;132:2850–70.
36. Kraus MF, Little DM, Donnell AJ, Reilly JL, Simonian N, Sweeney JA. Oculomotor function in chronic traumatic brain injury. Cogn Behav Neurol. 2007;20:170–8.
37. Thiagarajan P, Ciuffreda KJ, Capo-Aponte JE, Ludlam DP, Kapoor N. Oculomotor neurorehabilitation for reading in mild traumatic brain injury (mTBI): an integrative approach. NeuroRehabilitation. 2014;34:129–46.
38. Ciuffreda KJ, Han Y, Kapoor N, Ficarra AP. Oculomotor rehabilitation for reading in acquired brain injury. NeuroRehabilitation. 2006;21:9–21.
39. Jackowski MM, Sturr JF, Taub HA, Turk MA. Photophobia in patients with traumatic brain injury: uses of light-filtering lenses to enhance contrast sensitivity and reading rate. NeuroRehabilitation. 1996;6:193–201.
40. Bohnen N, Twijnstra A, Wijnen G, Jolles J. Tolerance for light and sound of patients with persistent post-concussional symptoms 6 months after mild head injury. J Neurol. 1991;238:443–6.
41. Vos PE, Battistin L, Birbamer G, et al. EFNS guideline on mild traumatic brain injury: report of an EFNS task force. Eur J Neurol. 2002;9:207–19.
42. Truong JQ, Ciuffreda KJ, Han MH, Such off IB. Photosensitivity in mild traumatic brain injury (mTBI): a retrospective analysis. Brain Inj. 2014;28:1283–7.
43. Howard RJ, Valori RM. Hospital patients who wear tinted spectacles—physical sign of psychoneurosis: a controlled study. J R Soc Med. 1989;82:606–8.
44. Bronstein AM. Vision and vertigo: some visual aspects of vestibular disorders. J Neurol. 2004;251:381–7.
45. Ciuffreda KJ. Visual vertigo syndrome: a clinical demonstration and diagnostic tool. Clin Eye Vis Care. 1999;11:41–2.
46. Cohen AH. Vision rehabilitation for visual-vestibular dysfunction: the role of the neuro-optometrist. NeuroRehabilitation. 2013;32:483–92.
47. Meehan 3rd WP, Bachur RG. Sport-related concussion. Pediatrics. 2009;123:114–23.
48. Meehan 3rd WP, Mannix RC, Stracciolini A, Elbin RJ, Collins MW. Symptom severity predicts prolonged recovery after sport-related concussion, but age and amnesia do not. J Pediatr. 2013;163:721–5.
49. Gibson S, Nigrovic LE, O'Brien M, Meehan 3rd WP. The effect of recommending cognitive rest on recovery from sport-related concussion. Brain Inj. 2013;27:839–42.
50. Ciuffreda KJ, Ludlam DP, Thiagarajan P, Yadav NK, Capo-Aponte J. Proposed objective visual system biomarkers for mild traumatic brain injury. Mil Med. 2014;179:1212–7.
51. Okonkwo DO, Tempel ZJ, Maroon J. Sideline assessment tools for the evaluation of concussion in athletes: a review. Neurosurgery. 2014;75 Suppl 4:S82–95.
52. Galetta KM, Morganroth J, Moehringer N, et al. Adding vision to concussion testing: a prospective study of sideline testing in youth and collegiate athletes. J Neuroophthalmol. 2015;35(3):235-241.
53. King D, Brughelli M, Hume P, Gissane C. Concussions in amateur rugby union identified with the use of a rapid visual screening tool. J Neurol Sci. 2013;326:59–63.
54. King D, Clark T, Gissane C. Use of a rapid visual screening tool for the assessment of concussion in amateur rugby league: a pilot study. J Neurol Sci. 2012;320:16–21.

Dental and Temporomandibular Joint Injuries

15

Mariusz Kajetan Wrzosek and David Alexander Keith

Background

General Considerations and Pertinent Dental Anatomy

Traumatic dental injuries are a common occurrence in young athletes, especially in contact sports. The child athlete presents with the unique situation of the mixed dentition, with both primary and adult teeth present at the same time. The athlete's continued growth must also be taken into account in treatment and long-term prognosis. The unique aspects of injuries to primary dentition and its effect on permanent dentition and long-term sequela will be discussed in the context of various injuries.

In the adolescent athlete a mixed dentition is often present. The child's deciduous dentition consists of 20 teeth with two molars, a canine, and a lateral and central incisor present in each quadrant of the upper and lower jaw. Children start to enter the mixed dentition stage at around 6 years of age as the central incisors and adult molars erupt, with this stage persisting into adolescence, typically until the age of 13 or 14, based on the eruption and gradual replacement of the primary dentition with adult teeth. The full adult dentition consists of 32 teeth, 8 per quadrant, including the adult molars which develop distal to (behind) the primary molars and start erupting at around 6 years of age, with the primary molars eventually replaced by the adult premolars erupting at 10–12 years of age. The mixed dentition phase poses unique challenges both from a diagnostic and treatment standpoint, since the longitudinal prognosis of teeth and impact of primary tooth injury on developing adult dentition must be taken into account (Fig. 15.1).

M.K. Wrzosek, DMD, MD • D.A. Keith, DMD, BDS (✉)
Department of Oral and Maxillofacial Surgery, Massachusetts General Hospital,
55 Fruit Street, Boston, MA 02114, USA
e-mail: mwrzosek@partners.org; dkeith@partners.org

M. O'Brien, W.P. Meehan III (eds.), *Head and Neck Injuries in Young Athletes*,
Contemporary Pediatric and Adolescent Sports Medicine,
DOI 10.1007/978-3-319-23549-3_15

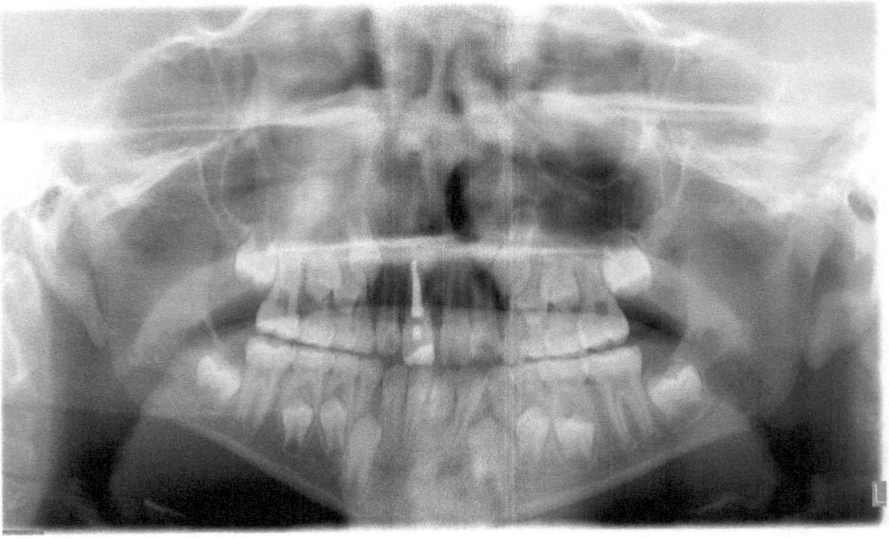

Fig. 15.1 Panoramic radiograph of 10 year old child in mixed dentition stage. The adult maxillary and mandibular incisors and first (6-year) molars are fully erupted in addition to the deciduous canines and molars. The second molars (12 year molars), canines, and premolars have not yet erupted, and can be seen developing behind the first molars and below the deciduous canines and premolars, respectively. Note the incomplete root formation of the molars and premolars at this age. Also note the endodontically treated maxillary right central incisor with radio-opaque material filling the root canal and a restoration of the previously fractured crown

Dental and Oral Injuries

Dentoalveolar injuries are the most frequent facial injury in children. Many of these are treated by the dentist or oral and maxillofacial surgeon in an outpatient office setting. Many traumatic injuries in young athletes involve head trauma so a thorough medical and neurological exam is necessary. Blunt trauma from an object, particularly in sports such as football, baseball, or hockey, is one of the most common mechanisms of injury [1–5].

Diagnosis

A careful oral examination should be performed in all dental and facial trauma cases. As with any trauma evaluation, the clinical history of the accident is very important. The oral injury may be a distracting injury, especially if a tooth is avulsed or displaced and there is a significant amount of hemorrhage from the oral cavity lacerations. It is important that this does not distract from the bigger picture of the trauma evaluation. Particularly in cases of significant force to the head, loss of consciousness and other injuries need to be addressed. Concussions, cervical spine injuries, and head trauma are discussed in separate chapters [1].

For the examination of the oral and maxillofacial region, the examiner should evaluate the soft tissue for any lacerations extraorally as well as intraorally and look for any missing, loose, or chipped teeth. It is also very important to evaluate the occlusion, since a malocclusion, or step-off in the occlusal plane, can reveal a mandible fracture or displaced teeth. All teeth should be accounted for. An attempt should be made at the scene to locate any avulsed teeth and these should be immediately replanted or properly transported in the appropriate storage medium if any attempt at replantation is to be made. Exposure of the root surface and severing of the neurovascular bundle at the tooth root apex leads to tooth necrosis, and prolonged avulsion greatly reduces the chance for a successful rescue. Ideally, if it can be accomplished safely, the avulsed tooth is transported in its original socket. If this cannot be accomplished safely, there are commercially available solutions for storing avulsed teeth, such as Hank's Balanced Salt Solution (HBSS). When such media are not available, avulsed teeth may be transported in pasteurized milk. If there is no alternative, teeth may be transported in saliva or saline. Chipped teeth and fractured crowns should prompt the clinician to look for intraoral lacerations since fragments can often become imbedded in soft tissues. In cases of missing teeth or fragments that cannot be accounted for, a chest radiograph is a prudent exam, especially in cases with significant trauma and loss of consciousness. Dental fragments can easily be aspirated and, if revealed on plain films, need to be retrieved. In cases of swallowed fragments, revealed on an abdominal radiograph, these usually do not require any treatment other than surveillance [1].

The radiographic examination is a critical component of the trauma evaluation. The panoramic radiograph is an excellent screening tool that will show the entire upper and lower jaw in one plane, as well as the entire dentition. Many patients already have a CT scan, especially if evaluated for head trauma in the emergency room. However, the mandible and lower teeth are often excluded in the window of the typical brain CT used to screen for intracranial hemorrhage. Even in cases where a face CT is obtained, the panoramic radiograph is still a helpful tool for several reasons. First, it will reveal mandible fractures and relative displacement, as well as all erupted and unerupted teeth, which are present in many adolescent athletes and children. The panoramic radiograph shows the entire dentition together in a single plane making evaluation much easier. It allows for evaluation of root formation and detection of root fractures, which will determine treatment. The radiograph can also determine the presence of foreign bodies and fragments of teeth imbedded in soft tissue [1] (Fig. 15.2).

An initial panoramic radiograph is also very useful since this radiograph is used as a baseline for future panoramic radiographs obtained during follow-up care. Individual radiographs of traumatized teeth should also be taken since they are much more sensitive than the panoramic radiograph in determining root fractures with minimal displacement. The radiographs can be taken at multiple angles to determine position and direction of luxations, as well as the relationship of injured primary teeth to underlying permanent dentition. In fact, with deep lacerations of the lips, it is often wise to take a periapical radiograph of the soft tissue to look for foreign bodies such as tooth fragments. An occlusal radiograph can be a useful

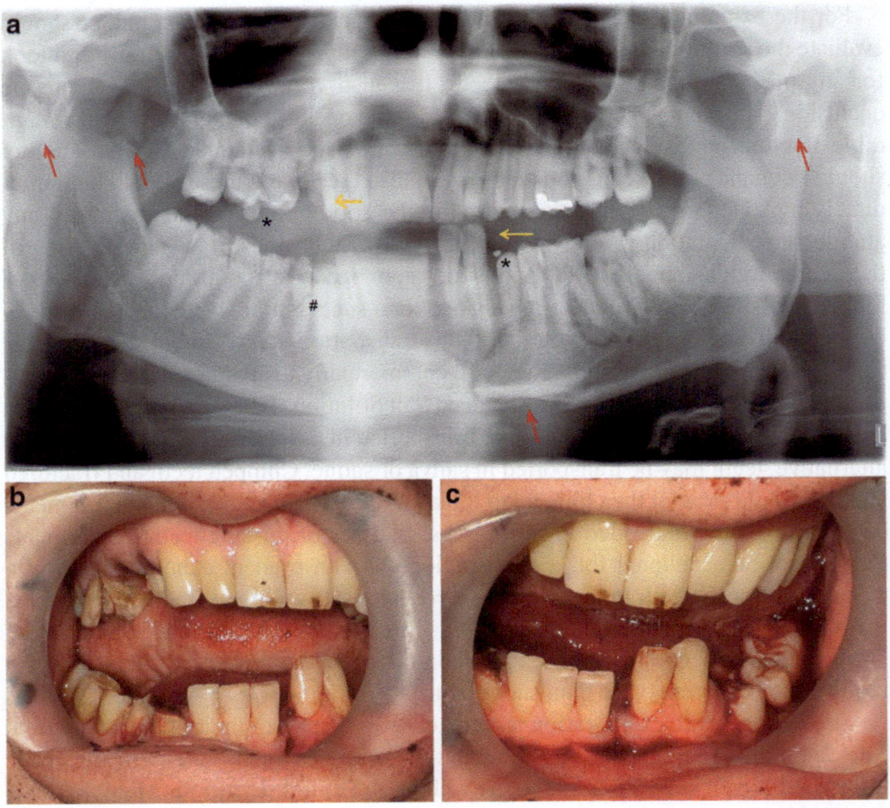

Fig. 15.2 (**a**) Panoramic radiograph of traumatic injury to the mandible with multiple findings. *Vertical arrows* point out mandibular fractures in the left parasymphysis region, bilateral condylar fractures, and right coronoid process fracture. The * points out tooth fragments. The # points out a root fracture of the right mandibular premolar. The *horizontal arrows* point out a stepoff in the occlusal plane corresponding to mandible fracture and displacement of the canine and lateral incisor in the mandible and fractured dental crowns in the maxilla. (**b**) and (**c**) show corresponding clinical photos of the stepoff in the occlusal plane in line of fracture and fractured teeth. Due to severity of mandibular injuries, the patient required surgery and open reduction with internal fixation of mandibular body fractures

supplement to determine the relationships of the anterior dentition to the developing permanent dentition [1, 5–7].

It is worthwhile noting that over the last few years, many dental and surgical offices have been equipped with low-dose conebeam CT scanners, which are increasingly used for evaluations, and provide an excellent 3D image of the dento-alveolar structures as well as a reconstructed panoramic view at a fraction of the exposure of a medical CT. This technology has enhanced the diagnostic capabilities of many local offices and clinics.

Types of Injuries

Injuries to teeth and surrounding structures can be subdivided into injuries affecting the hard tissue of the teeth alone such as chips and fractures of the crown; injuries of the dental pulp, such as crown fractures involving pulpal exposure; injuries to the surrounding periodontal support tissues and supporting bone; and finally injuries to the gingival and soft tissues of the oral cavity. In most instances there is injury involving multiple structures, combining these types of injuries. The treatment of particular injuries to the oral cavity and dentition depends on the type of dental injury and is discussed in the context of each injury [8, 9].

Oral Soft Tissue Injuries

Tongue lacerations are usually a result of bite injuries sustained in a collision or fall with chin trauma, resulting in the tongue being trapped between the teeth. The tongue and oral mucosa heal very quickly, and the resulting minor tongue lacerations often do not require suturing. However, temporary hemorrhage can occur and be significant since the tongue is very vascular, but this is usually self-limiting. When suturing is required, resorbable sutures such as plain or chromic gut are always used. The patient is also often treated with a course of topical antimicrobial chlorhexidine rinse and antibiotics if necessary.

Dental injuries are often accompanied by abrasions and lacerations of the surrounding gingiva. In the anterior maxilla and mandible, the vestibular frenum attachment in the midline is often torn and injured since it is easily mobile and friable. These wounds often require a few resorbable sutures. Gingival lacerations should be treated, especially if the gingiva is detached or stripped off the alveolar bone. The treatment usually involves interdental sutures to reapproximate the gingiva. This will allow for proper healing preserving soft tissue aesthetics. Gingival lacerations and injuries tend to heal very quickly, since oral mucosa has a very high turnover rate.

Lip lacerations often occur when the lip becomes trapped between the upper and lower teeth. These can be through-and-through lacerations with the teeth biting through the lip. Lip lacerations often require repair, especially in cases where the laceration crosses the vermillion border. Any lacerations should be carefully examined for the presence of tooth fragments or foreign bodies since these can become a nidus of infection. This is where a soft tissue radiograph can be useful to look for foreign objects. Thorough debridement and copious irrigation is necessary. The antibiotics of choice in oral injuries are typically penicillins, which have excellent oral microbial coverage. In cases of penicillin allergy, clindamycin is typically the preferred option (Fig. 15.3).

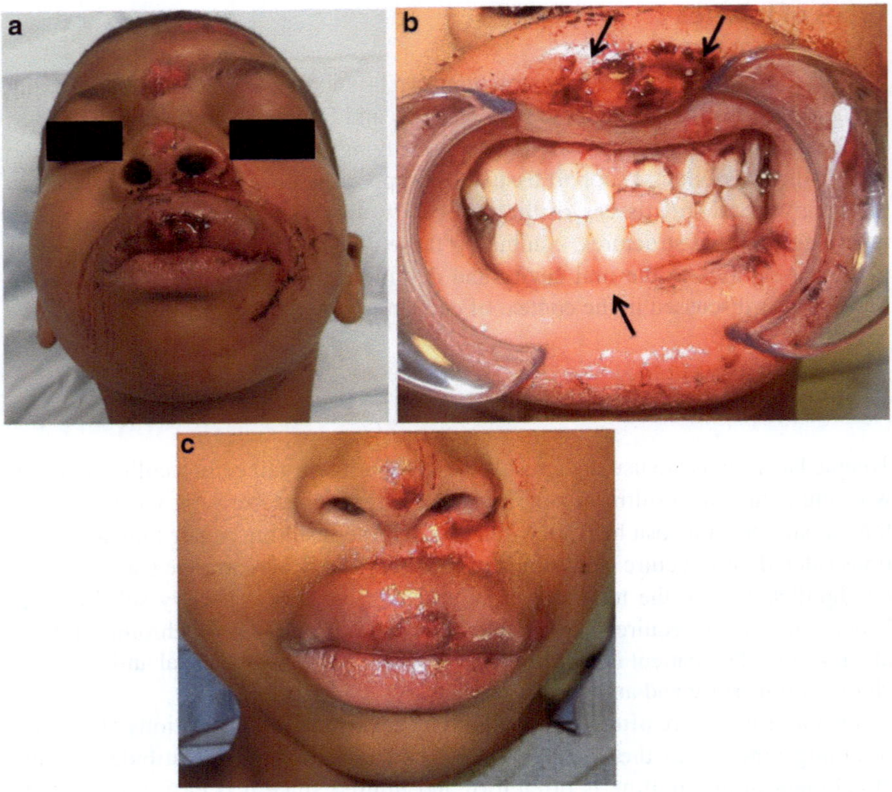

Fig. 15.3 (**a**) Example of a 9-year-old patient in a bicycle accident with soft tissue injuries and dental fragments within deep lip laceration. Patient suffered multiple abrasions, with a through and through upper lip laceration. (**b**) Multiple dental fragments from the fractured teeth are noted embedded in the soft tissue. (**c**) The wound was carefully debrided and irrigated prior to layered closure. The loose dental fragments were removed

Hard Tissue Injuries

Our discussion here will involve the various types of dental injuries, the treatment, and future sequela. All of these aspects are important principles for primary clinicians involved in the management of athletes, from the youth to professional levels, as well as for parents and for the athletes themselves. The treatment of these hard tissue dental injuries is based on the anatomy of the teeth and surrounding tissues, ranging from limited to severe injury of the crown and root to the displacement of teeth and injury of the periodontium and supporting bone. Treatment is guided by the severity of the anatomical components injured. The World Health Organization (WHO) has presented a widely accepted injury classification system that is based on anatomic considerations and accepted therapies of dental injuries and surrounding structures. The system, known as the Applications of International Classification of Diseases to Dentistry and

Stomatology (ICD-DA), was initially published in 1973 with the third edition published in 1994. It has been modified by Anderson and colleagues and is still widely used [8, 9].

Dental Injuries

Injuries of teeth can be described based on the component of the injured tooth. A fracture of a tooth can involve multiple layers of the crown of the tooth including the enamel and dentin, can extend into the pulp, and can involve the root. An uncomplicated crown fracture involves the enamel and dentin only and does not expose the pulp. This may be a simple chip of the enamel involving only the incisal edge of an incisor or a more substantial fracture involving both enamel and dentin. In the case of a fracture extending to the dentin, the tooth may exhibit increased sensitivity. Ellis classified these fractures as Type I (involving enamel only) and Type II (involving enamel and dentin) [9]. Treatment of an uncomplicated fracture typically involves composite bonding to restore form and aesthetics. If a large fragment is fractured, it should be saved and brought to the dentist since in certain cases it may be used and bonded to the remaining tooth. The definitive treatment and material will be determined by the restoring dentist based on the amount of missing tooth structure [1, 4, 5, 8, 9] (Figs. 15.4 and 15.5).

A complicated crown fracture involves exposure of the dental pulp. This type of fracture involving enamel, dentin, and pulp exposure was classified by Ellis as Type III [9]. This type of injury should be evaluated as soon as possible by a dentist since prognosis depends on factors such as age of the patient and stage of dental development, time of exposure, and amount of pulpal exposure. All exposed pulpal tissue will require treatment. In cases of small pulpal exposures in young patients that have incompletely formed root apices, the prognosis of pulpal survival is much better than in adults where the tooth root is completely formed and the apex (where the neurovascular bundle enters the tooth) is closed. Significant pulpal exposure in older patients will likely require endodontic therapy, with long-term prognosis to be determined by close follow-up on clinical and radiographic exams by the patient's dentist [7, 9].

The dental hard tissue injury can also extend into the root of the tooth. The crown-root fracture can extend into the cementum, or root structure, again with pulpal exposure (complicated) or without pulpal exposure (uncomplicated). An injury involving the root was classified as a Type IV fracture in the Ellis classification [9]. Fractures that extend past the gingival margin into root structure cause significant damage and may have a poor prognosis depending on the level of root fracture. If there is no pulpal exposure in certain cases, the mobile crown segment can be removed and the tooth restored. In cases of pulpal exposure in young patients with incomplete root formation, the dentist may be able to preserve pulpal vitality. In older patients, once root formation is complete, and there is a complicated (pulpal exposure) crown-root fracture, the tooth will require root canal therapy if it is restorable. These cases often require complicated restorative

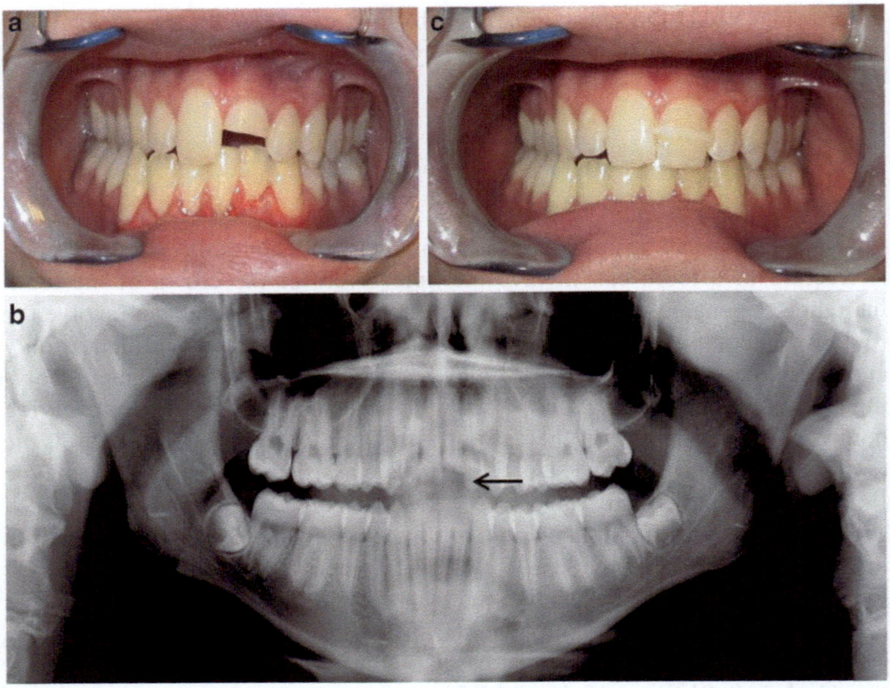

Fig. 15.4 (**a**) Sixteen-year-old patient with a crown fracture involving enamel and dentin of the maxillary left central incisor, sustained in an ice-skating accident. The patient saved the crown fragment. (**b**) Panoramic radiograph showing fracture. (**c**) It was provisionally bonded to the tooth in the emergency room reducing sensitivity and restoring esthetics. He later followed up with his dentist for definitive treatment

procedures, including full coverage crowns to fully restore function and aesthetics. In the extreme crown-root fracture, where the tooth is fractured along its vertical axis, the tooth is non-restorable and requires extraction. Often, complicated crown-root fractures also result in non-restorable situations or very difficult restorative situations where it may be more beneficial to extract and replace the tooth based on cost, prognosis, and risk and benefit discussion with the patient. Treatment planning of complicated fractures often requires endodontic treatment as well as involvement of the orthodontist to extrude the tooth to allow exposure of enough tooth structure for the dentist to restore the tooth. These decisions are based on the individual patient and involve multiple specialists and are beyond the scope of this discussion [4–23] (Fig. 15.6).

Although rare, accounting for about 7.7 % of injuries to the permanent dentition, a dental injury can involve an isolated root fracture. The most commonly affected teeth are the maxillary incisors since they are most exposed and most easily injured. These fractures are often detected on radiographic exam. The involved tooth may also be slightly extruded from the socket and luxated. The prognosis depends on the level of the horizontal root fracture. The best prognosis occurs in root fractures involving the apical (deepest) third of the root and the worst in cases near the

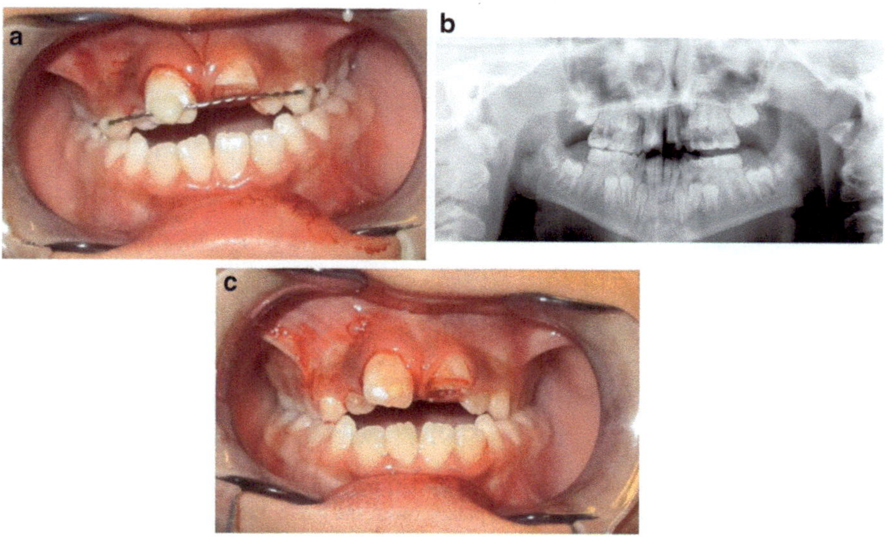

Fig. 15.5 (**a**) A 10-year-old boy involved in an ice-skating accident. Clinical presentation involving luxation and enamel and dentin fracture of the right central incisors and a complicated fracture of the left central incisors involving the dentin and pulp exposure of the left central incisor. (**b**) The panoramic radiograph shows the fractures and no other injuries. (**c**) Treatment involved splinting the slightly mobile right central incisor. The left central incisor will require additional treatment and restoration

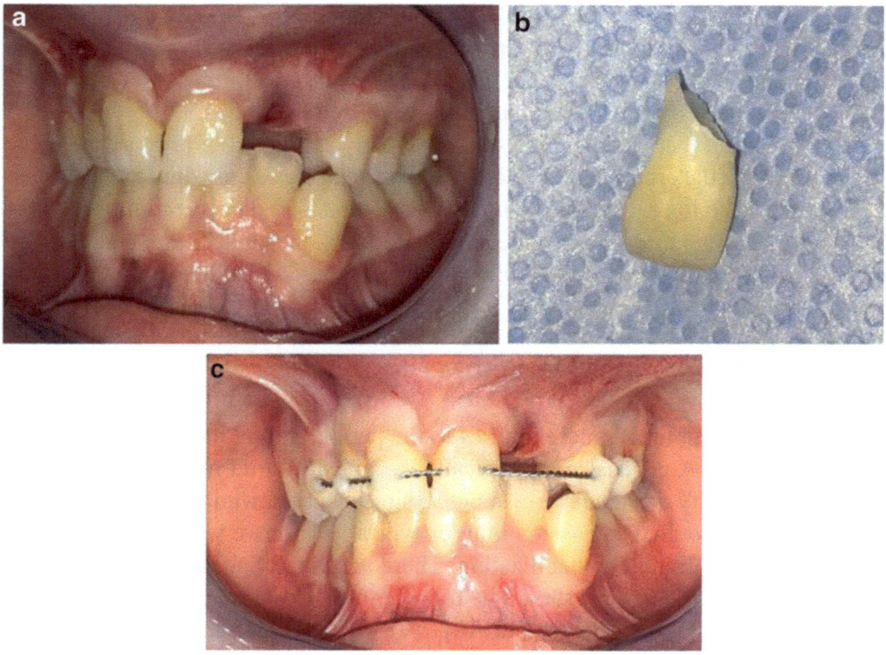

Fig. 15.6 (**a**) Complicated crown injury involving crown and root of the left maxillary lateral incisor, extending below the gingiva. (**b**) The fractured segment is nonrestorable due to root fracture being in the coronal segment and the oblique angle. (**c**) The adjacent subluxed teeth were splinted for 2 weeks. The remaining root will require extraction and eventually an implant will be placed

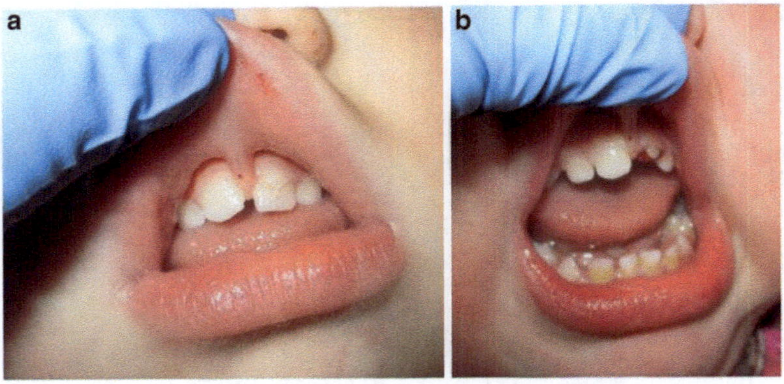

Fig. 15.7 (**a**) A 19-month-old with trauma to the left maxillary central incisor. The crown was fractured below the gingival margin with pulpal exposure and the tooth was nonrestorable. (**b**) The tooth was extracted due to significant fracture

coronal third. Fractures involving the most apical third of the tooth are typically stabilized with a flexible splint for 4 weeks. More coronal root fractures may involve longer splinting periods. These teeth need to be carefully monitored for pulpal necrosis and need for endodontic therapy by the patient's dentist [4, 5, 7, 20].

Primary teeth can sustain similar injuries to the permanent dentition. However, the age of the patient and time to planned exfoliation of the tooth also need to be considered prior to treatment. The priority is placed on preservation of the erupting or developing permanent dentition. Therefore, primary teeth are never replanted, and severely luxated primary teeth are often extracted [6] (Fig. 15.7).

It is important that parents understand that early extraction of primary teeth can sometimes alter the eruption of the adult teeth and can cause crowding in the permanent dentition, so long-term follow-up is important. A soft diet is recommended for at least a week as part of the treatment of all concussion, subluxation, and luxation injuries for symptom relief and to allow healing of the surrounding structures.

Injuries to Surrounding Structures

Concussion and subluxation are injuries to the periodontium, the supporting structure of the tooth. A concussion is typically sustained in mild trauma and is manifested by sensitivity and tenderness to percussion or biting, without displacement or loosening of the tooth. Concussion injuries typically improve with soft diet and do not require any splinting or stabilization. There are usually no radiographic abnormalities on exam. The injury should be followed for symptom resolution and vitality testing by the patient's dentist [15, 16].

Subluxation injury typically requires more force and involves loosening of the traumatized tooth without displacement. The tooth will be tender to touch and percussion. There will likely be no radiographic abnormalities since there is no displacement. If there is mobility of the tooth, it may need to be splinted with a

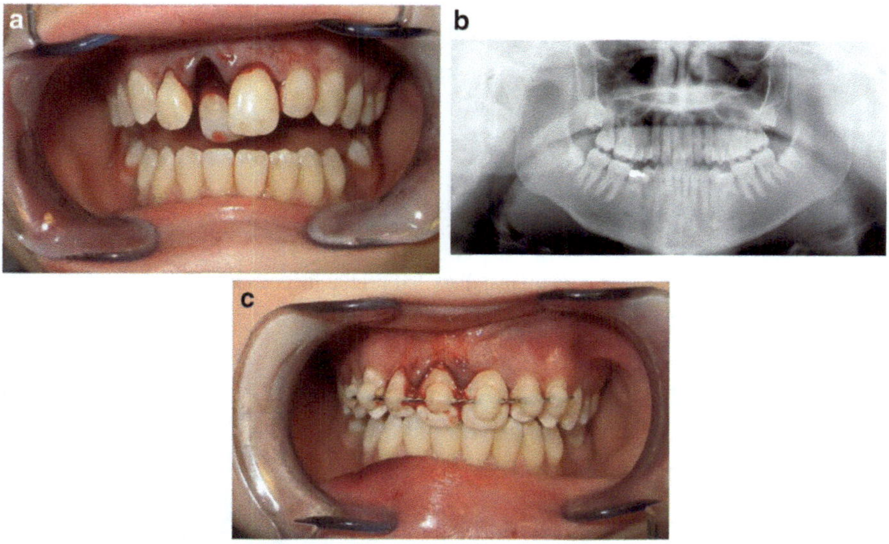

Fig. 15.8 Extrusive and palatal luxation of the maxillary right central incisor in a football injury without use of a mouthguard. (**a**) Initial presentation. (**b**) Panoramic radiograph shows no other bony or dental injuries, with the tooth displaced and out of the correct occlusal plane. (**c**) Since there was no alveolar bone fracture, the tooth was repositioned after administration of local anesthesia and splinted with a flexible composite-bonded splint

flexible composite bonded splint for 2 weeks. The patient should be placed on a soft diet for a week. This injury should also be followed for symptom resolution and vitality testing [11, 15, 16].

Luxation indicates a movement from the normal position. Luxation injury can be extrusive, lateral, or intrusive in nature. This typically occurs with significant force and is often associated with fracture of a tooth as well as the alveolar bone supporting the tooth. Splinting is typically required with a flexible splint for a period of 2 weeks. Extrusive luxation is displacement of the tooth outward or incisally out of the socket. Lateral luxation involves any lateral movement out of the occlusal arch, other than in an apical or coronal direction [16–18] (Fig. 15.8).

This type of injury often involves a fracture of the thin overlying alveolar bone cortex. Intrusive luxation defines apical displacement into the alveolar bone. Teeth that are extruded or laterally luxated are usually repositioned in the office under local anesthesia. In the case of intrusion, the tooth is pushed into the socket and can either be allowed to re-erupt or can be repositioned based on the patient's age. On occasion, significant intrusion may require orthodontic forces to reposition the tooth gradually. In teeth of older patients with complete root formation, intrusion injuries often lead to pulp necrosis and will frequently require endodontic treatment. Intrusion injuries in particular may have significant sequela in the future. In cases of primary dentition, depending on the child's age, luxation of a deciduous tooth may not require much force, since the roots of deciduous teeth are gradually resorbed by

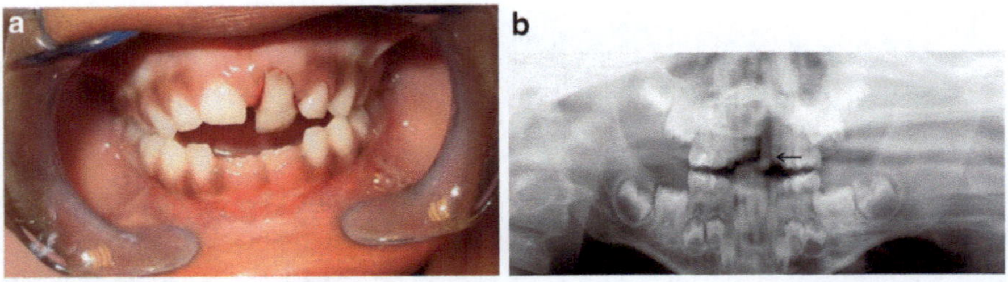

Fig. 15.9 (**a**) An example of a primary maxillary left central incisor luxated in a 5-year-old girl. (**b**) Panoramic radiograph shows degree of luxation and proximity of adult teeth, and short root. The tooth was extracted during the visit

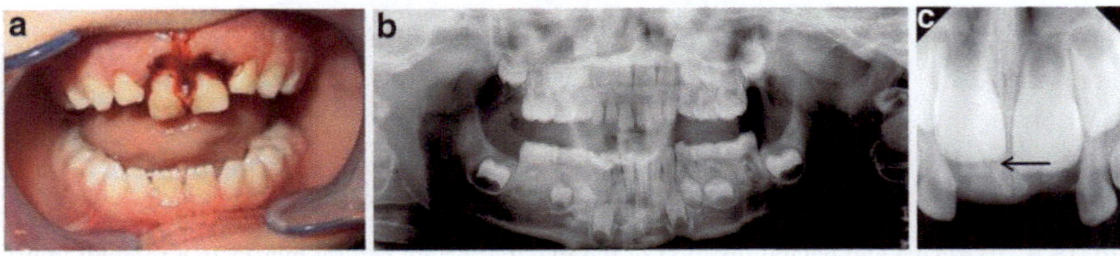

Fig. 15.10 (**a**) Extrusive luxation of primary central incisors in a 6-year-old. (**b**) Panoramic radiograph showing degree of displacement. Note the short roots of the primary incisors as a result of root resorption by the erupting permanent incisors. (**c**) The teeth were extracted. After extraction, a follow-up periapical radiograph in clinic shows a small residual root tip. This will resorb as the adult teeth erupt over the next year

the erupting permanent teeth. In these cases the primary teeth are often extracted [4, 6, 22] (Figs. 15.9 and 15.10).

After an intrusion injury, teeth have a higher risk of ankylosis or root resorption even years after the injury, so long-term surveillance by the patient's dentist will be required to monitor for such signs. In the case of a young patient where the adjacent dentition is still erupting, ankylosis may lead to dental crowding or malocclusion as the surrounding dentition develops and adjacent teeth erupt, while the ankylosed tooth can no longer move [4, 5].

In the case of the deciduous dentition, intrusion injuries may also damage the crowns of the developing adult teeth below the roots of the primary tooth. In certain scenarios, and depending on the degree of intrusion of the primary dentition, the injured primary teeth may require extraction. It is important to stress the long-term surveillance and follow-up of these injuries by the patient's dentist to monitor for these sequelae [18–20].

Avulsion

In the case of avulsion, the tooth is completely displaced out of the alveolar socket. In this case the periodontal fibers supporting the tooth and the neurovascular bundle at the apex are completely severed. The thin alveolar bone surrounding the tooth is often fractured since a significant amount of force is required for this type of injury.

Avulsion injuries account for about 15 % of traumatic injuries involving permanent teeth. The most frequently involved teeth in both the adult and primary dentition are the maxillary central incisors. These are the most prominent teeth in the dental arch for a long time, especially in young children since they are the first to erupt in the maxilla. These teeth typically erupt at around age of 6–7 and are particularly prone to avulsion within the first few years of eruption [7, 21].

Tooth avulsion is a true dental emergency, and the treatment and timeline are critical. Successful replantation of an avulsed tooth is inversely related to the time a tooth is out of the socket. The critical aspect is maintenance of the viability of the cells in the pulp and in the periodontal ligament, necessary for successful reattachment. In the best scenario, the tooth is immediately replanted in its socket. In case of avulsion at a sporting event, the best option is to gently rinse off the tooth and immediately replace into the socket, since time is the most critical factor in survival. Other factors impacting survival include the maturity and stage of root development and type of storage medium used to transport the tooth. Teeth reimplanted with the first hour have the best survival and least amount of complications. Andreasen and his colleagues performed extensive studies in dental traumatology and determined that over a period of 2 years, teeth reimplanted within less than 30 min of avulsion showed no resorption of roots, but in teeth that have been reimplanted after two or more hours, 95 % showed root resorption. Root resorption has been attributed to an inflammatory process and damage to the dental root during the extraoral period. A tooth reimplanted within 15–20 min has the greatest chance of successful replantation due to survival of the periodontal ligament cells [4, 5, 13–22].

In the case where it is impossible to reimplant the tooth immediately, the manner in which the tooth is handled is critical to survival. First, the tooth should be preserved in a moist environment to prevent the drying of the periodontal ligament cells present on the root. Handling of the root should be minimized and it should be kept moist at all times. The best storage medium is Hank's Balanced Salt Solution (HBSS) which is a physiologic solution with nutrients that will allow for survival of the periodontal and pulpal cells the longest and allows for the best prognosis. Use of cell culture media such as Viaspan has also been described as an alternative. In case HBSS is not available, milk is an alternative. Milk is readily available, has a pH that is compatible with cell survival, and provides a bacteria-free environment. The third best option is saline. As an alternative, the tooth can be stored under the tongue or under the lip if the patient is old enough to prevent swallowing or aspiration or in a wet saliva-soaked towel to maintain moisture. Storage in regular water is contraindicated since pure water is hypotonic and will cause lysis of any viable cells on the root surface [1, 7, 21].

After immediate replantation, the tooth must be splinted with a flexible splint for a period of 1–2 weeks if it has been stored in a physiologic medium and reimplanted within an hour or in a case of prolonged extraoral time (>60 min) splinted for 4 weeks. This period of fixation allows for reattachment of the periodontal ligament. The patient must be on a soft non-chew diet for this time. Patients are prescribed antibiotics for a period of one week, typically penicillin or clindamycin (in case of allergy), and topical chlorhexidine rinse. It is also critical that tetanus status be

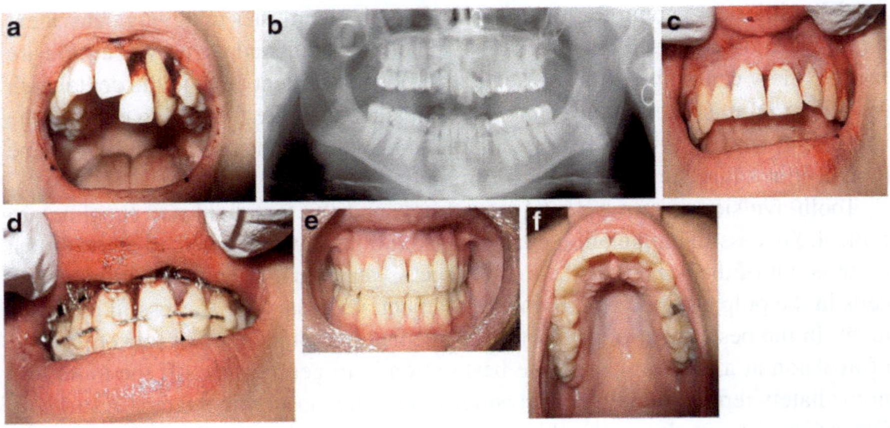

Fig. 15.11 (**a**) Clinical presentation of trauma case of young woman resulting in avulsed left maxillary lateral incisor and severely luxated maxillary central incisor. (**b**) Panoramic radiograph showing displacement of teeth and no mandibular fractures. (**c**) Treatment involved repositioning of teeth under local anesthesia. (**d**) The teeth required splinting with an archbar for alveolar bone fracture and segment mobility and flexible composite splint to stabilize the teeth. (**e**, **f**) The archbar and splint were removed at 4 weeks and at 2 months follow up; the patient was doing well with excellent stability of the teeth. Both teeth required root canal treatment by her dentist

updated. Delayed replantation has a poor long-term prognosis, since the periodontal ligament is not expected to heal, and the long-term outcome is usually ankylosis and root desorption. Replantation, however, does provide temporary restoration for aesthetic and functional reasons and will maintain the shape and height of the alveolar ridge [4, 5, 21] (Fig. 15.11).

In the case of avulsion and loss of a permanent tooth, or inability to replant the tooth in an athlete who has stopped growing, the best option to replace the missing tooth is a dental implant. The complete dental treatment of these injuries is beyond the scope of this book (Fig. 15.12).

Alveolar Fractures

In the scenario with a lateral luxation of a tooth, the alveolar bone overlying the root is often fractured and minimally displaced. In this case to allow for bony healing, the involved teeth are splinted for a period of 4 weeks with close follow-up. In the scenario where a larger alveolar segment containing several teeth is fractured, there will be mobility of the teeth as a unit. Since this is mostly a bone injury, it will require more rigid splinting for a period of 4 weeks. This is typically accomplished with an archbar and circumdental wiring for stability. Alveolar bone fractures and luxation and avulsion injuries often occur together, so additional splinting of teeth may be necessary [1, 4, 5] (Figs. 15.13 and 15.14).

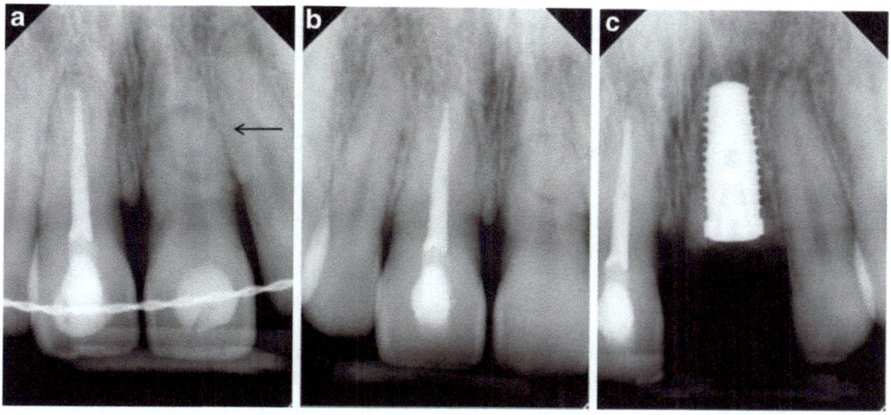

Fig. 15.12 (**a**) This patient sustained a luxation of right central incisor and root fracture at midroot of left central incisor. Note the completed root canal treatment on the right central incisor. (**b**) The left central incisor failed to stabilize after splinting, and demonstrated continued mobility. (**c**) The tooth required extraction and was replaced with a dental implant which restores function and cosmetics

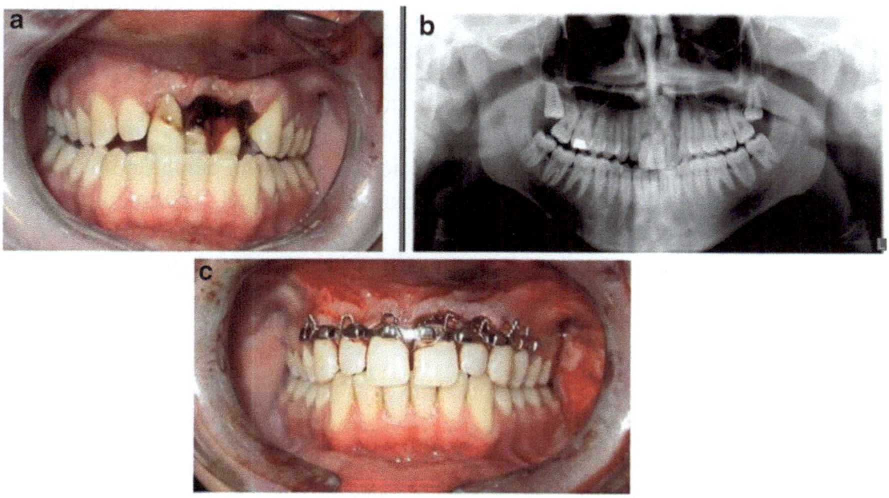

Fig. 15.13 (**a**) Luxation and alveolar fracture involving maxillary left central and lateral incisors. (**b**) Panoramic radiograph showing displacement of the teeth and a root fracture of the central incisor at mid root. (**c**) Treatment: the segment involving the teeth was grossly mobile due to the alveolar fracture required an archbar for stabilization due to mobility after reduction. An additional composite splint was applied due to root fracture of the right central incisor

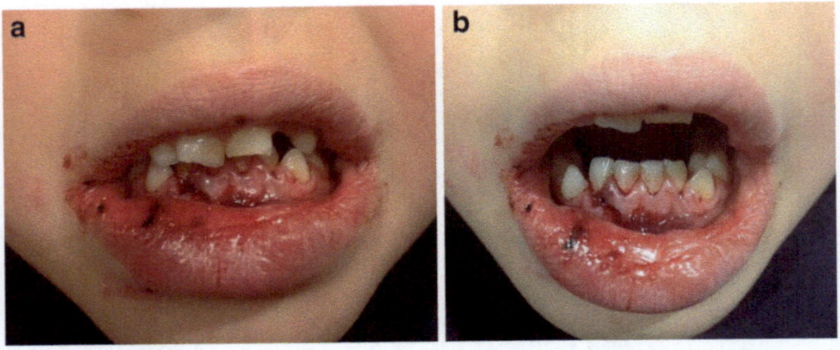

Fig. 15.14 (a) An alveolar fracture of the deciduous mandibular incisors in a 4-year-old patient. The four mandibular incisors were luxated as a unit. The teeth were repositioned under local anesthesia and splinted for a period of 4 weeks. (b) Note also the uncomplicated enamel fracture of the incisal edge of the maxillary left central incisor

Need for Long-Term Surveillance

In the case of any dental or alveolar process injury scenario, there is a need for long-term follow-up. Time is often needed to determine the vitality of teeth after a concussive injury or trauma. The vitality testing of traumatized teeth is often not reliable at the time of injury and must be repeated in the next weeks and months following the injury, since pulpal necrosis often takes time to manifest. These teeth will require endodontic (root canal) treatment to prevent infection. The surveillance is best performed by the patient's dentist who will maintain long-term records.

The guidelines for treatment of dental injuries are regularly updated and published by several professional dental associations involved in dental traumatology research including the International Association of Dental Traumatology, the American Academy of Pediatric Dentistry, and the American Association of Endodontists, with a list of website addresses to the most updated guidelines online, provided at the end of the chapter.

Protective Equipment

Injuries in various high school sports have led to safety protective equipment requirements by school sports groups—for example, the National Federation of State High School Associations (NFHS).

Many professional societies, including the ADA, have also made recommendation based on research into athletic injuries. One of the pieces of equipment that is commonly recommended in all contact sports or sports where potential facial injury can result is the mouthguard, which protects the dentition and oral soft tissues.

In 1962 the National Alliance Football Rules Committee required high school students to wear mouthguards and faceguards. The mouthguard wear rule went into effect in 1973 season and all high school, college, and professional football levels require the use of mouthguards. Currently mouthguards are required in organized hockey, football, and boxing matches in the USA. They are also recommended for many more sports, such as basketball, soccer, field hockey, racquetball, lacrosse, martial arts, and others where a potential for trauma from collisions or falls exists. According to Fonseca, an estimate of about 200,000 dental injuries is being prevented every year by the use of mouthguards [1, 24–27].

The mouthguard is designed to fit over the upper teeth and alveolar process, reaching into the vestibule, protecting the teeth and the entire alveolar ridge, as well as providing separation between the dental arches (and thus providing separation between the mandibular condyle and glenoid fossa), minimizing transmission of force to the TMJ in case of mandibular trauma. Ideally, the thickness of the mouthguard at the incisal edge of teeth should be about 4 mm to allow adequate force absorption.

There are several different types of mouthguards ranging from stock mouthguards, to boil-and-bite mouthguards, to custom-made laminated mouthguards fabricated by a dental professional. The stock mouthguards are usually the simplest and thinnest. They are purchased over the counter and come preformed by the manufacturer and are typically constructed from silicone or latex. They can often be loose fitting so the athlete needs to bite the teeth together to hold it in place. These are the least retentive. They are the least expensive and come ready to wear so use is common in organized sports. However, they tend to impede speech and breathing the most and are the least comfortable. They also offer the least amount of protection [1, 28, 29].

The second type of mouthguard is the thermoplastic or "boil-and-bite" mouthguard which has improved retention. This type is available over the counter in many athletic stores and is formed after placing in hot water and having the athlete bite into it, adapting it to the arch and the upper jaw. The retention and comfort is therefore improved, but it still may require adjustment. This type of mouthguard also comes as a shell and liner mouthguard, with a plastic or silicone outer layer and an inner liner that the athlete bites into for a few minutes after it is softened or relined with a soft curing mixed polymer. A bimaxillary mouthguard protector is also available, which covers both arches and holds the mandible slightly open and relaxed, allowing adequate breathing and air movement while rotating the condylar head and providing separation from the glenoid fossa, reducing transmission of force during mandibular trauma.

The third type of mouthguard is the custom fabricated guard, made by a dentist based on an impression of the athlete's teeth. Although this type is the most expensive, it can offer a superior fit and be appropriately adapted to cover the dental arch and oral soft tissues. The thickness can also be controlled by the thickness of the laminate used in fabrication and is usually the thickest, offering the most protection. In cases of athletes with a protrusive mandible and malocclusion, this type of mouthguard can also be fabricated to fit the lower jaw if necessary. The custom-made mouthguard is often the ideal mouthguard for an athlete in orthodontic treatment. The dentist will often keep the model so a replacement can be fabricated in case of loss or damage. It is also important to note that in adolescents who are growing, and in particular are in a mixed dentition stage, it may be necessary to provide a new mouthguard every season, as the dentition changes (Fig. 15.15).

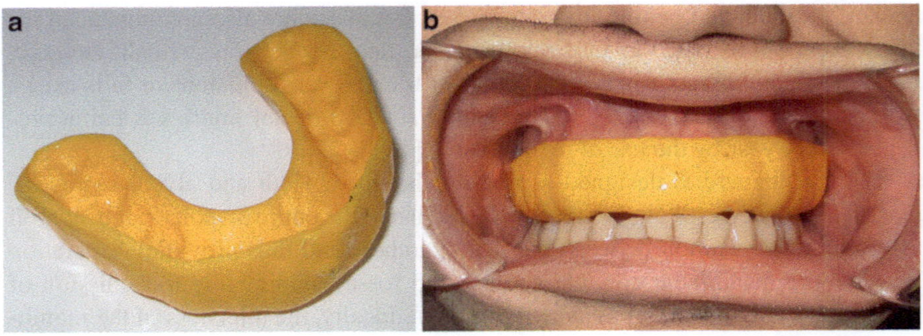

Fig. 15.15 (**a**) A custom fabricated mouthguard with extension covering the alveolar ridge. (**b**) Well-fitting custom mouthguard, with the entire crowns of the teeth and alveolar process protected

Multiple studies have been done studying protective equipment mandated by the leagues, including mouthguards. The evidence that mouthguards protect against dental and alveolar injuries is quite strong and has been independently verified by multiple studies in many sports by multiple independent researchers worldwide. Meta-analyses have shown that the risk of an oral and facial sports injury was 1.6–1.9 times higher when a mouthguard was not worn [26, 30–37].

While additional studies may further elucidate whether the superior fit of the custom-made mouthguard might prevent more traumatic brain injuries, there is no doubt that a mouthguard will reduce dental and many soft tissue injuries. Many dental schools and local dentists participate in programs in coordination with local schools to help provide adolescent athletes with mouthguards during sports seasons. In the end, the cost of a well-made mouthguard is minor compared to costs of treatment or tooth replacement over the life of the patient.

Temporomandibular Joint Injuries

If the force of injury is transmitted to the temporomandibular joints, patients can experience pain when chewing or upon wide opening or clenching. This is often due to localized trauma to the TMJ ligaments and retrodiscal tissues. The musculature involved with the TMJ includes the four muscles of mastication, the temporalis, masseter and lateral pterygoid involved in closing the mandible, as well as the medial pterygoid involved in opening and lateral excursions of the mandible. Symptoms experienced post injury can also involve muscle spasms and soreness involving these muscles.

The recommended treatment after TMJ trauma is joint rest, which includes a soft diet for several days, combined with anti-inflammatory medications, particularly NSAIDs. Warm heat application with a heat pack and gentle stretching and mobility exercises, in conjunction with a prescribed muscle relaxant if needed, help relax the musculature responsible for opening and closing the jaw [38].

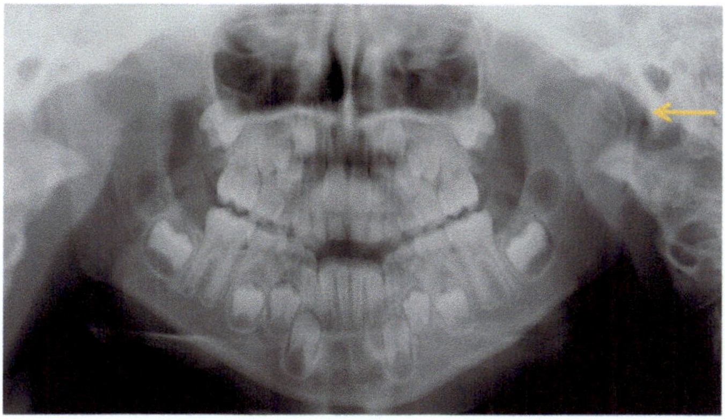

Fig. 15.16 Panoramic radiograph showing left condylar head fracture in an 8-year-old boy after a bicycle accident. The patient was treated with a soft diet and continued mobilization with close follow up at weekly intervals for first month. He maintained a normal range of motion and normal occlusion and has remained symptom free. Long-term follow up is required to be sure that the left mandible continues to grow at the same rate as the right mandible

Any continued dysfunction including pain, limitation of movement, or deviation on opening of the jaw should be further evaluated by a dentist or oral and maxillofacial surgeon, with at least a panoramic radiograph to evaluate for fractures. A change in occlusion typically manifested by patient's complaint of the "bite not feeling right" could be the result of a mandibular fracture and the patient should be referred for evaluation. It is important to note that patients may not always notice a change in occlusion immediately and may seek medical treatment at a later time when symptoms do not spontaneously resolve.

Fractures Involving the TMJ

Facial bone fractures are described elsewhere in the book, so we will limit our discussion to fractures involving the temporomandibular joint, as these are often detected based on the change in occlusion. Mandibular condylar fractures can result after trauma to the mandible or the chin. The mandible is the thinnest and therefore weakest at the condylar neck, which makes this a relatively vulnerable point. Since the mandible is a U-shaped bone, trauma to the anterior mandible is distributed posteriorly to the condyles and TMJs. Condylar fractures can be isolated or can be associated with other mandibular fractures. In particular, a mandibular angle or parasymphysis fracture is often associated with a contralateral condylar fracture. A blow to the midline of chin can result in bilateral subcondylar or intracapsular fractures. Although facial fractures in the pediatric population are relatively uncommon, the mandible is the second most frequently fractured bone after nasal bone fractures. Reports demonstrate that 20–26 % of facial fractures involve the mandible. In the young athlete as much as 40–60 % of these injuries involve the condylar process, which is a higher proportion than is seen in the adult [38–41, 45–50] (Figs. 15.16 and 15.17).

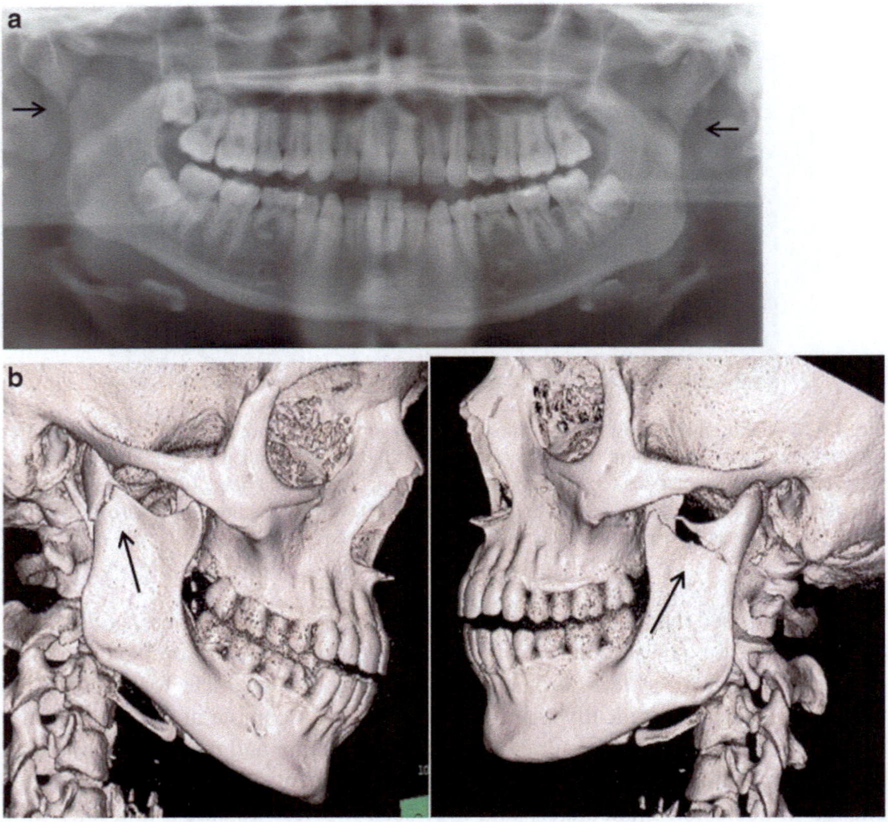

Fig. 15.17 (**a**) Bilateral subcondylar fractures sustained in trauma to the mandible in an ice-skating accident. (**b**) Corresponding *left* and *right* 3D CT images with *arrows* pointing to fractures

The clinical exam is particularly important in diagnosing potential TMJ and condylar injuries. After a general trauma and head and neck exam, the clinician should evaluate for additional clinical signs and symptoms. Evidence of trauma to the mandible and chin should prompt a more thorough TMJ and occlusal evaluation. Tenderness or swelling over the TMJ may indicate a TMJ injury or fracture and displacement of the condyle. New onset crepitus of the joint is highly suspicious of injury. Malocclusion without other cause such as a mandibular angle or body fracture is often indicative of condylar fracture, with occlusion on the ipsilateral side premature in the posterior dentition due to foreshortening of the ramus-condyle length as the condylar head buckles. As a result the patient can have a new onset facial asymmetry. A condylar injury is often accompanied with deviation of the mandible to the side of fracture as the patient opens, due to the unopposed pull of the medial pterygoid muscle of the unaffected side. In the scenario of unilateral fracture of the condyle, patients complain of their teeth not occluding on the unaffected side. Bilateral condylar fractures may also result in an anterior open bite and premature posterior contact at the molars. See Fig. 15.2. The external auditory meatus should also be carefully examined, as bleeding may indicate a fracture of the thin bone caused by a posteriorly displaced condyle. In this case, an otorhinolaryngology evaluation is indicated. The best imaging for suspected condylar fractures is a CT scan [40, 42, 45–49].

In general, the treatment of condylar fractures is conservative. Management of the subcondylar and intracapsular condylar head fractures is usually nonsurgical but requires special attention, especially in young patients. In children the condylar head is much more vascular than in an adult and cortex is thinner, which can make the condylar head more susceptible to fractures. With this increased vascularity and osteogenic potential, children and adolescents have an increased ability to regenerate and heal a fractured condyle. However, the condylar head fracture and associated hemarthrosis can lead to ankylosis in the growing child, which is why close follow-up is particularly important. In cases of condylar fractures with a malocclusion, a period of brief immobilization of 7–10 days has been suggested, followed by early mobilization and physical therapy and analgesics [39, 41, 43, 44].

Late complications involve malocclusion, temporomandibular joint dysfunction, growth disturbances, and ankylosis. Therefore, condylar fractures need to be monitored over time. In particular, children should be monitored for growth disturbances and development of facial asymmetry. These injuries and complications are best managed by an oral and maxillofacial surgeon.

Additional Factors

Timing of Elective Procedures

Adolescent athletes particularly in the 17–19-year-old range are in the age range where they suffer symptoms from erupting wisdom teeth, usually noted on regular dental evaluations. Many require the extraction of actively symptomatic and potentially problematic wisdom teeth. One important issue to consider is timing. In the immediate few weeks after extraction, while the athlete may feel well and back to his or her baseline function, it is important to note that bone healing takes several months and until the bone heals the mandible is weaker at the point of extraction. Therefore, those playing contact sports may be at an increased risk of a mandible fracture after the procedure in case of trauma to the mandible. It is best to follow the advice of the oral surgeon and recommended time frame of reduced activity in the postoperative period.

Tobacco Use by Athletes

When adolescents participate in team sports, they often emulate the behavior of athletes in professional sports. This is also a critical time to impress good habits and discourage harmful ones.

Although we focused our discussion on traumatic injuries to the dentition and maxillofacial region, it is worth noting the harmful effects of tobacco. Chewing tobacco has been featured prominently in professional sports, particularly football and baseball. While there is no immediate trauma to the athlete, the carcinogenic effects of chewing tobacco and associated higher risk of oral cancer and its devastating consequences have been clearly demonstrated by decades of scientific studies and clearly described by the literature. It is therefore worthwhile to bring this to the attention of parents and coaches to discourage the use of tobacco and educate the young athlete [28].

Conclusions

Dental Injuries in adolescent athletes are relatively common. These patients are often in the mixed dentition stage so severity of injuries and treatment depends on the types of tissues involved, ranging from contusions and abrasions of soft tissue to tooth displacement or fracture. Tooth avulsions and luxations require prompt treatment, since prognosis is often dependent not only on severity of initial trauma but on treatment in the immediate period. Prognosis is also dependent on tooth structures involved and requires attention by a dentist or specialist. Protective equipment is a requirement in many sports where potential for facial trauma exists, in particular the mouthguard which can protect both soft tissues and the dentition. Those involved in adolescent sports, including teachers, parents, and coaches, should be aware of the most common injuries and immediate first aid in the various scenarios.

Recommended Resources and Links to Guidelines Available Online

The American Association of Endodontists recently updated the guidelines for treatment of traumatic dental injuries available at their website at http://www.nxtbook.com/nxtbooks/aae/traumaguidelines/.

The American Academy of Pediatric Dentistry guideines
http://www.aapd.org/

The International Association of Dental Traumatology guidelines can be accessed at http://www.iadt-dentaltrauma.org/for-professionals.html.

http://www.academyforsportsdentistry.org/
http://www.dentaltraumaguide.org/

References

Trauma

1. Powers MP, Quereshy FA, Ramsey CA. Diagnosis and management of dentoalveolar injuries. In: Fonseca JF, Walker RV, Betts NJ, Barber HD, Powers MP, editors. Oral and maxillofacial trauma. 3rd ed. St. Louis: Elsevier Saunders; 2005. p. 427–77.
2. Meadow D, Lindner G, Needleman H. Oral trauma in children. Pediatr Dent. 1984;6(4): 248–51.
3. Nalliah RP, Anderson IM, Lee MK, Rampa S, Allareddy V, Allareddy V. Epidemiology of hospital-based emergency department visits due to sports injuries. Pediatr Emerg Care. 2014;30(8):511–5.

Dental Trauma

4. Andreasen JO, Andreasen FM, Bakland LK, Flores MT. Traumatic dental injuries: a manual. 2nd ed. Oxford: Blackwell; 2003.
5. Andreasen JO, Andreasen FM, editors. Textbook and color atlas of traumatic injuries to the teeth. 3rd ed. St. Louis: Mosby; 1994.
6. McTigue DJ. Introduction to dental trauma: managing traumatic injuries in the primary dentition. In: Pinkham JR, Casamassimo PS, Fields HW, McTigue DJ, Nowak A, editors. Pediatric dentistry: infancy through adolescence. 3rd ed. Philadelphia: WB Saunders; 1999. p. 213–24.
7. McTigue DJ. Introduction to dental trauma: managing traumatic injuries in the young permanent dentition. In: Pinkham JR, Casamassimo PS, Fields HW, McTigue DJ, Nowak A, editors. Pediatric dentistry: infancy through adolescence. 3rd ed. Philadelphia: WB Saunders; 1999. p. 531–45.
8. The application of the International Classification of Diseases to dentistry and stomatology, IDC-DA. 3rd ed. Geneva: World Health Organization; 1994.
9. Ellis RG, Davey EW. Classification and treatment of injuries to the teeth of children. 5th ed. Chicago: Year Book Medical; 1970.
10. Bakland LK, Andreasen FM, Andreasen JO. Management of traumatized teeth. In: Walton RE, Torabinejad M, editors. Principles and practice of endodontics. 3rd ed. Philadelphia: WB Saunders; 2002. p. 445–65.
11. Andreasen JO, Lauridsen E, Gerds TA, Ahrensburg SS. Dental trauma guide: a source of evidence-based treatment guidelines for dental trauma. Dent Traumatol. 2012;28(5):345–50.
12. Diangelis AJ, International Association of Dental Traumatology, et al. International Association of Dental Traumatology guidelines for the management of traumatic dental injuries: 1. Fractures and luxations of permanent teeth. Dent Traumatol. 2012;28(1):2–12.
13. Andreasen JO, Andreasen FM, Skeie A, Hjørting-Hansen E, Schwartz O. Effect of treatment delay upon pulp and periodontal healing of traumatic dental injuries—a review article. Dent Traumatol. 2002;18(3):116–28.
14. Lauridsen E, Hermann NV, Gerds TA, Kreiborg S, Andreasen JO. Pattern of traumatic dental injuries in the permanent dentition among children, adolescents, and adults. Dent Traumatol. 2012;28(5):358–63.
15. Lauridsen E, Hermann NV, Gerds TA, Ahrensburg SS, Kreiborg S, Andreasen JO. Combination injuries 1. The risk of pulp necrosis in permanent teeth with concussion injuries and concomitant crown fractures. Dent Traumatol. 2012;28:364–70.
16. Lauridsen E, Hermann NV, Gerds TA, Ahrensburg SS, Kreiborg S, Andreasen JO. Combination injuries 2. The risk of pulp necrosis in permanent teeth with subluxation injuries and concomitant crown fractures. Dent Traumatol. 2012;28:371–8.
17. Lauridsen E, Hermann NV, Gerds TA, Ahrensburg SS, Kreiborg S, Andreasen JO. Combination injuries 3. The risk of pulp necrosis in permanent teeth with extrusion or lateral luxation and concomitant crown fractures without pulp exposure. Dent Traumatol. 2012;28:379–85.
18. Robertson A, Andreasen FM, Andreasen JO, Norén JG. Long-term prognosis of crown-fractured permanent incisors. The effect of stage of root development and associated luxation injury. Int J Paediatr Dent. 2000;10(3):191–9.
19. Hecova H, Tzigkounakis V, Merglova V, Netolicky J. A retrospective study of 889 injured permanent teeth. Dent Traumatol. 2010;26(6):466–75.
20. Andreasen JO, Ahrensburg SS, Tsilingaridis G. Root fractures: the influence of type of healing and location of fracture on tooth survival rates - an analysis of 492 cases. Dent Traumatol. 2012;28(5):404–9.
21. Andersson L, et al. International Association of Dental Traumatology guidelines for the management of traumatic dental injuries: 2. Avulsion of permanent teeth. Dent Traumatol. 2012;28(2):88–96.
22. Malmgren B, et al. International Association of Dental Traumatology guidelines for the management of traumatic dental injuries: 3. Injuries in the primary dentition. Dent Traumatol. 2012;28(3):174–82.
23. Jaramillo DE, Bakland LK. Trauma kits for the dental office. Dent Clin North Am. 2009;53(4):751–60.

Mouthguards

24. National Federation of State High School Associations (NFHS) position statement and recommendations for mouthguard use in sports. http://www.nfhs.org/sports-resource-content/position-statement-and-recommendations-for-mouthguard-use-in-sports/
25. Harmon KG, Drezner JA, Gammons M, Guskiewicz KM, Halstead M, Herring SA, Kutcher JS, Pana A, Putukian M, Roberts WO. American Medical Society for Sports Medicine position statement: concussion in sport. Br J Sports Med. 2013;47(1):15–26.
26. Powell JW, Barber-Foss KD. Traumatic brain injury in high school athletes. JAMA. 1999;282(10):958–63.
27. ADA Council on Access, Prevention and Interprofessional Relations; ADA Council on Scientific Affairs.Using mouthguards to reduce the incidence and severity of sports-related oral injuries. J Am Dent Assoc. 2006;137(12):1712–20; quiz 1731.
28. Ranalli DN. Sports dentistry and mouth protection. In: Pinkham JR, Casamassimo PS, Fields HW, McTigue DJ, Nowak A, editors. Pediatric dentistry: infancy through adolescence. 3rd ed. Philadelphia: WB Saunders; 1999. p. 635–44.
29. Guevara PA, Ranalli DN. Techniques for mouthguard fabrication. Dent Clin North Am. 1991;35(4):667–82.
30. Winters J, DeMont R. Role of mouthguards in reducing mild traumatic brain injury/concussion incidence in high school football athletes. Gen Dent. 2014;62:34–8.
31. Cohenca N, Roges RA, Roges R. The incidence and severity of dental trauma in intercollegiate athletes. J Am Dent Assoc. 2007;138(8):1121–6.
32. Labella CR, Smith BW, Sigurdsson A. Effect of mouthguards on dental injuries and concussions in college basketball. Med Sci Sports Exerc. 2002;34(1):41–4.
33. Wisniewski JF, Guskiewicz K, Trope M, Sigurdsson A. Incidence of cerebral concussions associated with type of mouthguard used in college football. Dent Traumatol. 2004;20(3):143–9.
34. Newsome PR, Tran DC, Cooke MS. The role of the mouthguard in the prevention of sports-related dental injuries: a review. Int J Paediatr Dent. 2001;11(6):396–404.
35. Knapik JJ, Marshall SW, Lee RB, Darakjy SS, Jones SB, Mitchener TA, delaCruz GG, delaCruz GG, Jones BH. Mouthguards in sport activities: history, physical properties and injury prevention effectiveness. Sports Med. 2007;37(2):117–44.
36. Patrick DG, van Noort R, Found MS. Scale of protection and the various types of sports mouthguard. Br J Sports Med. 2005;39(5):278–81.
37. Mihalik JP, McCaffrey MA, Rivera EM, Pardini JE, Guskiewicz KM, Collins MW, Lovell MR. Effectiveness of mouthguards in reducing neurocognitive deficits following sports-related cerebral concussion. Dent Traumatol. 2007;23(1):14–20.

TMJ

38. Kademani D, Rombach DM, Quinn PD. Trauma to the temporomandibular joint region. In: Fonseca JF, Walker RV, Betts NJ, Barber HD, Powers MP, editors. Oral and maxillofacial trauma. 3rd ed. St. Louis: Elsevier Saunders; 2005. p. 523–68.
39. Kaban LB. Diagnosis and treatment of fractures of the facial bones in children 1943–1993. J Oral Maxillofac Surg. 1993;51(7):722–9. Review.
40. Lindahl L. Condylar fractures of the mandible. I. Classification and relation to age, occlusion, and concomitant injuries of teeth and teeth-supporting structures, and fractures of the mandibular body. Int J Oral Surg. 1977;6(1):12–21.
41. Amaratunga NA. The relation of age to the immobilization period required for healing of mandibular fractures. J Oral Maxillofac Surg. 1987;45(2):111–3.
42. Lindahl L. Condylar fractures of the mandible. III. Positional changes of the chin. Int J Oral Surg. 1977;6(3):166–72.

43. Dahlström L, Kahnberg KE, Lindahl L. 15 years follow-up on condylar fractures. Int J Oral Maxillofac Surg. 1989;18(1):18–23.
44. Gassner R, Tuli T, Hächl O, Moreira R, Ulmer H. Craniomaxillofacial trauma in children: a review of 3,385 cases with 6,060 injuries in 10 years. J Oral Maxillofac Surg. 2004;62(4):399–407.
45. Haug RH, Foss J. Maxillofacial injuries in the pediatric patient. Oral Surg Oral Med Oral Pathol Oral Radiol Endod. 2000;90(2):126–34.
46. Shaikh ZS, Worrall SF. Epidemiology of facial trauma in a sample of patients aged 1–18 years. Injury. 2002;33(8):669–71.
47. Silvennoinen U, Lindqvist C, Oikarinen K. Dental injuries in association with mandibular condyle fractures. Endod Dent Traumatol. 1993 Dec;9(6):254–9.
48. Zimmermann CE, Troulis MJ, Kaban LB. Pediatric facial fractures: recent advances in prevention, diagnosis and management. Int J Oral Maxillofac Surg. 2006;35(1):2–13.
49. Zachariades N, Mezitis M, Mourouzis C, Papadakis D, Spanou A. Fractures of the mandibular condyle: a review of 466 cases. Literature review, reflections on treatment and proposals. J Craniomaxillofac Surg. 2006;34(7):421–32. Epub 2006 Oct 19.
50. Hall RK. Injuries of the face and jaws in children. Int J Oral Surg. 1972;1(2):65–75.

Ear Injuries in the Athlete

16

Marcus Robinson and Anthony Luke

Introduction

As one of the five senses and a component of the oculo-vestibular system, the ear is critical to athletic performance. When functioning well, the ear is often not considered, but when an injury occurs, the results can be debilitating. Ear injuries common to the athlete are generally a result of trauma (auricular hematoma/cauliflower ear, perforated ear drum, barotrauma, or lacerations) or infection (otitis externa or acute otitis media). The following section describes pathophysiology, diagnosis, and management of these conditions, as well as nontraumatic hearing loss.

Auricular Hematoma and Cauliflower Ear

The auricle consists of fibrocartilaginous subunits including the helix, antihelix, concha, tragus, and antitragus. With repetitive shearing-type trauma to the ear, a hematoma may develop, typically situated in the space between the cartilage and its blood supply. Consequently, tissue necrosis may occur if the hematoma is not drained and the blood supply restored. Over time, the healing process produces disorganized fibrotic tissue that is structurally and cosmetically different from normal tissue and is known as cauliflower ear.

The repetitive, blunt trauma responsible for auricular hematoma/cauliflower ear is typically seen in sports such as rugby, wrestling, and mixed martial arts. In the

M. Robinson, BASc, MASc, MD, CCFP, Dip
Sport & Exercise Medicine, Calgary, Alberta, Canada

A. Luke, MD, MPH (✉)
Department of Orthopaedic Surgery, University of California, San Francisco,
1500 Owens Street, San Francisco, CA 94158, USA
e-mail: anthony.luke@ucsf.edu

M. O'Brien, W.P. Meehan III (eds.), *Head and Neck Injuries in Young Athletes*,
Contemporary Pediatric and Adolescent Sports Medicine,
DOI 10.1007/978-3-319-23549-3_16

initial 24 h after onset of the auricular hematoma, the lesion is tender, erythematous, and fluctuant to palpation. Following that, persistent lesions become firmer and less painful. When the lesion has progressed to cauliflower ear, there is typically no pain associated with the firm, fibrotic remodeled tissue. Rarely, infection may occur and an abscess develops. This may be associated with piercings in the affected area.

Treatment of auricular hematoma involves prompt drainage to allow for return of blood supply to the auricular cartilage. By 7 days, remodeling can already lead to permanent deformity. The procedure for drainage begins with the fundamental principles of informed consent and sterile technique. First, a regional auricular block is typically performed using a local anesthetic like 1 % lidocaine without epinephrine. For hematomas less than 48 h old and less than 2 cm in diameter, an 18 gauge needle is used to aspirate the contents. For larger (>2 cm) hematomas and those older than 48 h, incision and drainage are the preferred technique [1]. To do so, the base of the hematoma is first incised parallel to the helical curve. Then, the contents are evacuated and the lesion flushed with saline before closing with mattress sutures. Occasionally, a bolster is used to prevent re-accumulation into the space formerly occupied by the hematoma and to provide more support for cosmetic healing [2]. The bolster may be made from gauze or thermoplastic resin and sutured into place. Another bolstering technique involves the use of magnets [3]. For lesions older than 7 days, referral to a plastic surgeon is recommended.

Following a drainage procedure, the patient should be evaluated every 24–48 h to assess for re-accumulation of hematoma or signs of infection. Sutures should be removed in 7–10 days. Empiric antibiotic prophylactic treatment consists of oral levofloxacin for 7–10 days [4]

Athletes may return to play once the site has healed—generally about 7–10 days. Use of protective headwear to prevent recurrence is recommended.

Otitis Externa

Otitis externa refers to inflammation of the external auditory canal. It is most commonly seen in children aged 5–9 years [5]. Although inflammation can result from allergy or a primary dermatologic condition, it is most commonly associated with infection. In particular, *P. aeruginosa*, *S. epidermidis*, and *S. aureus* are the most common pathogenic organisms [6].

Risk factors for otitis externa include swimming (particularly lake swimming), traumatic removal of cerumen from the canal, use of in-ear devices like ear plugs or headphones, and prior history of dermatologic conditions like psoriasis or eczema.

The athlete with otitis externa will often complain of ear pain or itchiness and drainage (otorrhea). There may be apparent hearing loss but no constitutional symptoms of fever or malaise. Evaluation of the athlete for otitis externa involves visual examination with an otoscope. Generally, the canal appears erythematous, swollen, and full of debris. There should be no evidence of fluid behind the tympanic membrane.

Treatment of otitis externa begins with canal irrigation with sterile room temperature saline to remove cerumen and debris once an intact tympanic membrane is confirmed. (N.B. using cold or warm water for ear irrigation can activate the vestibulo-ocular reflex causing significant vertigo and nystagmus.) Following that, fluoroquinolone/glucocorticoid combination (e.g., Cipro HC) drops are applied four times daily for 7–14 days [7]. For moderate to severe pain, oral NSAIDs are appropriate.

If possible, athletes should refrain from exposing the canal to water until the infection has resolved. For competitive swimmers, pool training may resume within 2–3 days if ear plugs and cap are used. Athletes with a perforated tympanic membrane or those with persistent symptoms beyond 48 h of treatment should be referred to an otolaryngologist.

Acute Otitis Media

Acute otitis media (AOM) refers to an infection of the middle ear and manifests as otalgia and hearing changes. There may be associated or preceding upper respiratory tract infection (URTI) symptoms. Occasionally, a systemic response to the infection results in fever and increased heart rate.

Risk factors for AOM include age (most common between 6 and 18 months and between 5 and 6 years), attendance at daycare, exposure to smoke, lack of breastfeeding, and family history [8].

With the advent of pneumococcal vaccines, the incidence of AOM has decreased. Most cases of AOM now result from viruses (RSV, influenza, rhinovirus). In bacterial cases, *S. pneumoniae*, *H. influenzae*, and *M. catarrhalis* are most often identified as the culprit pathogens [9].

The hallmark of diagnosing AOM is visualizing a middle ear effusion and inflamed tympanic membrane with an otoscope. Inflammation of the tympanic membrane is characterized by erythema, bulging, opacity, and immobility.

Treatment of AOM depends on the severity of the infections and the presence of risk factors for the likelihood of bacterial infection or treatment resistance. For nonsevere illness with no risk factors, a watchful waiting approach is appropriate [10]. Analgesics should be administered for symptom control and the athlete should be reassessed in 48 h. For severe illness or the presence of risk factors including recent antibiotic use, recent AOM episode, or early AOM recurrence, oral antibiotic therapy is warranted [11]. For these cases, high-dose amoxicillin (80 mg/kg/day div q8h) for 5 days is used.

Referral to an otolaryngologist should be considered for athletes with more than three episodes of AOM in 6 months or more than four episodes in 12 months. If an effusion is present for more than 3 months, audiology may be appropriate. Return to play is based on the athlete's tolerance of his or her symptoms but should be restricted in situations in which rapid fluctuations in pressure are typical (e.g., diving) [12].

Recent evidence suggests that water precautions for those with tympanostomy tubes are not necessary [13]. Athletes may swim and generally participate in water sports without increasing the risk of middle ear infection.

Perforated Ear Drum

Injury to the tympanic membrane may occur as a result of infection or from a penetrating injury or direct blunt force to the ear. In the case of infection, the primary infection should be managed as outlined in the sections Otitis Externa and Acute Otitis Media. If a perforation develops, antibiotic drops should be used if there is evidence of infection, water in the ear canal should be avoided, and the patient should be referred to an otolaryngologist and for hearing assessment [14]. The same recommendations are applied in the case of a small perforation from mild trauma (e.g., using a Q-tip).

For suspected perforations resulting from significant blunt trauma to the ear or head, a more thorough examination is required once the principles of ATLS have been established. Symptoms of hearing loss, facial weakness, ataxia, or vertigo are concerning for significant middle or inner ear pathology. On physical examination, the integrity of the facial nerve should be examined and documented. Relevant visual inspection of the area includes otoscopy for signs of hemotympanum or ottorhea, tests for nystagmus, and inspection of the mastoid for ecchymosis. Finally, the Rinne and Weber tests are performed to establish the status of the athlete's hearing. If any of these tests are abnormal, the athlete should be removed from play and taken immediately for further evaluation.

Barotrauma, Deep Water Diving, and Surfing

Barotrauma refers to incongruence between the pressure in the middle ear and that of the surrounding atmosphere. The middle ear is bounded by the tympanic membrane from the outer ear; the oval and round window membranes from the inner ear; and the closed Eustachian tube from the nasopharynx. Pressure differences across the tympanic membrane are equalized with the flow of air when the Eustachian tube opens (as with swallowing). Dysfunction of the Eustachian tube leads to the inability to equalize pressures, which leads to bulging or retraction of the tympanic membrane. The sensation of tympanic membrane stretching in these cases may cause pain or a feeling of aural "fullness." Malposition of the tympanic membrane may also lead to hearing dysfunction.

Typically, barotrauma occurs when pressure differences are too rapid for the equalizing system to accommodate. This may happen with flying or diving and can range from mild discomfort to tympanic membrane rupture. Dysfunction of the Eustachian tube is another risk factor for barotrauma. With an upper respiratory tract infection (URTI), the Eustachian tube may become edematous and fail to open appropriately. Finally, fluid in the middle ear retards the speed of equalization and lowers the threshold for barotrauma in the cases of changing pressure differences.

Management of barotrauma begins with prevention. If the athlete is suffering from a URTI, antihistamines or decongestants may be used to limit the swelling of the Eustachian tube. Also, the use of repeated Valsalva maneuvers can speed equalization and limit discomfort. If a perforation and vertigo symptoms develop, the athlete can be managed with antibiotic drops, avoidance of water in the ear canal, and referral to an otolaryngologist [14].

Diving at depths greater than 30 m puts athletes at risk for decompression sickness, in which gas bubbles form in the inner ear [15]. This generally occurs on the ascent and leaves divers with feelings of vertigo, nausea, and tinnitus. The mainstay of management is with hyperbaric oxygen therapy.

Repeated exposure to cold water may lead to external auditory canal exostoses, also known as surfer's ear [15]. These bony growths are thought to develop secondary to stimulation of the periosteum of the external canal when blood flow is increased to area as a response to the cold. Buildup of the exostoses can obstruct the canal and increase the risk of cerumen impaction, infection, and hearing loss. Definitive treatment for symptomatic surfer's ear involves surgical excision.

Ear Lacerations

Lacerations to the outer ear of an athlete typically result from incidental contact from an opponent or sporting equipment.

In gathering the history of the incident, the physician should enquire about the mechanism of injury to assess for possible inner ear or concussive symptoms. This includes symptoms like vertigo, hearing loss, headache, visual changes, loss of consciousness, cognitive symptoms, and emotional symptoms. Details around the mechanism of injury can also help identify the likelihood of foreign bodies or contamination of the wound.

The physical examination begins with the principles of ATLS. Once stability is established, a more focused approach is warranted. Characterization of the wound is important for repair decision making. A screening neurologic examination plus otoscopic inspection should be performed to rule out concussion, basilar skull fracture, and inner ear pathology.

The general principles of laceration repair apply to ear lacerations, but there are also special considerations. Primary repair of ear lacerations can be performed within 24 h of injury. Following an auricular anesthetic block and/or local infiltration with 1% lidocaine without epinephrine, the wound is irrigated and minimally debrided of nonviable tissue [16]. Generally, nonabsorbable 6-0 sutures are used for simple lacerations that do not involve the cartilage. Repair with cartilage involvement is more technically challenging to achieve good cosmetic outcome.

Aftercare of an ear laceration repair includes consideration of the patient's tetanus immunization status, follow-up at 24–48 h to check for auricular hematoma, and suture removal in 7–10 days [17].

Nontraumatic Hearing Loss

Nontraumatic hearing loss in an athlete may be classified as conductive (deficiency in sound wave propagation to the inner ear) or sensorineural (deficiency in sound wave processing). As sound waves enter the external auditory canal, any obstruction can blunt signal intensity. Typically, obstructions result from cerumen buildup or swelling and debris from infection. In the middle ear, fluid collection secondary to infection affects the mobility of the tympanic membrane and signal transmission. Treatment for conductive hearing changes depends on the primary pathology (see above sections on outer and middle ear infections). Cerumen impaction causing hearing loss can be remedied with irrigation, ceruminolytic medications, or manual removal with a curette [18].

Sensorineural hearing loss in the general population has many possible etiologies including infection, Meniere's disease, labrynthitis, age-related degeneration, tumors, systemic causes, and exposure to loud noises. In addition, several medications, including oral aminoglycosides, are potentially ototoxic [19]. For travelling athletes on antimalarial prophylaxis, chloroquine should be suspected if hearing loss develops.

References

1. Riviello RJ, Brown NA. Otolaryngologic procedures. In: Roberts JR, Hedges JR, editors. Clinical procedures in emergency medicine. 5th ed. Philadelphia: Saunders Elsevier; 2010. p. 1178.
2. Mohamad SH, Barnes M, Jones S, Mahendran S. A new technique using fibrin glue in the management of auricular hematoma. Clin J Sport Med. 2014;24(6):e65–7.
3. Park TH, Chang CH. In response to: acute management of auricular hematoma: a novel approach and retrospective review. Clin J Sport Med. 2013;23:329.
4. Greywoode JD, Pribitkin EA, Krein H. Management of auricular hematoma and the cauliflower ear. Facial Plast Surg. 2010;26:451.
5. Sander R. Otitis externa: a practical guide to treatment and prevention. Am Fam Physician. 2001;63:927Y36–7.
6. Roland PS, Stroman DW. Microbiology of acute otitis externa. Laryngoscope. 2002;112:1166.
7. Kaushik V, Malik T, Saeed SR. Interventions for acute otitis externa. Cochrane Database Syst Rev. 2010;20, CD004740.
8. Pelton S. New concepts in the pathophysiology and management of middle ear disease in childhood. Drugs. 1996;52 Suppl 2:62–7.
9. Stephenson J, Martin D, Kardatzke D, et al. Prevalence of bacteria in middle ear effusions for the 1980s. Reprinted Bluestone C, Stephenson J, Martin L. Ten year review of otitis media pathogens. Pediatr Infect Dis J. 1992;11:S7–11.
10. http://www.topalbertadoctors.org/download/366/AOM_guideline.pdf
11. Lister P, Pong A, Chartrand S, Sanders C. Rationale behind high dose amoxicillin therapy for acute otitis media due to penicillin non-susceptible pneumococci: support from in-vitro pharmaco-dynamics. Antimicrob Agents Chemother. 1997;41(9):1926–32.
12. Nichols AW. Nonorthopaedic problems in the aquatic athlete. Clin Sports Med. 1999;18:395Y411, viii.
13. Rosenfeld RM, et al. Clinical practice guideline: tympanostomy tubes in children. Otolaryngol Head Neck Surg. 2013;149(1 Suppl):S1–35.
14. Orji FT, Agu CC. Determinants of spontaneous healing in traumatic perforations of the tympanic membrane. Clin Otolaryngol. 2008;33:420.
15. Cassaday K, et al. Ear problems and injuries in athletes. Curr Sports Med Rep. 2014;13(1):22–6.
16. Lammers R. Methods of wound closure. In: Roberts JR, Hedges JR, editors. Clinical procedures in emergency medicine. 5th ed. Philadelphia: Saunders Elsevier; 2010.
17. Up to date. Assessment and management of auricle (ear lacerations).
18. McCarter DF, Courtney AU, Pollart SM. Cerumen impaction. Am Fam Physician. 2007;75:1523Y8.
19. Roland PS, Stewart MG, Hannley M, et al. Consensus panel on role of potentially ototoxic antibiotics for topical middle ear use: introduction, methodology, and recommendations. Otolaryngol Head Neck Surg. 2004;130:S51.

Index

M. O'Brien, W.P. Meehan III (eds.), *Head and Neck Injuries in Young Athletes*,
Contemporary Pediatric and Adolescent Sports Medicine,
DOI 10.1007/978-3-319-23549-3